WHAT IF IT'S NOT ALZHEIMER'S?

WHAT IF IT'S NOT ALZHEIMER'S?

A CAREGIVER'S GUIDE TO DEMENTIA

THIRD EDITION

Edited by **Gary Radin** and **Lisa Radin**
Foreword by **Murray Grossman, MD, EdD**

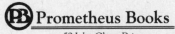 **Prometheus Books**
59 John Glenn Drive
Amherst, New York 14228

Published 2014 by Prometheus Books

Cover image © Media Bakery
Cover design by Grace M. Conti-Zilsberger

Unless otherwise indicated, all illustrations are by the authors of the chapters in which they appear.

The Best Friends™ Dementia Bill of Rights by Virginia Bell & David Troxel. Copyright © 2013 Health Professions Press, Inc.

Inquiries should be addressed to
Prometheus Books
59 John Glenn Drive
Amherst, New York 14228
VOICE: 716–691–0133
FAX: 716–691–0137
WWW.PROMETHEUSBOOKS.COM

18 17 16 15 14   5 4 3 2 1

Library of Congress Cataloging-in-Publication Data

What if it's not Alzheimer's? : a caregiver's guide to dementia / edited by Gary Radin and Lisa Radin ; foreword by Murray Grossman, MD EdD. — 3rd edition.
      pages cm
   Includes bibliographical references and index.
   ISBN 978-1-61614-968-0 (paperback) — ISBN 978-1-61614-969-7 (ebook)
     1. Dementia—Nursing—Handbooks, manuals, etc. 2. Dementia—Patients—Care—Handbooks, manuals, etc. 3. Caregivers—Handbooks, manuals, etc. I. Radin, Gary, 1969- II. Radin, Lisa, 1944-

RC521.W438 2014
616.8'30231—dc23

2014015843

Printed in the United States of America

*This book is dedicated to
our loving husband and father, Neil, and
to all those who walk in our footsteps
through the journey of FTD.*

CONTENTS

PART 1: A MEDICAL FOCUS

Chapter 1. The ABCs of Neurodegenerative Dementias
Martin Rossor, MD, FRCP, FMedSci   29

PART 2: MANAGING DAILY CARE

PART 3: CAREGIVER RESOURCES

PART 4: CARING FOR YOURSELF

Chapter 23. A Daily Break: Respite and Personal Care for the Caregiver
Vivian E. Greenberg, ACSW, LCSW

Chapter 24. From Loss to Life: Managing Emotions and Grief
Rev. David Cotton

FOREWORD

This is the third edition of *What If It's Not Alzheimer's? A Caregiver's Guide to Dementia*. This is important for many reasons. First, our knowledge of frontotemporal degeneration (FTD) and related conditions is advancing very rapidly. Treatments are being developed for FTD, and useful diagnostic tests are becoming available so we know who should be receiving these treatments. Second, non-Alzheimer's forms of neurodegeneration are recognized increasingly by clinicians, and this will lead to improved care for patients with FTD. FTD is the second most common form of dementia following Alzheimer's disease (AD) in those less than sixty-five years of age. Third, patients, families, friends, and a concerned public are increasingly interested in learning about FTD and related conditions. The public needs to participate in this remarkable progress, and this book will make it possible.

This volume also enhances the educational efforts of physicians, nurses, and other healthcare providers. Time for communication with patients is increasingly constrained by the pressures of delivering increasingly complex clinical care. Indeed, despite substantial progress in understanding FTD and related conditions, there is still limited information available to the public and medical professionals on this topic. This book fills this gap by covering the most critical educational issues related to FTD for the public as well as for clinicians who do not specialize in neurodegenerative disorders. We are improving our understanding of the clinical presentations of FTD, the ways in which FTD is diagnosed, the role of genetics in this condition, the microscopic pathologies found in FTD, and the treatments for this condition. Indeed, FTD is a family of conditions with heterogeneous presentations despite being caused by similar pathologies and inherited disorders, and this complexity is important to understand as we move forward.

Not only does this book capture the essence of these exciting advances, but it also conveys them in readily accessible language and places them in a context that patients and families will understand. By communicating this new knowledge so effectively, this book offers hope to patients and families that the prospects for improving their lives are brighter every day.

Murray Grossman, MD, EdD
Director, Penn Frontotemporal Degeneration Center
University of Pennsylvania Perelman School of Medicine

PREFACE

Over the past several years, I have spoken with hundreds of people living and working with frontotemporal degeneration (FTD). It is from caregivers, like Lisa and Gary Radin, that I have learned the most about how the approach one takes to this journey can shape the quality of the experience and determine the place the family will be when the journey comes to an end. The grace, strength, and even good humor with which many of these people have faced their challenges have taught me much about the human spirit, resilience, and love.

We know what this disease steals from our loved ones. The ability to focus: to take on a problem and think through a logical path to a solution, then to put that plan into action. The ability to communicate: to share information, feelings, and needs and, in turn, to really hear what another person is saying. The ability to know oneself: to understand one's own strengths and weaknesses and embrace our own unique take on life. The ability to connect: to be a part of a larger community that can find deeper meaning in the experiences that life presents to us.

Although the pace of research is encouraging, in 2014 we do not yet have the means to prevent these losses in the person diagnosed with the disease. However, it is clear that the most successful caregivers are those who call upon these very same qualities in themselves to manage their journey.

Focus. There is no denying that the task ahead of you is daunting. Learn all you can about the disease and the current options for care.

Communicate. Be a proactive partner in the care team. You know the patient best, and your perspective is critical to setting appropriate goals and preserving quality of life. In many cases you may need to educate medical professionals who have not had experience with this rare disease. You'll also need to listen carefully, even when the message is not one you want to hear.

Know Yourself. Play to your own strengths. Open yourself to asking for and accepting help from others who can complement these strengths. Don't lose sight of the person you care about, and why you are doing this. Above all, give yourself permission to make mistakes, and to need a break once in a while.

Connect. You do not need to face this alone. Join a support group. Take part in research. There is a vibrant community of families, researchers, and clinicians who are working together to build a better future that includes accurate diagnosis, effective treatments, and a cure. Connecting with this broader community can counteract the isolation you may find overwhelming at times. And it can give meaning and hope to the path you are on.

The tragedy of this disease is the loved one you are losing. The great hope is that you do not need to let FTD ruin the other things you value most in your life. The information in this book will provide you with the tools to know three critical things for the journey ahead: You are not alone. You are not helpless. And you need not cede all control to the disease. Use these tools as a source of strength to face the challenges ahead of you, and you will be honoring the person you are losing in the greatest way possible.

Susan L.-J. Dickinson, MS, CGC
Executive Director
The Association for Frontotemporal Degeneration

ACKNOWLEDGMENTS

Creating a book of this scope was no small task. However, in light of the monumental difference it could make in the lives of those caring for someone with frontotemporal degeneration (FTD), it was worth every minute. The idea of assembling the thoughts, knowledge, and expertise of this ensemble of talented professionals and caregivers was both exciting and overwhelming. The number of titles and credentials following the names of the writers in this book is impressive. They are experts who have dedicated their lives to caring and providing for people whose loved ones have FTD, as well as researching and contributing to the future care of FTD patients.

We also owe our gratitude to the many families, friends, and professionals, too numerous to mention, who supported us and cared for our loved one during the most difficult time of our life. You are truly at the source of our commitment to take our experience and turn it into something that will help others as they face the role of caregiving.

We are so grateful and thankful for the incredible generosity that each and every contributor has made to this endeavor. Their efforts go far beyond the writing of this book. They offer information, guidance, and hope for all those who come into contact with the challenges and reality of living with FTD.

We want to thank Murray Grossman, MD, EdD, for his ongoing encouragement to create this book and for his personal commitment to patients and families dealing with dementia. He is a role model for the medical profession. Jennifer Farmer, MS, CGC, has given spirit, knowledge, and many hours to ensure that we have included everything caregivers need to know and that all the contributors to this book have been well represented. She is an angel that descended upon this project. Helen-Ann Comstock is a pioneer in supporting, educating, advocating, and loving both caregivers and FTD patients in need in our region. Carol Lippa, MD, has proven time and again that caregivers and their loved ones deserve knowledge they can understand and take home into everyday life. Landmark Worldwide's transformative educational experience beginning with the Landmark Forum has allowed us to overcome our fears and create ongoing new possibilities for life. We also acknowledge the contributing authors, without whom this book would never have been possible: Kate J. Bowen; Richard J. Caselli, MD; Jeannette Castellane; Heather Cianci, PT, MS, GCS; Helen-Ann Comstock; Rev. David Cotton; Sharon S. Denny, MA; Susan L.-J. Dickinson, MS, CGC; Lisa Ann Fagan, MS, OTR/L; Paul L. Feldman, Esq.; Maribeth Gallagher, DNP, PMHNP-BC, FAAN; Rosalie Gearhart, RN, MS, CS; Vivian E. Greenberg, ACSW, LCSW; Murray Grossman, MD, EdD; Geri R. Hall, PhD, ARNP, GCNS-BC, FAAN; David J. Irwin, MD; Morris J. Kaplan, Esq., NHA; David S. Knopman, MD; Virginia M.-Y. Lee, PhD; Carol F. Lippa, MD; Amy P. Lustig, PhD, MPH, CCC-SLP; Lauren M. Massimo, PhD, AGNP-BC; Elisabeth McCarty Wood, MS; Bruce L. Miller, MD; Darby Morhardt, PhD, LCSW; Mary O'Hara, AM, LCSW; Katherine P. Rankin, PhD; Keith M. Robinson, MD; Martin Rossor, MD, FRCP, FMedSci; John Q. Trojanowski, MD, PhD; and Roy Yaari, MD, MAS.

In addition, we'd like to thank the Alzheimer's Association Delaware Valley Chapter, Pick's Support Group for its love, caregiver words of wisdom, and bravery in the face of fear; Fytie Drayton and Joyce Shenian, special caregivers and friends, who have given their blessing for this book and invaluable feedback and unconditional support to all those around them; all the caregivers who responded to our questionnaire; our close family and friends for their interest and support—especially Geri for her love and compassion and Vince for his ongoing patience, humor, and willingness to let us disappear as we worked for hours and even days at a time.

INTRODUCTION

It has been many years since our bodies have recovered from the incredibly challenging task of caring for a loved one, yet our minds still have vivid memories of the overwhelming experience. We are the wife and son of an intelligent, loving, and generous husband and father. We are the caregivers of a beautiful man who died at age fifty-eight after suffering from a neurodegenerative brain disease.

Our four years of providing in-home care unraveled a series of events that we discovered no one could ever be prepared for. Every day included the challenges of what doctors to consult, where to go for financial assistance, who could provide us with support, how to get information, and when we would ever deal with the loss. We were driven to find answers to questions that would help us understand, cope, and manage and put us on a path to learn everything we could from every source we could find. Finding almost nothing, the only answer we did see to make it through was to pave our own road.

What If It's Not Alzheimer's? A Caregiver's Guide to Dementia is a map of the road we traveled. It is a collection of information addressing everything we had to confront and conquer while caring for our loved one. Medical professionals and experienced caregivers, many of whom are renowned for their work, write the pages of these chapters. Some are the same people we personally sought out and from whom we asked advice. Providing the information that every caregiver seeks, this volume encompasses all the facts that would take monumental efforts to gather together.

Giant steps are being taken in this book to direct focus on the group of brain disorders known collectively as frontotemporal degeneration (FTD). This classification of progressive, neurodegenerative illnesses, along with other non-Alzheimer's diseases, have been overshadowed or even eclipsed by the dominance of funded research and awareness campaigns for Alzheimer's disease. Although concentration on Alzheimer's disease over the past twenty-five years has provided significant medical developments and needed public attention, it is critical that we continue to acknowledge and bring focus to other degenerative conditions that affect the brain.

The medical profession has been distinguishing dementia illnesses in greater depth in recent years. As a result, diagnosis has led to other dementias as clinical observations rule out Alzheimer's. For this reason, the medical community and our ever-growing caregiving society must educate itself and disseminate the distinctions that will provide better treatment and care to those afflicted with FTD and related disorders.

Non-Alzheimer's disorders are often considered rare; however, they are not actually that uncommon. It could be said that FTD is often misdiagnosed and under-recognized. This is also true of the numerous other non-Alzheimer's disorders, which present both subtle and not so subtle differences from Alzheimer's disease. This guidebook presents both caregiver advice and information along with medical discussion and experience specifically targeted at FTD but absolutely relevant to other dementias. We also think it is equally useful and informative to the healthcare community by presenting insight into caregiver daily needs as well as a comprehensive perspective on medical care.

Too many people struggle with unanswered questions, little direction, and no diagnosis, sometimes for as long as years. Others are misdiagnosed with personality and psychological conditions, only to later find out there is a neurodegenerative condition that is the cause of the illness. For this reason, the information that follows will be useful to caregivers who are moving down the road and to professionals who are directing them.

For you, the caregiver, we understand what lies ahead. It is a difficult time and certainly an emotional one. Your commitment to provide the best quality of life for your loved one is recognized. And we know that the time and energy it takes is unparalleled. Be strong, be fearless, and, most of all, keep on loving the one you care for as well as yourself.

This book is our ongoing mission to take our experience and make a difference in the lives of those who are now suffering with FTD. Read these pages one by one. Use each chapter in every way you can to provide the knowledge and power that will sustain you in your time of caregiving.

EDITORS' NOTE

We wrote this with the intention of providing accurate and timely information. We have addressed this subject matter with care and concern for caregivers and respect for healthcare and other professionals. There is a great amount of detail from numerous sources, and we have attempted to organize it in a manner that allows you to reference relevant information at any time.

We acknowledge that there are many different types of relationships involved in caregiving, but for the purposes of literary clarity we may not have been able to mention all people in the text. Those afflicted with neurodegenerative illnesses and their caregivers are both men and women. To simplify reading, we use only one pronoun (i.e., he or she) at a time and switch continually throughout the book.

Note that the term *frontotemporal degeneration* (FTD), which this book uses as the most current term to describe the group of frontotemporal syndromes, may be referred to as *frontotemporal dementia* by resources that have not yet adopted this nomenclature.

Information at the time of publishing can be considered correct and current; however, due to ongoing research, new practices, changes in law, and so on, additional information and facts will arise over time and may change. This book is for informational purposes only and is not intended to provide medical or legal advice. Health conditions and treatments are unique to every individual, and medical or other professionals should be consulted for each individual circumstance.

PART 1

A MEDICAL FOCUS

CHAPTER 1

THE ABCs OF NEURODEGENERATIVE DEMENTIAS

Martin Rossor, MD, FRCP, FMedSci

WHAT IS DEMENTIA?

The most common cause of dementia is Alzheimer's disease (AD), which has dominated our thinking about neurodegenerative disorders and even determined the definition of the term *dementia* itself. It is clear, however, that there are many other causes of dementia. Before discussing these it is first necessary to consider what is meant by dementia and the history behind it.

The term *dementia* refers to a clinical syndrome, a combination or pattern of clinical features. Thus, dementia is not a disease but rather a syndrome that can be associated with many different underlying diseases. In this sense it is similar to heartburn or headache, which is caused by many different things and could require many different treatments. Therefore, the statement that somebody has dementia is an inadequate diagnostic formulation: One must always try to determine the cause by appropriate investigations.

With the syndrome dementia, impairment of cognitive function is widespread. It can involve, in different combinations, memory for events; memory and understanding of facts, language, thinking, and reasoning; and perception of the world. Identifying patients with this combination of cognitive impairment was particularly important in the days before imaging (e.g., MRI and CT). It was important to distinguish patients with a localized deficit from those with more widespread problems. Cognitive function in the brain is modular, and particular areas of the cerebral cortex are specialized for particular functions; for example, our ability to remember day-to-day events is critically dependent on the hippocampus, which is found on the inside of the temporal lobes. (See figure 1.1.)

THE BRAIN

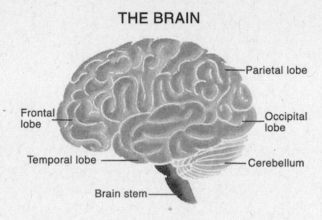

Figure 1.1. Illustration of the major areas of the brain.

What the Different Parts of the Brain Do

Cerebrum: This is the term for the major part of the brain. The cerebrum is responsible for many aspects of thinking, including memory, problem solving, language function, personality, mood, and response to different sensory signals from the world around us. It also plays a role in movement and in feeling the senses. It is highly developed in humans but more rudimentary in animals.

Cerebellum: This part of the brain coordinates, smoothes out, and balances movement to enable us to stand, walk, and use our arms.

Frontal lobe: This part of the brain controls our ability to use words and speech (the left side) and determines how we react to situations. The frontal lobes are also important for problem solving, mood, judgment, inhibiting impulses, and for individual personality.

Parietal lobe: This part of the brain enables us to interpret sensory input such as pain, temperature differences, vibration, and touch. The left parietal lobe is involved with planning complex movements, and the right parietal lobe is important for our sense of direction.

Occipital lobe: This part of the brain interprets what we see.

Temporal lobes: The temporal lobes are crucial for formation of new memories (remembering). This part of the brain is nearly always involved in Alzheimer's disease and may be involved in frontotemporal dementia (FTD). The left temporal lobe is also important for understanding what we hear.

Brain stem: This connects the brain with the spinal cord. Without the brainstem, we would not be able to move or feel anything. This area is also important for automatic reflexes such as breathing.

Our language functions are critically dependent on areas of the left frontal and temporal cortex in right-handed people. Patients with a discrete abnormality, such as a loss of language or dysphasia, by implication would have a focal or localized damage to the cerebral cortex. If this were of sudden onset, it would likely be a stroke, but if it were of slow onset, then it would likely be a tumor and thus require invasive and potentially dangerous investigation and surgery. On the other hand, a patient with widespread deficits would likely have a disease more diffusely affecting the cerebral cortex, such as Alzheimer's disease, and further investigation could be avoided. Historically the terms *senile* and *presenile dementia* were used merely to refer to dementias coming on late or early in life. These were most likely to be Alzheimer's disease, but again this was not a specific diagnosis as such.

More recently the definition of dementia has been made more precise. The necessity for more than one cognitive domain to be involved remains critical to the definition; however, memory, and particularly our ability to remember day-to-day events (episodic memory), has to be affected for dementia to occur. Alzheimer's disease, in which episodic memory is the most salient deficit, is the most common dementia disorder. In addition to memory impairment, there has to be at least one other domain of cognitive impairment, such as language, thinking, or perception. Furthermore, the cognitive impairment has to be significant enough to interfere with social or employment functions. In other words, the patient must be quite severely impaired. More recent definitions of dementia give less prominence to memory as causes of dementia other than Alzheimer's disease are increasingly recognized.

The different degenerative diseases that can cause the dementia syndrome tend to affect different areas of the cerebral cortex. Since different areas of the cortex are specialized for different functions, the disease will tend to have characteristic patterns of deficit. This is most apparent early in the disease.

As the disease progresses, the patterns become more similar as dysfunction becomes more severe and more widespread. Clearly, as we move toward earlier diagnosis, which is essential to successful management of these diseases in the future, we will attempt to diagnose them before a patient fulfills the criteria for dementia. For example, a patient with early Alzheimer's disease may present with mild memory deficit, but this alone is not sufficient to fulfill the criteria for dementia. Similarly, many patients with frontotemporal dementia may have preserved memory early in the disease but demonstrate quite profound behavioral and personality changes. For these reasons, many specialists now believe we should begin to move away from the term *dementia* and to speak in terms of specific patterns of cognitive impairment and the relationship to presumed underlying diseases. The term *mild cognitive impairment* (MCI) has been introduced to describe patients with cognitive problems that are not severe enough to justify the term *dementia*.

FRONTOTEMPORAL DEGENERATION

Frontotemporal degenerations (FTDs) compose the main topic of this book, and the clinical and pathological details are discussed in the following chapters. However, the key feature of this group of disorders is the involvement by a variety of disease processes of the frontal lobes and the front part of the temporal lobes of the brain. It is this characteristic distribution or topography of the degenerative process that determines the clinical features of early personality change and language and speech impairment. There are many different underlying diseases that can present as frontotemporal degeneration. Some of these are quite specific, such as Pick's disease. Pick's disease was identified even earlier than Alzheimer's disease. Arnold Pick in Prague described two patients with prominent behavioral and language impairment. Intriguingly, it was Dr. Aloysius "Alois" Alzheimer who again applied his expertise with the microscope to the examination of the brain and demonstrated some abnormal inclusions subsequently referred to as Pick bodies. These are now known to be deposits of tau protein. The tau protein that is deposited in Pick's disease is the same as that found in the neurofibrillary tangles of Alzheimer's disease, but is deposited in a different way. Senile plaques are not a feature of Pick's disease.

The term *Pick's disease* has been somewhat confusing, since it has been used both as a general clinical term, essentially the same as frontotemporal degeneration, as well as a very specific pathological disease. Increasingly it is used in the latter sense.

Corticobasal degeneration (CBD) is another disease of abnormal tau. Typically it affects the parietal lobe and causes major difficulty with motor skills but can affect the frontal and temporal lobes, causing FTD.

Some cases of FTD show deposits of a protein TDP-43 found in another degenerative disorder, motor neuron disease or Lou Gehrig's disease, also known as amyotrophic lateral sclerosis (ALS). FTD can run in families, and most of the gene abnormalities have now been identified.

It is the early behavioral and personality changes and/or changes in language and speech that define this group of patients. Their memory for day-to-day events may be strikingly preserved when compared with Alzheimer's disease, and they very rarely if ever get lost until late in the disease. Three prototypic clinical syndromes have been described in association with FTD: a frontal behavioral syndrome, progressive nonfluent aphasia, and semantic dementia. The frontal syndrome is characterized by behavioral abnormalities. Patients become socially disinhibited, with some becoming apathetic. There may be changes in eating and sexual behavior. The term *frontotemporal degeneration* is sometimes confined to this behavioral group. Progressive nonfluent aphasia refers to patients with speech-production difficulties. Early on, they have excellent comprehension and may write well despite speaking with difficulty. As the disease progresses, they can become mute. *Semantic dementia* refers to patients with impairment of semantic memory. This term refers to our knowledge of meaning. Verbal semantic memory is our memory for the meaning of words, and visual semantic memory is our memory for the meaning of objects that we see. Semantic memory contrasts with our memory for day-to-day events, referred to as episodic memory. Patients with semantic memory speak fluently, but their speech is empty of meaning and they have major difficulty understanding language. With this condition there is loss of tissue in the temporal lobes.

DEMENTIA WITH LEWY BODIES

Dementia with Lewy bodies (DLB) has been increasingly identified as an important cause of dementia in the elderly. In some studies it is believed to be the cause of dementia in up to 20 percent of the patients over sixty-five years of age. Under the microscope, the brains of people with DLB show the senile plaques of Alzheimer's disease but far fewer neurofibrillary tangles. By contrast, they show the brain-cell changes that are normally associated with Parkinson's disease, that is, a protein deposit referred to as a Lewy body, named after its original discoverer.

Patients with DLB more closely resemble patients with Alzheimer's disease than those with FTD. There is a characteristic clinical triad that favors the diagnosis, namely fluctuation in the cognitive impairment, hallucinations, and Parkinsonian syndrome.

The fluctuations in cognitive impairment can be quite dramatic and last from minutes to days. In between times, the family will often feel that the patient is normal, at least early in the disease. The hallucinations are very frequent, and patients often retain insight. They are normally of people and animals. The people may often be familiar to them and distressingly may be deceased relatives or friends. The hallucinations are rarely threatening and rarely speak to the patients. They commonly accompany misidentifications of objects in their environments. For example, an abnormally hanging curtain may be seen as a figure that then takes the form of a more definite hallucination.

The Parkinsonian syndrome is very similar to that seen in patients with classical Parkinson's disease. There is a gradual slowing of movement and of rigidity, but the tremor or shakiness of classical Parkinson's disease is less often seen. A significant proportion of patients with Parkinson's disease, particularly the elderly, will develop cognitive impairment as the disease progresses. The features are similar to DLB, but when the dementia follows a diagnosis of Parkinson's disease it is referred to as Parkinson's disease dementia.

ALZHEIMER'S DISEASE

It is often claimed that there is an epidemic of Alzheimer's disease. The disease has always been with us, but since it is a disease of old age, the numbers of cases have increased with the aging of the population. The real increase, however, has been due to current diagnosis, whereas thirty years ago many patients would simply have been diagnosed as suffering from senile dementia.

Alzheimer's original case was a lady of only fifty-one years of age who presented with dementia. Alzheimer examined her brain after death using the newly available silver stains. He was thus able to demonstrate the two

characteristic microscopic features of Alzheimer's: senile plaques and neurofibrillary tangles. Senile plaques are now known to reflect deposits of an
abnormal protein, beta-amyloid, within the brain but not within the neurons
or brain cells themselves; this is thought to be a key event in the causation of
the disease. Neurofibrillary tangles are now known to be abnormal deposits of
another protein within the cell itself. This protein is tau, the microtubule-associated protein. Microtubules are the building blocks of the internal skeleton
of brain cells and are essential to maintain the integrity of the extensive and
complex wiring within the brain. If tau loses its function, then microtubules
become unstable, and one can see the collapse of the cytoskeleton as neurofibrillary tangles.

Since Alzheimer's first case was a middle-aged lady, it was assumed
that this was a rare early onset or presenile dementia. However, studies in
the United Kingdom in the 1960s demonstrated that the majority of elderly
patients with dementia, which had previously been called senile dementia,
were in fact suffering from Alzheimer's disease.

The key clinical feature of Alzheimer's disease is an early impairment
of episodic memory, our memory for day-to-day events. Patients may have
difficulty recalling what has happened to them; they forget to do things; they
may misplace items; they repetitively question; and as the disease progresses,
they may get lost. We all experience memory lapses from time to time, but it
is the inexorable progression that identifies the patient with early Alzheimer's disease. After a period of a few years, other features supervene, with
increasing difficulties with language and perception of the world. This pattern
reflects the early involvement of the hippocampus, as explained previously,
and other parts of the temporal lobe by the disease process.

VASCULAR DEMENTIA

It used to be thought that impairment of blood supply to the brain was the main
cause of dementia. It was believed that hardening of the arteries, or atheroscle-
rosis, led to a reduced blood flow. This has been disproved. While blood flow
may be reduced in dementia, this is a consequence of the nerve-cell loss rather
than a cause. What can cause dementia is recurrent large or small strokes and
nerve-cell damage from disease in the small arteries to the central parts of the
brain, called small-vessel disease or Binswanger's disease.

Patients with strokes can have significant problems with cognitive impairment, such as a patient with a right-sided paralysis accompanying loss of language or dysphasia. Multiple strokes can give rise to widespread cognitive impairment, but due to motor abnormalities, it is usually obvious that these are strokes and such patients rarely come to attention because of the cognitive impairment alone. Occasionally, a stroke in particular areas of the cerebral cortex or in the center of the brain (in the thalamus), can result in quite-widespread cognitive impairment.

Much more common are the consequences of high blood pressure, smoking, and diabetes in patients with dementia. These conspire to cause thickening and damage to the very small arteries that supply the center of the brain with oxygen and result in little ministrokes or lacunas together with more diffuse damage to the central white matter of the brain. These patients often present with cognitive impairment or dementia. They tend to be characterized by cognitive slowing and often have problems with recall but not with recognition memory. Gait disturbance, which can resemble Parkinson's disease with shuffling, is quite common. This is an important group of patients to identify. Careful management of risk factors such as blood pressure, cholesterol, and blood sugar are important and may slow progress. In addition, many patients with Alzheimer's disease have coincidental vascular disease, and it is believed that the vascular disease may exacerbate the Alzheimer pathology changes.

OTHER DEGENERATIVE DISEASES

Alzheimer's disease, frontotemporal degeneration, and dementia with Lewy bodies are the three main groups of degenerative diseases causing dementia, that is, diseases with direct and progressive loss of brain cells. There are other degenerative diseases that can cause dementia, such as Huntington's disease and progressive supranuclear palsy or Steele Richardson syndrome, but with these there are often other neurological abnormalities such as problems with walking. Creutzfeldt-Jakob disease (CJD) is a very distressing and rapidly progressive degenerative disorder that can lead to death in a matter of months. In all of the degenerative dementias, the underlying disease process tends to affect particular areas of the brain or particular groups of cells. It is this selective vulnerability that determines the early clinical features. These are very important diagnostic clues for the neurologist and psychiatrist.

OTHER CAUSES OF DEMENTIA

The causes of dementia and/or less severe cognitive impairment are innumerable. Many of the causes give rise to cognitive slowing or mild cognitive impairment rather than the panoply of severe dementia. However, as patients are presenting earlier, it is important to undertake very careful investigation and consideration of the full differential diagnosis. Patients with a frontal meningioma, a benign tumor, can still present late with slowly progressive personality change and emerging dementia. Chronic infections such as tuberculous meningitis can also give rise to cognitive impairment, as can HIV disease.

Drug-induced dementia is an important group to consider. The elderly in particular can be quite sensitive to side effects of many medications. Sleeping tablets are notorious for causing memory lapses. Alcohol also can cause cognitive impairment, and the history is not always obvious. In some patients with poor nutrition and very high alcohol intake, Korsakov's syndrome occurs with a very severe memory deficit. Depression is another important cause to consider. Many patients with depression will complain of their memory and can be shown to have a genuine cognitive slowing. In severe, untreated depression this can resemble Alzheimer's disease. The clinical situation is complicated by the fact that depression is common in early Alzheimer's disease. Therefore, even if there is improvement in cognition following a trial of an antidepressant, the patient may still go on to progress to a clinically definite Alzheimer's disease. If in doubt, such a patient should always have a trial of an antidepressant.

INVESTIGATIONS

Since dementia is a clinical syndrome and not a disease, full investigation is required for each patient. Much information is obtained by a careful history from the patient and from the partner or family members. An assessment of the pattern of the cognitive impairment, both by bedside testing and by more detailed assessment of neuropsychological function, will provide the likely diagnosis in the majority of cases. Neuroimaging or brain scanning, of which magnetic resonance imaging (MRI) is the most useful, will exclude many of the secondary causes of dementia such as tumors and strokes. A variety of blood tests and occasionally an electroencephalogram (EEG) will complete the investigation. Some patients will require more intensive investigation such as examination of the cerebrospinal fluid.

The majority of patients will have an underlying degenerative disease, whether it is Alzheimer's disease, frontotemporal degeneration, or dementia with Lewy bodies. As such, many of the investigations are essentially normal, but this can be difficult for the patient and family to understand. Normal means that many other abnormalities have been excluded. Neither brain scans nor the other investigations can provide a definitive diagnosis of the underlying degenerative disease. This can only be established with certainty by examination of brain tissue. However, with careful clinical assessment, supplemented by investigations, a diagnosis can be made with approximately 80 percent accuracy. The 20 percent of uncertainty tends to be in identifying other degenerative diseases rather than missing a major reversible cause. Increasingly, MRI scans can demonstrate tissue loss, which is common among degenerative diseases, and in a characteristic distribution, as in FTD. The pattern of atrophy, for example, in the semantic dementia type of FTD characteristically is a very focal involvement of the front part of the temporal lobe.

Recently it has been possible both to image beta-amyloid and to measure it in the cerebrospinal fluid obtained by lumbar puncture. This is proving valuable for excluding Alzheimer's disease in someone with the clinical features of FTD.

Finally, it is important to remember that our classification of diseases is there to help manage patients. We classify patients and their problems either at the level of the clinical presentations (memory impairment or dementia); damage to an organ (frontotemporal lobar degeneration or strokes); or at a molecular level, in terms of specific DNA mutations in familial disease or particular abnormal proteins that are deposited.

Which classification we choose to use when we determine that changes in cognition are abnormal is determined by what is helpful to us as clinicians and patients to manage these distressing problems.

Table 1.1. Frontotemporal Degeneration and Alzheimer's Disease: Similarities and Differences

FEATURES	FRONTOTEMPORAL DEGENERATION	ALZHEIMER'S DISEASE
Age at which disease generally occurs	• common between 40 and 70 years of age	• common over 65 years of age
Brain areas affected	• frontal and temporal lobes	• starts in the medial temporal area, usually in the hippocampus • spreads to other areas of the brain
Pathologic features	• loss of nerve cells • no amyloid plaques • tau protein tangles seen in certain FTDs, but different from AD tangles	• loss of nerve cells • amyloid plaques • tau tangles
Clinical features	• varying personality and behavior changes, from apathy to hyperactivity • loss of empathy toward others; lack of proper social conduct • memory is preserved early on • language difficulty • compulsive eating and oral fixations • repetitive actions	• begins with memory loss • loss of ability to learn new information • inability to orient oneself to time and place • later, personality and behavior problems develop • possible hallucinations and delusions in later stages

CHAPTER 2

WHAT IS FRONTOTEMPORAL DEGENERATION?

A Clinical Perspective

Murray Grossman, MD, EdD

INTRODUCTION

Frontotemporal degeneration (FTD) is a progressive neurodegenerative condition that typically begins in the fifth or sixth decade of life, although cases have been reported with an onset as young as twenty-one years of age and as old as eighty-five years of age. Community-based epidemiologic studies establishing the frequency of this condition in the population are rare, although it appears that FTD is as common as Alzheimer's disease (AD) up to sixty-five years of age. FTD differs from AD in that the frequency of AD, but not FTD, increases thereafter with age. There are many other features that distinguish between FTD and AD, and these will be noted below when the clinical features of FTD are described. There do not appear to be any geographic or sociodemographic risk factors associated with FTD. There is no evidence that head trauma, consumption of particular foods, or exposure to a substance in the environment is a risk factor for the development of FTD.

In large clinics, the estimated frequency of FTD ranges from 5 to 20 percent. Estimates suggest that between 2 and 13 percent of autopsy series of demented patients in large hospitals have frontotemporal lobar degeneration (FTLD), the pathologic condition that causes clinical FTD in about 80 percent of cases. There are several forms of FTLD pathology. Perhaps the most common form is an accumulation of microscopic pathology showing TDP-43

(FTLD-TDP). This is also the most common pathology in amyotrophic lateral sclerosis (ALS, also known as motor neuron disease or Lou Gehrig's disease), and up to 10 percent of FTD patients with FTLD-TDP pathology may also have ALS. Another common condition causing FTD is FTLD-tau, where the accumulation of microscopic tau is associated with Pick's disease as well as movement disorders such as corticobasal syndrome and progressive supranuclear palsy. There are several other, less common pathologies such as FTLD-FUS.

The vast majority of patients with FTD are sporadic, that is, without any evidence of a family history of an inherited neurodegenerative disease. However, careful ascertainment with a three-generation family history suggests that about 25 percent of patients with FTD have a high-risk or medium-risk family history consistent with an inherited disorder. Among these patients, about 80 percent or about 20 percent of all FTD patients—have a genetic mutation that can be defined. The three most common inherited disorders are a mutation of microtubule-associated protein-tau (*MAPT*) on chromosome 17, a mutation of progranulin (*GRN* [the official abbreviation is *GRN*, and *PGRN* is a synonym that is widely used outside this book]) on another portion of chromosome 17, and a hexanucleotide repeat expansion in an open reading frame on chromosome 9 (*C9orf72*). The latter is also frequently associated with ALS. Moreover, 5–10 percent of cases with a repeat expansion of *C9orf72* occur spontaneously and without any evidence of a family history of disease.

This chapter focuses on the clinical features of FTD. First, I will discuss the major clinical presentations, including changes in cognition, language, and affect. Some of the neurological changes associated with FTD also will be described. Following a description of these initial clinical presentations, the natural history, prognosis, and diagnosis of this condition will be addressed.

CLINICAL PRESENTATION

The Syndromic Approach to Frontotemporal Degeneration

FTD typically presents with one of two clinical syndromes, although there are some less common presentations that will be mentioned below as well. The two most common clinical presentations include primary progressive aphasia (PPA), and a disorder of social comportment and executive functioning (planning, organization, and dual tasking) known as behavioral variant frontotemporal degeneration (bvFTD). A related but less common presentation involves PPA or bvFTD occurring together with ALS, a form of motor weakness that can affect the face, arms, and/or legs. Other forms of FTD involve an involuntary motor disorder. Some cases have a disorder of eye movements and axial rigidity with gait disturbance known as progressive supranuclear palsy (PSP) or lateralized involuntary movements together with apraxia (difficulty with gestures) and visual-perceptual-spatial difficulty known as corticobasal syndrome (CBS).

Primary Progressive Aphasia

Aphasia is a central disorder of speech and language that can affect oral and written comprehension and production. In aphasia, there is no deafness, blindness, muteness, or peripheral disorder that can explain the language deficit. Components of language can be impaired in isolation or in combination with other language processes, depending on the portion of the brain that is compromised in FTD. Unlike a stroke or head trauma, this form of aphasia is progressive in nature. Finally, this form of aphasia is said to be primary because there is no other obvious cause of progressive aphasia such as a brain tumor or hydrocephalus. Hence the name primary progressive aphasia (PPA).

There are several variants of PPA. One form of progressive aphasia is known as the semantic variant of PPA (svPPA). Another name for this condition is semantic dementia. The dominant clinical features of this variant of PPA is difficulty with naming and impaired comprehension of single words and objects. The difficulty with single-word comprehension may begin with isolated vocabulary terms but will gradually involve larger portions of the vocabulary over time. A (lost) word will not be able to be described by patients with svPPA except in the most vague manner. This is because the mental representation of the meaning of word is progressively degraded. Sometimes very general words will be substituted for the target word (e.g., *bird* or *animal* for the intended word *robin*). Difficulty with single-word comprehension and retrieval will be evident in both oral communication and writing. As this condition progresses, there appear to be increasing problems with comprehension of objects, and patients with svPPA may be capable of using only their own familiar objects (e.g., a coffee cup or a brush) in a familiar context like their home. Difficulty with reading may be most pronounced for sight vocabulary terms that cannot be sounded out, such as *who* or *choir*. Repetition is accurate.

Speech remains relatively fluent, sentence production appears to be grammatically well formed, and comprehension of grammar appears to be relatively preserved. In autopsy series, the most common pathology associated with svPPA is FTLD-TDP.

Another form of language difficulty commonly seen in FTD is the nonfluent/agrammatic variant of PPA (naPPA). Another name for this condition is progressive nonfluent aphasia (PNFA). In this form of PPA, comprehension and expression of single-content words is relatively preserved, although these patients may develop some naming difficulty. The major problem in naPPA is a disorder of speech fluency. This is due in part to the patient's limited access to grammatical forms such as the small grammatical words that allow us to construct a sentence. Without these grammatical components, speech is disjointed and effortful. At first, patients use simplified grammatical forms, and over time there are many frank grammatical errors. This grammatical deficit appears to affect both expression and comprehension. Patients with naPPA thus have difficulty determining who did what to whom in a sentence. Oral and written utterances may have grammatical errors. In oral expression, some naPPA patients may have a disorder known as apraxia of speech. This involves poor coordination of the motor speech apparatus, so that patients produce many speech sound errors. The most common form of pathology associated with naPPA is FTLD-tau.

A third form of PPA is known as the logopenic variant of PPA (lvPPA). This is also known as progressive mixed aphasia. Speech in these patients may be slower but is often grammatically well formed. Comprehension of objects is largely preserved, although there may be some difficulty with word comprehension. However, these patients may produce frequent sound substitutions (phonemic paraphasic errors) in their speech. Their short-term memory for verbal material also can be extremely limited, resulting in difficulty repeating phrases and multisyllabic words. lvPPA is often associated with the same pathology seen in Alzheimer's disease.

Disorders of Affect and Social Comportment

Another major clinical presentation of FTD involves a disorder of social comportment and personality. This is known as the behavioral variant of frontotemporal degeneration (bvFTD). These patients are noteworthy for inappropriate social conduct. They seem insensitive to the norms governing social interactions and personal behavior in society. Initially, patients with bvFTD appear to make some odd or inappropriate statements or voice unusual opinions that are out of character for their previous personality. Over a short period of time, however, it becomes clear that this approach to social interactions is not restricted to a single event but reflects a broad underlying loss of appropriate behavior. Comments emerge that are disinhibited and may be blurted out without any sensitivity or consideration of context. These may involve comments on body habits or inappropriate joking. There is a loss of social graces and a frank rudeness.

These patients lack empathy for difficulties that others may be encountering. This lack of empathy is not restricted to strangers but also involves spouses and other family members with whom there is greater familiarity and intimacy. This results in a coldness and emotional distancing that is unusual for family members. There appears to be little insight into the intentions of others, and the patients appear to be entirely self-centered. These patients also can develop complex rituals and obsessions. They may collect unusual objects such as toilet paper rolls or develop pseudo-religious or pseudo-political beliefs. The may sing or whistle. There may also be simpler repetitive behaviors such as clapping and tapping. These changes can result in risky behavior. For example, there can be great susceptibility to monetary scams.

This stark change in personality can have consequences in other domains. Patients can appear to be hypersexual. This can manifest itself as promiscuous sexual encounters with strangers or inappropriate and unsatisfied sexual demands of spouses. Subtler manifestations of hypersexual behavior may include a fetish associated with a movie star, a focus on sexual jokes, and inappropriate sexual comments that seem disinhibited and out of context.

Another form of disinhibited behavior can involve an inappropriate attraction to small shiny objects or fire. At times this can be manifested as shoplifting or pocketing attractive artifacts from friends' houses.

Inappropriate rage responses can also be seen in these patients. This involves sudden, unexpected outbursts of angry behavior that rarely can become violent. The provocation can be minimal or even imagined in nature. Regardless of the perceived slight, these patients can produce a verbal tirade that sometimes can be difficult to quell. The patients do not appear to understand the reason for physical restraint.

Hyperoral behavior can be quite common in these patients. This can range from the disinhibited consumption of large volumes of food to oral exploration of inedible objects. Obsessive dietary preferences can emerge and the diet may become restricted to highly idiosyncratic choices of food substances. These changes in oral behavior can be accompanied by radical changes in weight.

There can be important changes in goal-directed behavior. Patients may appear to be profoundly apathetic. They have difficulty initiating the simplest behaviors spontaneously. Even significant prompting by a loved one for participation in a previously enjoyed hobby or avocation can yield no response. Patients may be content to literally do nothing all day. This disorder of motivation and apathy can affect all realms of human behavior, resulting in an akinetic state or mutism. Incontinence may emerge early in this context because of limited motivation to use the bathroom.

Dysexecutive Syndrome

A form of cognitive difficulty overlapping with a social disorder is a limitation in executive functioning. Executive resources include selective attention and control over inhibition, task switching, and planning and organizing. Difficulties with control over attention and inhibition can emerge as perseveration or repeatedly performing the same activities. This can also be manifested as echolalia or mindlessly repeating a phrase that has just been uttered. Echopraxia, or mindlessly repeating a gesture, also can be seen. Patients are distracted quite easily and can have difficulty refocusing their attention. Patients also can become environmentally dependent or perceptually bound. This involves thoughtlessly incorporating objects in the environment into ongoing activities. Task switching involves the ability to alternate between ongoing cognitive or physical activities in a flexible and organized manner. This can limit productive behavior since performance is restricted to the execution of simple tasks. Each event or thought has to be initiated anew, and patients consequently can appear to be quite sluggish and slow in their performance of activities, including familiar activities of daily living. Considerable guidance is needed, even for overlearned activities such as bathing. These kinds of difficulties can limit judgment and interfere with management of personal finances.

Working memory involves the ability to manipulate a relatively small amount of information held in short-term memory over a brief period of time. Working memory is involved in a large number of ongoing cognitive activities such as the comprehension of a conversation or a movie. Limitations in working memory can result in reduced enjoyment of previously appreciated activities such as watching TV or reading a book.

Activities in our complex society often require planning and organizing. This may be the heart of the concept of executive resources and include activities such as performing two or more tasks interchangeably. In this context, patients can execute complex activities when guided by others in a step-by-step manner, or when constrained by the environment. When performing activities spontaneously and without constraint, however, the patients can appear remarkably impaired. This can result in the phenomenon of a patient being quite incapacitated in the performance of multistep activities in the real world, without evidence for difficulties during a highly constrained medical or psychiatric examination. Disorganization in conversational exchanges results in tangential thoughts and comments, difficulty maintaining a topic of conversation, and frequent interruptions of ongoing speech and conversation of others.

These clinical features are described in isolation for the sake of clarity. It is important to understand that they may also co-occur. svPPA thus may occur with a disorder of social comportment, particularly a rigid and cold personality with obsessive, complex rituals. naPPA may co-occur with an apathetic and passive personality and poor organization. Combinations of language and social difficulties are less common at the onset of the disease and are more likely to be seen together in an individual as the disease progresses.

Unusual Clinical Manifestations of FTD

Corticobasal Syndrome

Corticobasal syndrome (CBS) is a rare condition allied to FTD. Early descriptions of CBS often emphasized the movement disorders associated with the condition, such as gait instability, body stiffness, brief and lightning-like movements known as myoclonus, a cramping posture of a hand or a foot known as dystonia, and an impairment in the voluntary control of limbs (so-called alien hand syndrome). Typically these are lateralized. More recently, it has become clear that CBS patients often present with cognitive or social difficulties, and these cognitive and social difficulties can dominate the clinical condition throughout some or all of the course of the disease. There may be problems with language such as impaired naming or effortful speech. Visual-perceptual-spatial functioning may be disturbed. These visual-spatial-perceptual impairments may interfere with the ability to locate objects in space, or limit the ability of an individual to negotiate space without tripping or falling down stairs. Patients may be able to identify individual attributes of a visual array such as the color or the size of an object. However, they cannot assemble this fragmented information into a coherent whole. These visual-perceptual problems can become severe enough to cause a form of visual agnosia or difficulty comprehending the visual appearance of objects.

Many patients develop limb apraxia or difficulty executing learned motor skills. Oftentimes this involves the inappropriate use of implements. A tool may be held in the wrong way or may be used at the wrong angle. Under rare circumstances, gestures may not be understood. Simple calculations also may become difficult, and there may be an impairment interpreting the meaning of objects that are palpated (so-called cortical sensory loss). Infrequently there can be a language deficit. This includes naPPA or an isolated speech disorder such as apraxia of speech. A majority of patients appear to have a form of pathology known as corticobasal degeneration (CBD) associated with CBS, although many patients have an unusual variant of the pathology associated with Alzheimer's disease when examined at autopsy.

Progressive Supranuclear Palsy

Progressive supranuclear palsy (PSP) is another condition that is associated with a disorder of voluntary movements. In this case, the most characteristic disorder is involves a limitation of eye gaze. Eye gaze is slowed at first so that there is early disturbance of the rapid eye movements or saccades that we ordinarily use to examine our visual environment. Typically vertical gaze is disturbed before lateral gaze, resulting in difficulty with walking since the floor can be easily seen and difficulty with eating since food on a plate cannot be easily seen. Eventually the eyes become frozen in the midline.

A second motor problem associated with PSP is rigid, stiff posture. This inflexibility, together with down-gaze difficulty, results in frequent, early falls.

Cognitive difficulty in patients with PSP often involves a limitation in executive functioning. This includes a deficit in planning and mental organization. There can also be apathy and a deficit of limited initiation. Patients with PSP also can have difficulty with language, including naPPA and apraxia of speech.

Amyotrophic lateral sclerosis with frontotemporal degeneration

Another unusual presentation of FTD involves the cognitive difficulties described above joined with a disorder of the motor system known as amyotrophic lateral sclerosis (ALS, motor neuron disease or Lou Gehrig's disease). The onset of the motor problems may precede or follow the onset of the cognitive difficulties. ALS is a motor disorder associated with weakness and reduced strength but preserved sensation. This is associated with fasciculations or flickering of muscles under the skin. There may be a loss of muscle bulk. Deep tendon reflexes can become very brisk. Weakness can affect muscles of the head, resulting in difficulty with speech and swallowing. ALS typically progresses relatively rapidly over three to five years, although there are certainly exceptions. Traditional thinking has been that ALS is purely a motor disorder, but it is increasingly recognized that up to 50 percent patients with ALS have cognitive deficits in addition to a motor disorder. About 10 percent of patients have ALS associated with a form of FTD—either bvFTD or PPA. The remaining individuals with cognitive difficulty have a milder, less progressive form of cognitive difficulty known as ALS-Mild Cognitive Impairment (ALS-MCI). These patients may have deficits in executive functioning or social functioning or language.

Natural History

FTD is a progressive neurodegenerative condition. Patients will worsen over time in the cognitive domains where they have difficulty. The trajectory of decline over time, however, is not linear. Instead, there appear to be three clinical phases of progression that involve different rates of change in various domains of functioning.

During the initial or mild stage of FTD, there can be a relatively prolonged period of subtle but insidious change. The subtle changes that do emerge over time are typically restricted to the domain of difficulty that brought the patient to medical attention in the first place. For example, there may be subtle and progressive decline in single-word and object comprehension as well as naming difficulty in patients with svPPA. Patients with naPPA a can have insidiously increasing difficulty with grammatical comprehension and expression. Patients with bvFTD can have worsening of personality and social comportment. It is only under very unusual circumstances that progressive change evolves rapidly during the early course of FTD. A rapid change should call to question the diagnosis of FTD, although the emergence of ALS often is associated with more rapid change. Intercurrent events such as the development of pneumonia or a urinary-tract infection should be investigated in the setting of rapid decline. Similarly, the absence of change over a prolonged period of time should raise questions about the underlying diagnosis. A "phenocopy" is an individual who resembles the characteristics of FTD but does not progress over time, raising the possibility that the patient may have a psychiatric condition rather than a progressive neurodegenerative condition.

The second or moderate stage of FTD involves a more rapidly emerging series of changes over a briefer time course. During this phase of the condition, qualitatively different kinds of language, cognitive, and behavioral changes can emerge. For example, a patient presenting with svPPA can begin having difficulty with social comportment and demonstrate a rigid personality. A patient with naPPA can begin to show apathy and poor judgment. A patient with a disorder of social comportment can begin to demonstrate language impairments.

At a functional level, patients in the moderate stage of FTD become increasingly dependent on others for instrumental activities of daily living. This can involve increasing dependence on others for more complex, multistep, day-to-day care needs, such as grooming and dressing, that previously may have been performed independently. Patients thus may require verbal guidance, prompting, and even some direct assistance to complete activities such as bathing.

The severe stage of FTD is characterized functionally by dependence on others for virtually all activities of daily living. This can include toileting, feeding, bathing, and basic mobility. Language, cognitive, and personality disorders can be quite extensive.

In the severe stage of disease, because patients are quite dependent on others for daily needs, there is increased risk of morbidity and mortality associated with meeting these needs. One example is that difficulty with independent feeding can result in aspiration of food into the lungs. This can cause chemical pneumonia, a frequent cause of death among FTD patients. The issues leading to aspiration are multifactorial. There can be difficulty coordinating the orofacial musculature. Patients can also be easily distracted from concentrating on a fundamental activity that previously had been automatic. For example, attention is needed to swallow food in a safe manner. Patients also may not appreciate the need to swallow and instead can continue to place food in the mouth in an unregulated manner.

Another example of morbidity in the severe stage of FTD is concerned with the role of mobility and frequent postural adjustments to avoid decubitus ulcers or skin breakdown in the form of bedsores. As part of normal mobility, we frequently adjust our posture so that our body's weight does not rest for long periods of time on the same portions of our skin. In apathetic patients with limited initiation, reduced motivation and poor planning, there may be long periods of time where they do not adjust posture and remain dependent on the same portions of skin. This limits blood circulation to the area and causes death to skin tissue. Skin breakdown results in infection that can spread to the bloodstream.

Patients with FTD can become incontinent quite early in the course of their condition because of apathy or poor insight. Incontinence can be associated with infection if there is incomplete bathing. Urinary-tract infections can develop (particularly in women), which can spread to the kidneys and bloodstream if not treated appropriately.

Prognosis

The time course over which these changes evolve is highly variable and difficult to predict. Average survival is about seven years from the onset of symptoms. Under rare circumstances, there can be relatively rapid decline over the course of eighteen months. This form of FTD is often associated with motor neuron disease. Some clinical impressions are that younger patients tend to progress more rapidly, although there are no data to support this observation. On the other hand, the natural history can be quite prolonged in some individuals, particularly where there are no other health-related comorbidities.

Several studies have related the specific, pathological cause of FTD to prognosis. However, the results of these studies have been contentious, and the precise role of various pathological entities remains to be resolved. Some have claimed that the particular aphasic or behavioral syndrome contributes to prognosis, but again this is controversial. Nevertheless, there appear to be some neurological changes that can have a reliably negative impact on prognosis. One relatively common change is concerned with gait. Deteriorating balance and gait stability can result in frequent falls. This may be due in part to poor postural adjustment associated with axial rigidity. Frequent falls increase the risk for fractures of the hip, vertebrae, or skull that can have profound and wide-ranging consequences for prognosis. In addition, patients can develop a subdural hematoma, a collection of blood between the brain and the skull that can result from closed head injury. One protective factor for the patient appears to be education—the more years of education, the better the prognosis.

MEDICAL INVESTIGATIONS

A variety of disorders can mimic FTD. It is important to detect these because some are treatable. Serum studies looking for B12 deficiency, reduced thyroid functioning, and other age-related disorders of metabolism should be performed.

A structural MRI image of the brain is necessary to rule out several conditions that can mimic FTD. For example, the accumulation of small strokes oftentimes can be detected only by MRI. Similarly, subtle forms of hydrocephalus require exclusion by MRI and possibly lumbar puncture. Other conditions that can potentially mimic FTD also can be excluded by MRI, including closed head injury, subdural hematoma, and a brain tumor or other forms of cancer. FTD itself is associated at times with focal atrophy or shrinkage of brain regions such as the frontal and temporal lobes of the brain. Oftentimes, the panel of medical investigations is within normal limits and atrophy on MRI is too subtle to provide reliable confirmation of a diagnosis of FTD. Under these circumstances, a functional neuroimaging study such as a positron emission tomography (PET) scan or a single proton emission computed tomography (SPECT) scan can be useful. New forms of functional MRI are being developed that are very sensitive to deficits in brain activity. These investigations can demonstrate focal reductions in gray-matter functioning in an anatomic distribution of the brain that corresponds to the patient's clinical difficulties. Preliminary work suggests that the profile of protein in the cerebrospinal fluid may be informative for diagnosis, such as a low level of tau in the cerebrospinal fluid. While several experimental procedures for diagnosing FTD are currently under development, there is no known definitive diagnostic test for FTD short of the direct examination of the brain with a biopsy or at autopsy. In chapter 8 the diagnostic criteria for FTD based on neuropathology findings are presented.

Under unusual circumstances, inflammation of the small arteries bringing blood to the brain can result in reduced brain perfusion and microscopically sized areas of ischemia or stroke. This can interfere with brain functioning, despite the absence of gross neurologic changes associated with larger strokes. Lymphoma, a collection of malignant cells in the cerebrospinal fluid that bathes the brain, can suppress brain functioning in a manner that mimics FTD. Finally, there may be unusual, slow-growing infections associated with meningoencephalitis that can affect the fluid around the brain. To identify these conditions, it is necessary to perform a lumbar puncture so that the cerebrospinal fluid bathing the brain can be directly examined to search for these conditions.

Unusual forms of partial complex seizures can mimic FTD in some circumstances. This may be detected only with a careful history and an EEG.

It is reasonable to obtain some blood tests that rule out metabolic conditions that can mimic FTD, including thyroid-function tests, B12 level (possibly supplemented by methylmalonic acid and homocysteine), liver-function tests, and other routine blood chemistries. Infections such as Lyme disease and syphilis should be omitted with blood tests. Blood tests can be performed to rule out systemic inflammatory conditions, too.

A lumbar puncture is important to obtain under some circumstances as well. In individuals who are immunocompromised or there is other evidence of a systemic condition, when there is a significant travel history, in individuals with a more rapid rate of progression, and in other circumstances, it is important to examine the cerebrospinal fluid for infectious diseases, evidence of inflammation, and cytopathology.

One issue to keep in mind is that these diagnostic studies are important for ruling out conditions that can mimic FTD. Only research studies are currently available to make a definitive diagnosis of FTD. Currently, the diagnosis of FTD is made by an experienced clinician, and imaging, blood, cerebrospinal fluid, and other tests are administered to rule out conditions resembling FTD.

TREATMENT AND MANAGEMENT

Treatment and management of FTD has immense potential. However, there have been few systematic clinical trials of medications or observations of behavioral interventions that have been well studied. In this context, management and treatment often is based on rational approaches derived from the principles of medical therapeutics. These issues are addressed in detail in chapter 5 this book. Commonsense safety precautions for the patient and the family should be implemented, and these are described in part 2 of this book.

Disease-modifying treatment trials are now beginning. These treatments are so important because they represent our best hope for a cure for FTD. Some of these involve medications and other substances that directly target the underlying factors that cause FTD, including tau and TDP-43. Some disease-modifying treatments target other protein products associated with these pathologies. Other hypothetical strategies for treatment also are being developed. These treatments are developed in animal models of disease, and they can be tried in humans following safety trials.

Symptomatic treatment can take the form of neurotransmitter supplementation. Medications borrowed from other conditions—such as Alzheimer's disease, Parkinson's disease, and depression—may contribute to clinical slowing of progression. However, one recent, multisite, double-blind, placebo-controlled trial did not demonstrate any benefit for FTD patients from memantine. Other symptomatic treatments are directed at specific complaints, such as the treatment of hallucinations, depression, fatigue, anxiety, and hypersexual behavior. Some substances may alter the natural history of FTD, although these have not been tested empirically. These include antioxidants, such as vitamin E, and nonsteroidal anti-inflammatory agents. It is important to discuss medications with a physician before initiating a treatment trial, particularly because some medications can worsen clinical functioning. For example, the behavioral and social disorder seen in FTD can be worsened by the class of cholinesterase-inhibitor medications typically used for Alzheimer's disease.

There are also behavioral interventions that may be beneficial. There is very reasonable evidence supporting the claim that physical activity and mental activity are quite beneficial in healthy aging and neurodegenerative conditions. Indeed, some evidence suggests a synergistic relationship between physical and mental activity that, when performed daily, is more beneficial than the sum of each.

Management of the environment can be very beneficial to patients as well. This includes strategies for optimizing communication to help aphasics and removal of provocative stimuli from patients with a social and behavioral disorder. Patients with a social disorder benefit from a relatively structured daily curriculum of activities. This is addressed in greater detail in other chapters of this book.

SUMMARY

The care of patients with frontotemporal degeneration is demanding on families and friends. Some of this burden can be eased with better understanding of the condition. The goal of this chapter was to characterize FTD in a manner that will familiarize families and friends with some of the clinical features of this condition. This should help explain previous experiences that may have been misinterpreted, such as understanding that unusual behavior is not willful but is a component of the disease process. Moreover, it is important to be able to understand what the future may hold. Also, this chapter helps family and friends appreciate the complexity of diagnosis for this group of conditions through an understanding of the various clinical presentations and lack of a specific diagnostic test. Because this group of conditions has only recently been defined, more research is needed to determine the underlying cause or biology along with treatment and management.

CLINICAL CRITERIA FOR FTD

Consensus criteria have been developed for behavioral variant FTD and for the various forms of primary progressive aphasia. These are provided below.

Criteria for Behavioral Variant FTD (Rascovsky et al., 2011)

I. Neurodegenerative Disease

The following symptom must be present to meet criteria for bvFTD.

  A. **Shows progressive deterioration of behavior and/or cognition by observation or history** (as provided by a knowledgeable informant).

II. Possible bvFTD

Three of the following behavioral / cognitive symptoms [A–F] must be present to meet criteria. These symptoms should occur repeatedly, not just as a single instance.

A. Early behavioral disinhibition (one of the following symptoms [A.1–A.3] must be present):

A.1. Socially inappropriate behavior
A.2. Loss of manners or decorum
A.3. Impulsive, rash, or careless actions

B. Early apathy or inertia (one of the following symptoms [B.1–B.2] must be present):

B.1. Apathy
B.2. Inertia

C. Early loss of sympathy or empathy (one of the following symptoms [C.1–C.2] must be present):

C.1. Diminished response to other people's needs and feelings
C.2. Diminished social interest, interrelatedness, or personal warmth

D. Early perseverative, stereotyped, or compulsive/ritualistic behavior (one of the following symptoms [D.1–D.3] must be present):

D.1. Simple repetitive movements
D.2. Complex, compulsive, or ritualistic behaviors
D.3. Stereotypy of speech

E. Hyperorality and dietary changes (one of the following symptoms [E.1–E.3] must be present):

E.1. Altered food preferences
E.2. Binge eating, increased consumption of alcohol or cigarettes
E.3. Oral exploration or consumption of inedible objects

F. Neuropsychological profile: executive/generation deficits with relative sparing of memory and visuospatial functions (all of the following symptoms [F.1–F.3] must be present):

F.1. Deficits in executive tasks

F.2. Relative sparing of episodic memory

F.3. Relative sparing of visuospatial skills

III. Probable bvFTD

All of the following symptoms [A–C] must be present to meet criteria.

A. Meets criteria for possible bvFTD

B. Exhibits significant functional decline (by caregiver report or as evidenced by Clinical Dementia Rating [CDR] or Functional Activities Questionnaire [FAQ] scores)

C. Imaging results consistent with bvFTD (one of the following [C.1–C.2] must be present):

C.1. Frontal and/or anterior temporal atrophy on CT or MRI

C.2. Frontal hypoperfusion or hypometabolism on SPECT or PET

IV. bvFTD with Definite FTLD Pathology

Criterion A and either Criterion B or Criterion C must be present to meet criteria.

A. Meets criteria for possible or probable bvFTD

B. Histopathological evidence of FTLD on biopsy or at postmortem

C. Presence of a known pathogenic mutation

V. Exclusion Criteria for bvFTD

Criteria A and B must be answered negatively for any bvFTD diagnosis. Criterion C can be positive for possible bvFTD but must be negative for probable bvFTD.

A. Pattern of deficits is better accounted for by other nondegenerative nervous-system or medical disorders.

B. Behavioral disturbance is better accounted for by a psychiatric diagnosis.

C. Biomarkers strongly indicative of Alzheimer's disease or other neurodegenerative process.

Criteria for Primary Progressive Aphasia (Gorno-Tempini et al., 2011)

INCLUSION: Criteria 1 through 3 must be answered positively for a PPA diagnosis

1. Most prominent clinical feature is difficulty with language (word-finding deficits, paraphasias, effortful speech, grammatical and/or comprehension deficits)
2. These deficits are the principal cause of impaired daily living activities (e.g., problems with communication activity related to speech and language, such as using the telephone)
3. Aphasia should be the most prominent deficit at symptom onset and for the initial phases of the disease.

EXCLUSION: Criteria 1 through 4 must be answered negatively for a PPA diagnosis

1. Pattern of deficits is better accounted for by other nondegenerative nervous-system or medical disorders (e.g., neoplasm, cerebrovascular disease, hypothyroidism, etc.)
2. Cognitive disturbance is better accounted for by a psychiatric diagnosis (e.g., depression, bipolar disorder, schizophrenia, preexisting personality disorder)
3. Prominent initial episodic memory, visual memory, and visuo-perceptual impairments (e.g., inability to copy simple line drawings)
4. Prominent initial behavioral disturbance (e.g., marked disinhibition, emotional detachment, hyperorality, or repetitive/compulsive behaviors)

Nonfluent Variant PPA

I. Clinical Diagnosis of Nonfluent Variant PPA

At least one of the following core features must be present:

1. Agrammatism in language production
2. Effortful, halting speech with inconsistent distortions, deletions, sub-

stitutions, insertions, or transpositions of speech sounds, particularly in polysyllabic words (often considered to reflect "apraxia of speech")

At least two of three of the following other features must be present:

1. Agrammatism in comprehension: impaired comprehension of syntactically complex sentences
2. Spared single-word comprehension
3. Spared object knowledge

II. Imaging-Supported Nonfluent Variant Diagnosis

Both of the following criteria must be present:

1. Clinical diagnosis of nonfluent variant PPA
2. Imaging must show one or more of the following results:
   a.   Predominant left posterior fronto-insular atrophy on MRI
   b.   Predominant left posterior fronto-insular hypoperfusion or hypometabolism on SPECT or PET scan

III. Nonfluent Variant PPA with Definite Pathology

Clinical diagnosis (Criteria 1 below) and either Criterion 2 or Criterion 3 must be present:

1. Clinical diagnosis of nonfluent variant PPA
2. Histopathological evidence of a specific pathology (e.g., FTLD-tau, FTLD-TDP) on biopsy or at postmortem
3. Presence of a known pathogenic mutation

Semantic Variant PPA

I. Clinical Diagnosis of Semantic Variant PPA

Both of the following core features must be present:

1. Poor confrontation naming (of pictures or objects), particularly for low-familiarity or low-frequency items
2. Impaired single-word comprehension

At least three of the following other diagnostic features must be present:

1. Poor object knowledge, particularly for low-frequency or low-familiarity items
2. Surface dyslexia and/or dysgraphia
3. Spared repetition
4. Spared motor speech (no distortions) and grammar

II. Imaging-Supported Semantic Variant PPA Diagnosis

Both of the following criteria must be present:

1. Clinical diagnosis of semantic variant PPA
2. Imaging must show one or more of the following results:
   a. predominant anterior temporal lobe atrophy
   b. predominant anterior temporal hypoperfusion or hypometabolism on SPECT or PET scan

III. Semantic Variant PPA with Definite Pathology

Clinical diagnosis (Criteria 1 below) and either Criterion 2 or Criterion 3 must be present:

1. Clinical diagnosis of semantic variant PPA
2. Histopathological evidence of a specific pathology (e.g., FTLD-tau, FTLD-TDP) on biopsy or at postmortem
3. Presence of a known pathogenic mutation

Logopenic Variant PPA

I. Clinical Diagnosis of Logopenic Variant PPA

Both of the following core features must be present:

1. Impaired single-word retrieval in spontaneous speech (speech fluency interrupted by word-finding pauses) and confrontational naming
2. Impaired repetition of sentences and phrases

At least three of the following other features must be present:

1. Speech (phonological) errors in spontaneous speech and naming
2. Spared single-word comprehension and object knowledge
3. Spared motor speech (no distortions)
4. Absence of frank agrammatism

II. Imaging-Supported Logopenic Variant Diagnosis

Both criteria must be present:

1. Clinical diagnosis of logopenic variant PPA
2. Imaging must show at least one of the following results:
   a. predominant left posterior perisylvian or parietal atrophy on MRI
   b. predominant left posterior perisylvian or parietal hypoperfusion or hypometabolism on SPECT or PET scan

III. Logopenic Variant PPA with Definite Pathology

Clinical diagnosis (Criterion 1 below) and either Criterion 2 or Criterion 3 must be present:

1. Clinical diagnosis of logopenic variant PPA
2. Histopathological evidence of a specific pathology (usually AD in this case) on biopsy or at postmortem
3. Presence of a known pathogenic mutation.

AUTHOR'S NOTE

This work was supported in part by grants from the United States Public Health Service (AG017586, AG032953, AG015116, NS044266, AG038490, and the Wyncote Foundation 35867). This work would not have been possible without the support of the patients and the families for whom I care. Their strength and insight continually inspire me.

BIBLIOGRAPHY

Rascovsky, K., J. R. Hodges, D. Knopman, et al. "Sensitivity of Revised Diagnostic Criteria for the Behavioural Variant of Frontotemporal Dementia." *Brain* 134 (2011): 2456–77.

Gorno-Tempini, M. L., A. E. Hillis, S. Weintraub, et al. "Classification of Primary Progressive Aphasia and Its Variants." *Neurology* 76 (2011): 1006–14.

CHAPTER 3

THE ROLE OF GENETICS

A Piece in the FTD Puzzle

Elisabeth McCarty Wood, MS

It was once thought that genetics pertained only to very rare diseases, often affecting children. Now we are constantly reminded that genetics has a much more prominent and complex role in common conditions such as cancer, diabetes, and Alzheimer's disease. The media routinely provides the public with information about the identification of genes linked to diseases and encourages individuals to pay attention to their family medical history. Also, as researchers focus on discovering the underlying causes of specific conditions, they are looking more and more to genetics. This is true for frontotemporal degeneration (FTD) also. As researchers try to determine what causes FTD, some are actively engaged in attempts to identify specific genes that are linked to it. By understanding genetics, one can learn more about the biological basis of the condition, and this knowledge can be used to investigate novel treatments.

The goals of this chapter include:

- explaining the importance of obtaining family-history information
- providing a brief introduction to genetics and patterns of inheritance
- discussing the genetics of FTD
- reviewing the utility and goals of genetic testing and genetic counseling

OBTAINING A FAMILY MEDICAL HISTORY

When a physician or healthcare provider is evaluating a patient for a diagnosis of FTD or a similar neurodegenerative condition, information regarding the family history can help determine a diagnosis. Thus, a detailed family history is a valuable diagnostic tool. It is worth the time and effort to contact relatives and obtain the most accurate details of family structure and medical information. A complete family history that describes structure and health history contains a lot of information. It is important to document the information in a meaningful way that is accessible and easy to read. Geneticists and genetic counselors create a pedigree, which is a graphic description of family structure and health history, to record information collected from patients and families. Determining the quantity and quality of information to collect can be difficult. It is generally recommended to research at least three generations of relatives, which includes:

- first-degree relatives: children, siblings, and parents
- second-degree relatives: half siblings, aunts, uncles, nieces, nephews, grandparents, grandchildren
- third-degree relatives: cousins

The type of medical information to obtain on relatives can include:

- vital status (living or deceased): age (date of birth); age at death; cause of death; autopsy
- health history: birth defects; mental retardation; deafness, blindness; chronic illness; cancer; neurological conditions (e.g., epilepsy, migraines, strokes, multiple sclerosis, movement disorders); mental illness (e.g., bipolar disorder, schizophrenia, OCD); dementia (Alzheimer's disease, senility)
- pregnancy, miscarriages, stillbirths, and infertility
- individuals with previous genetics evaluation
- environmental exposures: radiation, alcohol or drug abuse, tobacco
- ages of diagnoses

When going back and obtaining medical information from previous generations, keep in mind that many of the medical terms we use today, such as *FTD* and *corticobasal syndrome*, were previously not used. Therefore, many individuals with neurodegenerative conditions would have been told that they had *dementia* or *senility*. In such cases, it can be useful to try to gather more descriptive information. For example, it is useful to ask if the individual had problems speaking as a first symptom, or if he had a personality or behavior change. It is also important to try to determine an estimate for the age of onset. Another way to determine diagnosis in deceased relatives is to inquire about autopsy. If an individual had an autopsy, oftentimes the autopsy records (as well as other records, MRI reports, and brain biopsies) can be requested. These records can be most informative. Confirmation of diagnoses with medical records from previous evaluations and laboratory studies is also crucial. The family medical history or pedigree can be a powerful diagnostic tool to a clinician evaluating a patient. The pedigree can be utilized as a diagnostic tool in the following ways:

- to establish pattern of inheritance
- to identify individuals in the family who are at risk for the condition
- to determine strategies for genetic testing
- to help screen for medical risks (such as cancer and heart disease)

Family-history information needs to be respected and treated appropriately by healthcare providers and individual family members. Contacting relatives and asking about personal information is not an easy task. Navigating through the complex interpersonal relationships and personalities in a family can be emotionally difficult and stressful. This is a give-and-take process; it is important to state your intentions or reasons for collecting the information. Offer to recontact family members with information that you learn about your loved one's diagnosis and how it may affect them. Respect an individual's right to privacy. If you go through the effort of obtaining a family history, be sure to document the information clearly and secure it in a location that is accessible to other family members and future generations.

INTRODUCTION TO GENETICS AND INHERITANCE

Deoxyribonucleic acid (DNA) is a chemical that is the most basic unit of genetic information. Chromosomes are highly organized structures containing DNA in long strands. (See figure 3.1.) Most cells in our body contain a complete set of forty-six chromosomes, or twenty-three pairs. The chromosomes are numbered 1 to 22 (largest to smallest) and the twenty-third pair are the sex chromosomes, which determine gender (two X chromosomes = female, or one X and one Y chromosome = male). We inherit our chromosomes at the time of conception: one set of twenty-three from our mother and one set of twenty-three from our father. As we grow from a single cell into a complex human being, our chromosomes are copied into each new cell. Genes are specific subunits or groups of DNA along the chromosomes. Just as our chromosomes come in pairs, so do our genes. Each gene codes for a protein (or chemical) that has a specific function in the body.

The following analogy can be illustrative. One can think of a gene as a long word. Every letter in the word is a piece of DNA. Just like words, genes must be "spelled" or have the correct DNA code to function properly. There are two types of "misspellings" that can occur in our DNA. One type includes words with multiple spellings but with the same meaning or a misspelling that is silent and allows the word to still be read correctly. For example, the word *theater* is sometimes spelled as *theatre*. Despite this alteration, you still understand the word and its meaning. This type of alteration of the DNA code is called a polymorphism. The second type of misspelling involves changes to the word that alter the meaning or make the word unreadable. For example, if the word *good* were changed to *gxod*, one would not be able to make sense out of *gxod*. This type of misspelling or change in the DNA code is called a mutation. Mutations alter the function of the gene and are often associated with disease.

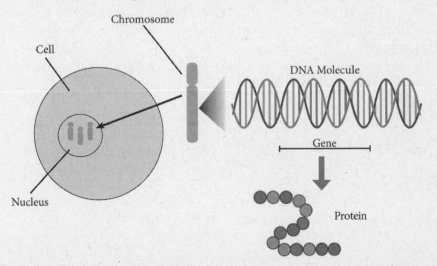

Figure 3.1. This is an illustration of DNA, chromosomes, genes, and proteins that are discussed in the text.

Inherited conditions can be passed on in families in different ways. Autosomal dominant conditions affect males and females equally, and only one gene of the pair needs to be abnormal for the individual to have the condition.

Autosomal dominant conditions are passed from an affected individual to offspring with a 50 percent chance. (See figure 3.2.) The word *autosomal* means the gene that causes the condition is on a numbered chromosome (1 to 22), not one of the sex chromosomes (X or Y). When examining a family history for an autosomal-dominant condition, oftentimes one will identify multiple individuals in each generation with the condition. If an individual did not inherit the abnormal gene, then she cannot pass it on.

Autosomal-recessive conditions affect males and females equally, but both copies of the disease gene need to be abnormal for the individual to have the condition. Autosomal-recessive conditions can be passed on when each parent is a carrier for the condition, and their offspring have a 25 percent risk of inheriting the condition. Carriers have one abnormal copy of the gene but do not have clinical symptoms and are not at increased risk to develop the condition. A family history of a recessive condition can reveal multiple individuals in a single generation (brothers and sisters) with the condition or, in the case of small families, there may be no other affected individuals. Autosomal-recessive conditions also appear more frequently among individuals with the same ethnic background or among individuals who marry within the same family. Other types of inheritance include conditions that are linked to the sex chromosomes (X-linked) or those that are only passed on through maternal transmission. At this time, the known genetic forms of FTD all follow autosomal-dominant inheritance.

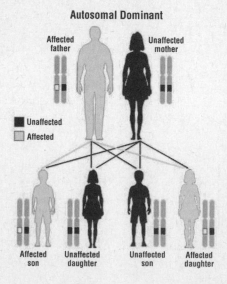

Figure 3.2. Features of autosomal-dominant inheritance. The condition appears in multiple individuals and in successive generations. Any offspring of a parent with the mutation has a 50 percent risk of inheriting the mutation. Individuals who did not inherit the mutation will not develop genetic disease and cannot pass it on to their own children. Males and females are equally likely to have the condition. *Image adapted from the US National Library of Medicine.*

Based on genetic research, we now appreciate that not all genetic conditions are caused by a single gene and show a clear pattern of inheritance when one examines the family tree. Rather, many conditions, especially neurodegenerative conditions, are likely caused by changes in multiple genes that create a susceptibility or increased risk for the condition, combined with environmental influences (e.g., head trauma, infection). Conditions that are caused by both genetic and environmental influences are called multifactorial. (See figure 3.3.) Often, multifactorial conditions are seen in multiple family members but without a specific pattern to the inheritance. However, these conditions can also appear in just one individual. Understanding the genetic contributions to multifactorial conditions can be useful to researchers in trying to identify treatments. Also, knowledge of the genetics can help individuals learn more about their risk for developing a condition.

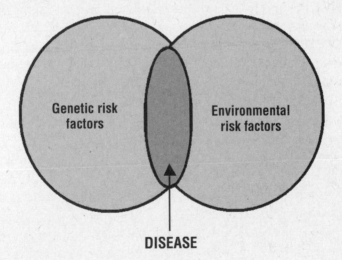

Figure 3.3. Multifactorial Inheritance. Many diseases, including FTD, may be caused by a combination of genetic and environmental factors.

GENETICS OF FTD

When looking at the family histories from patients with FTD, there appears to be three main types: hereditary, familial, and sporadic. (See figure 3.4.) While family history alone cannot predict or eliminate the chance of an underlying genetic cause, it can provide some guidance. Hereditary family histories are the most likely to have a genetic cause. About 15 percent of individuals with FTD have a strong family history that includes multiple relatives with FTD, ALS, dementia, and/or other related neurodegenerative diseases (see figure 3.5). Hereditary family histories often reflect the principles of autosomal-dominant inheritance, as the disease is passed from parent to child through the generations (see figure 3.2). About 25 percent of individuals with FTD have at least one other family member with a neurodegenerative condition or dementia but do not reflect such a strong pattern as seen in the hereditary category; this type of family history is called familial. Some familial cases will have an identifiable genetic cause, but the majority will not. It is possible that multifactorial inheritance (figure 3.3) may apply to some familial cases, but research is ongoing to discover environmental and genetic risk factors that may contribute to a familial history of neurodegenerative conditions. The majority (about 60 percent) of individuals diagnosed with FTD do not have a known family history of the disorder or any other neurodegenerative conditions; these families are typically referred to as sporadic. Individuals unaware of their family-history information are often also included in this category. Gene mutations are rare in sporadic cases. It can be difficult to assign a family history as being definitively hereditary, familial, or sporadic; these categories are meant as a general guide. Discussing an individual's family history in detail with a genetics professional can provide a greater level of interpretation and insight regarding the likelihood of a genetic cause.

Beyond family history, there are some other clinical clues that may help identify a possible genetic cause. In some cases of hereditary FTD, the age of onset may be younger (twenties, thirties, and forties) than for those with sporadic disease—and it may progress more rapidly. The presence of both FTD and ALS in a single individual or family history may also indicate a possible genetic risk. However, as has been described in other chapters, the clinical features of FTD are variable and cannot be used to definitively predict the presence or absence of a genetic cause. The only way to confirm a genetic cause is through genetic testing.

Researchers have been collecting blood and tissue samples from individuals with FTD and related conditions to determine the specific genetic causes for this group of diseases. This has led to the identification of several different genes connected to hereditary FTD. There are three genes that account for the majority of hereditary cases: the chromosome 9 open reading frame

72 (*C9orf72*) gene, the microtubule-associated protein tau (*MAPT*) gene, and the progranulin (*GRN*) gene. *C9orf72*, *MAPT* and *GRN* are inherited in an autosomal-dominant fashion, which means that each first-degree relative of the patient (siblings and offspring) has a 50 percent chance of having the same disease-causing gene mutation and thus developing the disorder.

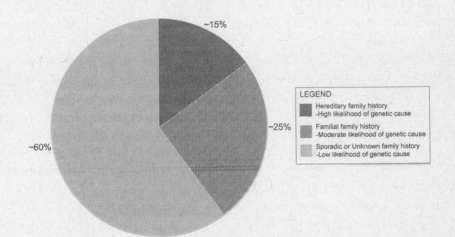

Figure 3.4. Family history and genetic causes of FTD. About 15 percent of all FTD cases are hereditary, reflecting a strong history of disease that suggests an autosomal-dominant pattern of inheritance. The majority, but not all, will have an inherited genetic cause. About 25 percent are familial, meaning that there is at least one other relative with a known neurodegenerative condition. Some individuals in the familial category will have a genetic cause, but not the majority. About 60 percent of FTD is either sporadic, meaning that there is no family history of FTD or neurodegenerative disease, or the family-history information is simply unknown. There is a low likelihood that an inherited genetic factor is responsible for the disease in these cases.

MAPT:

The *MAPT* gene is on chromosome 17 and codes for the protein tau. Mutations in *MAPT* are responsible for about 20–30 percent of hereditary cases of FTD, and about 5–10 percent of all FTD cases. Abnormal amounts of the tau protein have been described in neuropathology (brain tissue) and cerebro-spinal-fluid (fluid that surrounds the brain) investigations among individuals with FTD, Alzheimer's disease, and other neurodegenerative conditions. For more detailed information about the role of tau in pathology and brain cells, refer to chapter 8. In short, all patients with FTD due to *MAPT* mutations will have tau-positive autopsy findings (also known as FTLD-tau); however, not all tau-positive autopsy findings are due to a hereditary genetic cause. The families that were originally linked to the *MAPT* gene (commonly referred to as tau) were given a more specific diagnosis called frontotemporal dementia with Parkinsonism (FTDP-17). This condition was clinically described by the presence of dementia and/or Parkinsonism, frontal and/or temporal atrophy of the brain, as well as two or more similarly affected family members consistent with an autosomal-dominant pattern of inheritance. *MAPT* mutations have also been found in PSP and CBD, but these cases are rare.

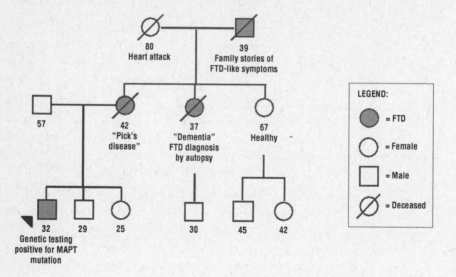

Figure 3.5. Example of a hereditary family history of FTD. This sample pedigree reflects the principles of autosomal-dominant inheritance in a family with a *MAPT* mutation. A well-constructed family history is often crucial for providing the appropriate genetic counseling to patients and family members.

Many different disease-causing mutations have been found in the *MAPT* gene. Some families have unique mutations that have only been described once. However, there are a few mutations that have been seen in multiple families around the world. In such cases, where the same mutation is seen in different families, specific phenotypic (clinical) features have been compared.

These types of studies are called genotype/phenotype correlations. Such information can be useful for counseling families about the associated clinical findings and prognosis when a known mutation is identified. For example, some mutations are associated with a more rapid progression of the condition, while other mutations have a longer duration of disease.

Many polymorphisms have been described in the *MAPT* gene that are not directly linked to disease, although there are some specific patterns of polymorphisms, called *haplotypes*, that have been implicated by association with FTD. Research on these haplotypes is ongoing, but such research does not have clinical or diagnostic implications at this time. Polymorphisms and ongoing genetic research for FTD are discussed in more detail at the end of this section.

GRN:

Through studying families that had autosomal-dominant inheritance of FTD but no mutations in the *MAPT* gene, researchers discovered mutations in a second gene that can cause FTD: progranulin (*GRN*). *GRN* mutations account for about 20–30 percent of hereditary FTD, and 5–10 percent of all FTD cases.

The *GRN* gene is also found on chromosome 17, and it codes for the progranulin protein. The fact that both *MAPT* and *GRN* are found on chromosome 17 is most likely a coincidence. Progranulin is a growth-factor protein, which means it plays a role in activities such as development and wound repair and is found in many different body tissues. At this time, the reason why or how progranulin mutations cause the development of FTD is unknown.

Clinical phenotypes of *GRN*-related FTD have been well described. One interesting finding is that even within the same family, the age of onset can vary greatly. Ages of onset can vary from the thirties to the eighties, with an average age of onset in the late fifties to early sixties. The reason for this variability is not known but suggests that there may be other factors, genetic or environmental, that can affect the onset of disease. Clinical features also vary. Behavioral and language symptoms are common, and like *MAPT*-related FTD, patients may have Parkinsonian features. It's not uncommon for members of the same family to have different presentations and clinical diagnoses. Because of the variability in onset age and clinical features, it may be more difficult to interpret a family history as being suggestive of a genetic cause. For this reason, it is encouraged that any patient or family member with concerns about family history seek the advice of a genetics professional, such as a genetic counselor.

Unlike *MAPT* mutations, in which the gene is directly connected to the disease protein seen in the brain tissue, individuals with *GRN* mutations have accumulation of a different protein, called TDP-43. The currently used term for diagnosis at autopsy would be FTLD-TDP (formerly, this diagnosis may have been written as FTLD-U). Not all patients with FTLD-TDP pathology have *GRN* mutations. For more on the TDP-43 protein and pathology findings in hereditary forms of FTD, please see chapter 8.

C9orf72:

For many years, researchers knew there must be another significant hereditary cause of FTD, but it was not until 2011 that this most recent discovery was made. The *C9orf72* gene was identified as a genetic cause of not only FTD but also amyotrophic lateral sclerosis (ALS). Individuals with the *C9orf72* gene mutation can develop FTD, ALS, or features of both; the diagnoses can also vary within a family. *C9orf72* is now considered to be the most common genetic cause of FTD, accounting for 40–50 percent of hereditary FTD and 5–20 percent of all FTD cases. It is also the most common genetic cause of ALS. Unlike *GRN* and *MAPT* mutations, which are more strongly associated with having a hereditary or familial family history, *C9orf72* mutations have been found in a small (less than 5 percent) of sporadic family histories.

The *C9orf72* mutation is a specific type of genetic change called a hexa-nucleotide repeat expansion. The term *hexanucleotide* refers to a specific segment of six (hexa-) units of DNA (nucleotide): GGGGCC. Everyone has the *C9orf72* gene, in which this GGGGCC segment is supposed to repeat a small number of times. However, a mutation occurs when the repeat grows too large, known as an expansion. In *C9orf72*, a repeat size of thirty or more GGGGCC segments is considered to be a disease-causing mutation. Twenty or fewer repeats is considered normal. Research is ongoing to better under-stand the significance of having 21–29 repeats. Research is also ongoing to explain why some individuals with an expansion develop FTD, some develop ALS, and still others develop both conditions.

The clinical features of FTD due to the *C9orf72* expansion do not differ greatly from nongenetic FTD. Behavioral symptoms are common, as are lan-guage and other classic FTD features. Due to the strong association with ALS, there is a significantly increased risk of the development of ALS. The age of onset is similar to *GRN*, in that the average age of onset is in the mid to late fifties, but the reported range of onset ages varies from the thirties to the eighties. This age-dependent, reduced penetrance may explain why some patients with FTD due to *C9orf72* may appear not to have a family history of disease, as it is possible that other relatives with the mutation died before ever developing disease symptoms. Also similar to *GRN*, *C9orf72*-related FTD and FTD-ALS has TDP-43 positive pathology upon brain autopsy.

Other Genetic Findings for FTD:

Besides *C9orf72*, *GRN*, and *MAPT*, there are other more rare genetic causes of FTD. For example, the valosin-containing protein gene (*VCP*) is a rare cause of hereditary FTD. *VCP* mutations are associated with a specific condition called inclusion body myopathy with Paget disease of the bone and FTD (IBMPFD). Affected individuals may develop FTD, inclusion body myopathy, and/or Paget disease; ALS due to *VCP* mutations has also been described. Another gene, called *CHMP2B*, was identified on chromosome 3 in several families with hereditary FTD. *CHMP2B* is considered to be a very rare case of FTD. The *TARDBP* gene, which is responsible for making the TDP-43 protein, has been extensively studied and is believed to be a potential, although rare, cause of hereditary FTD. The *FUS* gene is more commonly associated with rare forms of hereditary ALS, but it is also considered a potential but very rare cause of genetic FTD.

It is likely that research will continue to discover new genetic contributions to FTD, such as risk factor or susceptibility genes, that may continue to shed additional light on the causes of FTD. For example, genetic studies are investigating the potential significance of single-nucleotide polymorphisms, also known as SNPs. As described earlier in this chapter, polymorphisms are common changes or variations present in more than 1 percent of the general population. SNP-based research is focused on the idea that these small genetic variations, while not disease-causing, may have a small biological effect. It's possible that a SNP, or even a combination of SNPs, may directly or indirectly modify factors such as disease risk, age of onset, prognosis, or underlying pathology. Any additional insight that SNPs could offer would have important clinical research implications for both genetic and nongenetic forms of FTD.

GENETIC COUNSELING AND GENETIC TESTING

Genetic counseling is a communication process between an individual (or the family) and a healthcare provider with special training in genetics. Some of the activities in a typical genetic-counseling session are:

- construction of a pedigree and analysis for patterns of inheritance and genetic risk
- education about natural history, genetics, and inheritance of condition
- discussion of recurrence risk for inherited and multifactorial conditions
- discussion of benefits and limitations of genetic testing
- psychosocial support for individuals and families coping with a diagnosis

A genetic counselor can also be an important ally in advocating healthcare needs for patients and families.

Genetic testing can be extremely complex. Not all tests are 100 percent diagnostic, and often there are ethical and social concerns that influence one's decision whether or not to undergo genetic testing. Genetic testing for FTD is available in both research and clinical settings. There is an important distinction between research-based genetic testing and clinical or commercial genetic testing. Research testing is not a diagnostic test. There is no guarantee of a result that will be of benefit to the patient. Usually the goal of research testing is to advance scientific knowledge about the condition. This research is usually conducted in academic laboratories. A study coordinator or physician should review the details of the study and obtain informed consent from the patient and/or family members for participation. You should be provided with an informed-consent form that has been approved by an Institutional Review Board (IRB) at the university or hospital where the research is being performed. Clinical or commercial genetic testing is a diagnostic test. The patient receives an official result from the test, and this result becomes part of the medical record. The testing is performed in a laboratory that has been approved for this type of diagnostic testing to ensure the integrity of the results.

Such laboratories are located in hospitals, universities, biotechnology companies, and commercial laboratories. Often, clinical genetic testing is offered only after the patient and family have received genetic counseling to explore the benefits and limitations of testing.

Clinical genetic testing for FTD is available as part of a diagnostic workup in individuals with suspected FTD. However, this test will not be useful to all individuals, as the majority of FTD is unlikely to have a genetic cause. For those individuals concerned about a possible genetic cause, genetic testing can be a useful tool. If the genetic test detects a known disease-causing mutation, this result would confirm the diagnosis in the individual as well as define the inheritance risk for the family. It's important to note that if the genetic test does not detect a mutation, it does not mean that the clinical diagnosis is incorrect; it just means for the specific gene or genes included in the test, there was no genetic mutation detected. A genetics professional, such as a genetic counselor, can help explain the results provided by genetic testing, as well as discuss the implications of the result for both the patient and the family.

For patients with hereditary family history of FTD that test negative (no mutations) for the currently identified FTD genes, it would be important to discuss further testing options. There is still ongoing genetic-research analysis to discover new genetic causes and factors. In some cases, it may also be appropriate to consider genetic testing for other forms of dementia that may have been misdiagnosed as FTD. Another option to consider is DNA banking. For a fee, a commercial DNA-banking service will save a sample of an individual's DNA in a carefully regulated laboratory, thus enabling the sample to be used in the future. This is of particular value should new genetic causes of FTD be identified after the individual has died, as the family would still be able to pursue testing using the banked sample. Many individuals who do not have symptoms of FTD but either have a known disease-causing mutation in their family or believe that they are at increased risk for FTD based on family history, have expressed an interest in genetic testing so that they can learn if they inherited the genetic cause. Presymptomatic or predictive genetic testing is not a new concept in coping with neurodegenerative conditions. Such testing has been offered to individuals at risk for Huntington's disease, familial Alzheimer's disease, and other genetic conditions. For the vast majority of these conditions, FTD included, there is no treatment. Therefore, an individual who has the presymptomatic genetic testing may learn that he inherited the disease-causing gene mutation, but he would not have any available medical options to prevent the development of FTD. Genetic counseling for the at-risk individual is paramount.

Many clinical centers and laboratories require that the individual go through a formal protocol of pre- and post-test genetic counseling along with psychiatric evaluation. This offers the individual an opportunity to discuss his motives for testing; explore the possible result outcomes, anticipated reaction, and coping strategies; develop a support system; and discuss the risks associated with receiving a diagnosis (such as an adverse psychological outcome and insurance or employment discrimination). Concerns about the possibility of genetic discrimination are common and should be carefully considered. A federal law was passed in 2008, called the Genetic Information Nondiscrimination Act (GINA), which provides protection against discrimination in the health-insurance and employment settings. However, this law does not provide protection other kinds of policies, such as life or long-term-care insurance. Also, it is important to have the specific genetic abnormality or mutation in an affected family member documented to confirm the diagnosis before testing at-risk individuals. If a genetic mutation is not known in the affected family member, testing in other relatives has a great risk of being uninformative. Genetic testing for untreatable conditions is not recommended for at-risk children under the age of eighteen because they are not able to provide informed consent, and giving a child a genetic-status label may do great harm. For families that have a known genetic mutation, there may be reproductive options available, such as preimplantation genetic diagnosis, to reduce or eliminate the risk of passing the disease-causing gene to the next generation. Individuals who carry or are at risk for carrying a FTD gene mutation can learn more about these options through a genetic counselor, an obstetrician, or another type of fertility specialist with experience in genetics.

Genetic counselors have master's level training in human or medical genetics or genetic counseling and are certified by the American Board of Genetic Counseling. To locate a genetic counselor, inquire at your local medical center or contact the National Society of Genetic Counselors via the Internet at www.nsgc.org and use the "Find a Genetic Counselor" resource to identify someone near you.

DISCUSSING GENETIC ISSUES WITH YOUR FAMILY

Genetic issues present a difficult dichotomy within a family. Your genes are what make you unique: no one else in the world has the same exact combination of genes that you do. Yet you share 50 percent of your genes with each of your first-degree relatives (parents, siblings, and children). So any genetic issue is both extremely personal and common to all blood relatives.

For this reason, discussing genetic risk can be extremely difficult, even within the most supportive families. When the disorder in question is an adult-onset, progressive, neurological disease like FTD, the issues can be even more complicated. The patient's siblings are often raising their own families and are at the prime of their careers. The patient's children may be too young to understand genetic issues, may be considering marriage and a family of their own, or may already be raising their own children. None of these individuals will want to hear that they might be at risk for the disorder that is afflicting their loved one.

What can a caregiver do regarding communicating potential genetic risk to family members? To what extent is this your responsibility? While there is no one answer for every circumstance, here are some general guidelines and tools to help.

- Meet with a genetic counselor or have a serious discussion with your neurologist about the patient's family history and the likelihood that FTD might be inherited in the family. This is especially important if you have a high level of concern based on family lore about older relatives. This professional can help separate fact from "fiction" and, if there is valid reason for concern, they will devise a plan to get more information.
- If the patient's children are under the age of eighteen, there is no rush to have the discussion. Because FTD does not present a risk this early in life, no clinician would perform a genetic test on a minor; the policy is to test only adults who can understand the complicated issues involved and thus give truly informed consent. As with all complex, emotional issues, it is best to follow a child's lead, letting him know that you welcome his questions and making a judgment call as to how much information he is ready to know at any given time.

- Broach the subject with adult members of the immediate family. Chances are that if there is some family history, these people have been wondering about heritability but did not want to broach the subject themselves. Perhaps they were worried about appearing to have selfish concerns about the future, when you were dealing with the daily demands of your loved one. Opening the door to the topic will give them permission to pick up on the discussion, if they want to.
- There are different ways to introduce the topic. You could share copies of a letter from the neurologist that states the possibility that FTD may be a genetically inherited condition within the family. Use the exercise of researching the family history to introduce the topic with relatives who may have more information about ancestors. Share this book. Remember, it is OK that you do not have the answers to all of the questions; often it can be comforting just to know that others in the family have the same concerns.
- People within the family may react very differently to the subject. Some will want to talk about it; others may be scared and get angry. This is normal, and you should remember that they are not reacting to you but to the threat of FTD. The best you can do is to let them know that there is a support network and professionals who can help them find answers if and when they want to.
- Different members of the family will choose different paths to address this risk. Some will ignore it; some will want to discuss it with family; still others will pursue professional advice in private. It is important to know that a geneticist or a genetic counselor will hold each individual's consultation in the strictest confidence. Information is not shared with other family members without an individual's consent.
- You may not know which course each of your relatives takes. All that is important is for you to know that you opened the door to let each of them address it in his or her own way.

CONCLUSION

Genetics is a crucial piece of the FTD puzzle. Research has made great progress in identifying FTD-associated genes and scientists are continuing to study the connection between these genes and the development and progression of

FTD. To determine the cause of sporadic FTD, there is a great challenge to understand the complex interactions of genetic, environmental, and pathological factors. Genetic-testing options continue to expand and are proving to be a valuable tool for families and individuals with FTD. Genetic counseling is essential to help identify and accurately interpret risk, provide education, and explore the benefits and limitations of genetic testing.

RESOURCES

Genetic Alliance, Inc.: www.geneticalliance.org
The alliance supports individuals with genetic conditions and their families, educates the public, and advocates for consumer informed public policies.

Genetic Information Nondiscrimination Act: www.ginahelp.org
This site provides detailed information on the importance of genetic information and the scope and limitations of the protections provided by GINA, a federal law that addresses the concern of genetic discrimination in employment and health insurance.

National Human Genome Research Institute: www.genome.gov
The National Human Genome Research Institute leads the Human Genome Project for the National Institutes of Health, conducts cutting-edge research in its laboratories, and supports genomic science worldwide. This site contains useful information for the layperson about the Human Genome Project, genetic research, and genetic conditions and testing.

National Society of Genetic Counselors, Inc.: www.nsgc.org
The NSGC is the national professional organization for genetic counselors. Use the "Find a Genetic Counselor" link to find a genetic counselor by either geographic location or field of specialty. This site also has educational information and resources to help individuals and families collect and store their family-history information.

Understanding the Genetics of FTD: A Guide for Patients and Their Families
    A booklet written by the University of Pennsylvania and available through the Association for Frontotemporal Degeneration (AFTD): www.theaftd.org/ frontotemporal-degeneration/genetics.

US Surgeon General's Family History Initiative: www.hhs.gov/familyhistory
    A Web-based program titled "My Family Health Portrait" is available as a free download through the Family History Initiative. This site also contains resources and frequently asked questions pertaining to family history risks for many different health conditions.

CHAPTER 4

FINDING THE "A" TEAM

Creating a Collaboration of Health Professionals

Carol F. Lippa, MD; and Kate J. Bowen

Identifying the right physician or healthcare team can be a challenging experience regardless of the underlying medical condition. The situation is even more complicated when there are specialized needs because an individual has a cognitive or behavioral disorder. Frontotemporal degeneration (FTD) patients seldom have the insight to seek medical help on their own. Many would deny a problem even if their physician brought up the issue. For this reason, they are usually brought to medical attention by a caregiver. The caregiver needs to find the right physician and then persuade the often-unwilling individual to be assessed by the healthcare team. This can be one of the hardest things a caregiver has to do. Due to the reluctance of many FTD patients to cooperate with medical assessments, it is worth making an extra effort ahead of time to find the best physician for the problem.

SEEKING OUT A QUALIFIED SPECIALIST

Most individuals have a primary-care physician. A phone call or an office visit to this doctor is a good place to start. Few, if any, primary-care physicians will be comfortable making or confirming the diagnosis of FTD and managing the condition, since it is not common. Do not be surprised if your family doctor has not heard of it. Although primary-care physicians often lack the know-how to manage a patient with FTD, they may know a specialist or a cognitive-disorders center that they have confidence in and work well with. This approach will most likely enable you to gain access to experts experienced with FTD while maintaining a friendly relationship with the primary-care physician.

If the affected individual does not have a primary-care physician, most regions within the United States are associated with local branches of the Alzheimer's Association. These branches maintain listings of local physicians whom they recommend for the assessment of cognitive disorders. The Association for Frontotemporal Degeneration (AFTD) also maintains a list of medical centers with FTD-specific programs throughout the United States and Canada. Local medical centers, hospitals, adult/senior day programs, nursing homes, and other referral centers may also be able to guide you to a capable, cognitive-focused physician. Do not be afraid to take advantage of the Internet for physician recommendations and research. Online forums, blogs, social media, and personal postings about FTD can help you learn from others' mistakes and point you in the right direction. However, it is recommended that the user be sure the electronic resources are legitimate. One way to do this is to use websites associated with academic centers, such as medical schools.

Questions often arise regarding the type of medical specialist— neurologist, psychiatrist, or geriatrician—that is best qualified to care for the individual with FTD. In general, the neurologist has particular expertise in determining the specific dementia subtype an individual has. If you are wondering whether an individual has FTD, Alzheimer's disease, or another condition, a neurologist may be the specialist to seek. The psychiatrist has particular expertise in the management of behavioral symptoms. If there are behavioral problems that make the individual unsafe (e.g., agitated, destructive, aggressive, violent, severely depressed, or out of touch with reality) a psychiatrist may be of benefit. Psychiatrists are also helpful if the individual has had major side effects or a lack of response to medications that doctors have prescribed for behavioral problems. However, some patients are reluctant to be evaluated by psychiatrists due to the stigma attached to it; in these cases, cognitive neurologists may be an option. Geriatricians are often recommended for older dementia and Alzheimer's disease patients with numerous other medical problems. However, the younger age of many FTD patients makes selection of a geriatrician inappropriate for some individuals. Also, experience with Alzheimer's disease does not necessarily qualify a physician to manage patients with FTD because the underlying biology of the two diseases is different.

Before committing yourself to one specialist, be aware that many exceptions to these general guidelines exist. Some neurologists are very adept at handling behavioral problems and some psychiatrists are good at arriving at the correct diagnosis. The most important quality in a specialist is that you are comfortable with the level of care that he or she can provide. It is more important to ensure that the physician has a clinical interest in FTD, cognition, or degenerative diseases. You want the individual to be knowledgeable and skilled in handling the problems that arise and interested in the caregiver and the patient.

Another issue to consider when selecting a physician is his or her willingness to discuss the patient in the patient's absence. With the exception of those with primary progressive aphasia (PPA), patients with FTD lack insight into their condition. It is often difficult for caregivers to bring up the extent of cognitive loss or behavioral problems when the patient is present in the exam room, for fear of embarrassing him or her or making him or her defensive. Doctors have different policies about discussing the patient when the patient is not present. Most physicians believe that information should be shared between the patient, caregiver, and doctor. The majority of doctors will discuss the situation briefly with family members if you indicate the need to do so. If there is a need to discuss the patient in his or her absence, ask about the doctor's policy on this ahead of time.

The presence of coordinated care or support services is also important. If diagnostic studies are needed, is there someone who can coordinate the visits to minimize the number of trips the patient needs to make to the hospital? If you need extra help or are unable to handle the individual in his or her current home setting, is there a social worker available? If the patient is falling or has problems with movements, you may wish to identify a program with physical or occupational therapy (see chapters 6, 11, and 12 for more information). In general, physical therapists are effective when the person has trouble with falling, walking, or balancing. A program with an occupational therapist should be targeted when upper-extremity function is involved, including feeding, dressing, and bathing (for more information, see chapters 10 and 13).

If you truly cannot find a physician who meets your FTD requirements, or if you are comfortable with your current specialist even though he or she has minimal FTD experience, the AFTD offers educational resources for physicians who have limited exposure to FTD. These services are in the form of written information, live webinars, previously recorded talks, and the Partners in FTD Care online forum. This resource also includes updates on the current state of the disease, provides a forum to share physician expertise and experiences, and acts as an overall guide for physicians in diagnosis, progression, and treatment. Refer your physician to the AFTD website for more information.

PREPARING TO VISIT THE DOCTOR

To get the most out of the appointment, prepare for the encounter ahead of time. Before the appointment, you may wish to look up facts about FTD on websites or read about the disease so you are knowledgeable. It is wise to call the physician's office prior to your visit to feel out the situation. You might want to ask if the doctor has other patients with this condition or if he or she has an interest in this area. Find out if the office recommends bringing any specific documents and if it is preferred to have forms completed prior to the visit.

When preparing for the visit, obtain copies of reports from blood work, EEGs, and neuropsychological testing. If specialized studies (MRI, DAT, amyloid or traditional [FDG] PET scans) have been done, bring copies of the studies, including copies of the actual image discs. If possible, have all reports delivered in advance and call the office to be sure that they have arrived. Do not assume that your doctor will have automatically forwarded copies of the old records.

If you predict your loved one will become agitated, upset, or embarrassed at your explanation of symptoms during the visit, prepare a short journal of anecdotal evidence. Provide examples of the major changes, such as abnormal behaviors or changes in speech, dating back as far as possible. Include this information among the stack of imaging and diagnostic reports you provide the physician to help make the visit run smoothly.

If possible, plan to bring a family member or a friend to the appointment for support. The typical behaviors associated with the disease may be uncomfortable for you to recount. Those with FTD may not acknowledge their condition and may suggest such symptoms are nonexistent, igniting self-doubt when relaying information. Bring someone else who knows the affected individual. Encouragement from a close friend or relative who has witnessed symptoms will help to increase your confidence, allowing you to provide the physician with as much information as possible to make an accurate diagnosis. Also, bringing another person the patient trusts will help convince him or her that there are issues to address.

THE DOCTOR'S EXAMINATION

During the appointment, the doctor will take a detailed personal medical history and family history. If the disease runs in the family, be sure to make the physician aware that this is a concern. Provide the physician with a list of all cognitive or neurological disorders (Alzheimer's disease, dementia, Parkinson's disease, motor neuron disease, etc.) and psychiatric disorders (bipolar disorder, depression) that have been diagnosed in your family. If your family members did not see a specialist, misdiagnoses are possible because some doctors are less familiar with FTD and may have incorrectly categorized the symptoms. Also, make note of any family members with a history of criminal behavior starting later in life (most ordinary criminals show criminal behavior throughout their life).

In addition to taking a medical and family history, the doctor will do a general physical examination, mental-status examination, and general neurological examination. Do not have a patient with FTD go to the appointment alone without a caregiver or other informant present. The physician will most likely want to order additional tests and may want to repeat some of the tests that have already been done. He may recommend blood work, genetic tests, an MRI, a cerebrospinal fluid (CSF) examination, or metabolic imaging (PET or SPECT scans).

In centers where there is a multidisciplinary approach to patient care, a nurse, physical therapist, neuropsychologist, or other healthcare professionals may be involved with the individual's care. In these cases, it is crucial to be sure there is good communication among the team members. Make sure that there is a system in place so that all the healthcare professionals on the team receive copies of all reports, and that the patient's primary-care physician also receives copies.

During your initial appointment, you will want as many of your questions answered as possible. Bring a prepared list of questions and topics to discuss with the doctor. If there are behavior problems, be sure to bring them up. Caregivers are also frequently anxious about prognostic information. This is often not discussed unless the caregiver brings it up. Other topics you may want information on include support groups, educational materials, tools to explain the disease to your children, clinical trials, safety strategies (i.e., driving, falling, roaming), and legal and financial planning.

FOLLOW-UP AFTER VISITING THE DOCTOR

After the appointment, you may still be unsure if this is the right doctor for you. Do you think the doctor is interested and knowledgeable about this problem? It is important that you get peace of mind from the physician and medical team. Were your questions answered? Was the problem treated seriously? Did he address safety issues? Were blood work and imaging studies recommended to rule out conditions that mimic FTD? Were the CSF and genetic results reviewed? This is crucial. If the affected individual hasn't had a workup, and your doctor does not think a workup is warranted, you need another doctor. If you answered "yes" to the aforementioned questions but are still not satisfied, do not hesitate to get a second opinion.

Over time, a number of tests will be ordered and reordered. Changes in the studies can be as important diagnostically as the original results. As the caregiver, you should keep copies of all diagnostic studies. Develop an organized folder system to maintain all medical documents, with detailed information including the type of test, when it took place, where it occurred, which doctor wrote the order, and the results. If MRI scans are done, you should keep a copy of the discs in addition to the reports. These can be easily obtained if requested at the time of the study; you are entitled to copies of these tests. Also, when there is an upcoming physician appointment, call the office ahead of time to be sure that all new reports and discs or electronic copies were received. It is surprising how often the results have not been received or reviewed.

After the initial appointment and verification of diagnosis, you may ask yourself, am I interested in clinical trials? In general, an institution with ongoing research programs may have active clinical expertise and clinical trials in your area of need. Many caregivers are interested in clinical trials for medications that help FTD. Unfortunately, because the disease is uncommon, most pharmaceutical companies are not funding large-scale clinical trials for FTD. Additionally, some clinical trial sites are reluctant to engage in studies of FTD because of the small pool of FTD patients and the difficulty in recruiting enough subjects. Do not be discouraged, because with the increased awareness of FTD, more opportunities will arise. Studies to further the understanding of the disease as well as symptomatic trials are examples of potential research involvement. If this is of interest to you, be sure to express your interest in clinical trials to your physician. How involved is the physician in research and clinical trials? Will the latest treatments and innovative interventions be an option?

Keep in mind, you will want a program where the physicians and staff are interested in patients outside of their candidacy as a clinical-trial subject. If the site offers clinical trials, are the claims too good to be true? Centers that make great promises about the effectiveness of medications for the type of symptoms FTD patients experience are often illegitimate. If you wish to select a center because it offers clinical trials, do your research to be sure that the studies it offers are legitimate. The Alzheimer's Association and the AFTD provide listings of various studies that are in progress and recruiting participants. Also, clinicaltrials.gov, a service of the US National Institutes of Health, offers a comprehensive registry of all clinical studies regulated by the Food and Drug Administration (FDA).

SUMMARY

Spending time to identify the right physician or program is often worthwhile when dealing with someone with FTD. Use your primary-care physician and local resources to help guide you. FTD is less common than Alzheimer's disease, and few doctors are familiar with the issues that these patients experience. Make an effort to find a specialist with an interest in the area and get the most out of the first appointment by having results of prior testing organized and questions listed. As a bottom line, if you don't feel satisfied with the doctor or program, look for someone or someplace else.

CHAPTER 5

THERAPEUTIC INTERVENTIONS

Medical Therapy Options

Richard J. Caselli, MD; and Roy Yaari, MD, MAS

GOALS OF THERAPY

Treatment of frontotemporal degeneration (FTD) and other degenerative diseases that produce dementia aims to maximize the patient's quality of life and help families succeed in their roles as primary caregivers. The two broad categories of management are pharmacotherapy (medications) and lifestyle changes. Chapter 16 addresses nonmedical interventions.

PHARMACOTHERAPY

There are six categories of symptomatic disease management to consider in treating dementia. These categories are: prevention (drugs that prevent or delay the onset, and that slow the progression), intellectual decline (e.g., memory loss), behavioral problems (such as hallucinations or depression), sleep disorders (e.g., insomnia), commonly associated problems (e.g., Parkinsonism), and abrupt decline. Currently, there are few medications specifically approved for use in patients with dementia (and the few that exist are approved for Alzheimer's disease, not for FTD), so many such applications are considered "off-label," that is, not sanctioned by the Food and Drug Administration (FDA). Nonetheless, patients, their families, and their healthcare providers require management strategies and tools. Medications are an important part of the clinical armamentarium, even if many uses are off-label.

PREVENTION

It should be said at the outset that there are no highly effective preventive agents. This is largely a category for future hope. Still, if dementia onset could be delayed or progression of mild disease slowed, it would provide an enormous impact on our public health system. "In the land of the blind, the one-eyed witch doctor is king," and unfortunately, in the absence of an effective therapy, the desperate need for hope gives many theories more media attention than they are due. There have been numerous reports that any of the following may offer some hope for prevention or disease slowing: gingko biloba, aerobic exercise,[1] mental exercise,[2] vitamin A,[3] vitamin C,[4] vitamin E,[5] flavanoids,[6] omega-3 fatty acids,[7] vitamin B12,[8] vitamin B-complex supplements,[9] folate,[10] curcumin,[11] reduced caloric intake,[12] the Mediterranean diet,[13] moderate amounts of red wine (which contains resveratrol),[14] cholesterol-lowering agents,[15] antihypertensives,[16] insulin-sensitizing agents,[17] anti-inflammatory agents,[18] and hormonal therapies.[19] None of these therapies has withstood rigorous clinical testing, and there are now studies that have shown that several of these are indeed ineffective at best and possibly exacerbating at worst, including gingko;[20] NSAIDs; [21] vitamin E, [22] vitamin B12, and folate;[23] hormonal therapy;[24] and statins.[25] Healthy diets (low-fat and Mediterranean), physical exercise, and mental activity (which can be operationally defined many ways) remain reasonable recommendations that seem generally safe and help to promote general health whether or not they are ultimately proven to have a differential effect on preventing dementia.

INTELLECTUAL DECLINE

This is the category in which drugs specifically approved for use in patients with dementia actually exist. To date, however, all have been approved by the FDA for use exclusively in patients with Alzheimer's disease. There are no medications approved for use in FTD or other forms of dementia, so use in non-Alzheimer cases is again off-label and borrowed from the Alzheimer experience.

Two classes of drugs that have been approved for use to enhance memory and related intellectual skills are the cholinesterase inhibitors[26] and the

N-methyl-D-aspartate (NMDA) receptor antagonist memantine.[27] Three cholinesterase inhibitors are currently used for the treatment of mild to moderate AD: donepezil (Aricept®), galantamine (Reminyl®, Razadyne®), and rivastigmine (Exelon®). Tacrine (Cognex®) was the first acetylcholinesterase inhibitor approved by the United States FDA for AD, but it is no longer recommended due to its side-effect profile, which includes hepatotoxicity. Donepezil[28] is a once-a-day medication. Rivastigmine[29] has also been shown to inhibit butyrocholinesterase, the clinical significance of which remains unclear (and has a higher incidence of nausea than the other two currently used cholinesterase inhibitors). It is also now available as a transdermal patch, which may offer greater convenience for some patients. Galantamine[30] also binds to nicotinic receptors, the clinical significance of which remains unclear. As a class, these agents have demonstrated measurable, though modest, effects on cognition, activities of daily living, and global measures of functioning versus placebo in clinical trials.[31] For the most part, treatment goals focus on delaying worsening of these clinical features, although some patients experience temporary modest improvement. In some patients, these agents can have modest beneficial effects on some behavioral symptoms as well, but they are not a substitute for more effective therapies in patients with severe behavioral problems.

Although generally well tolerated, the main adverse effects are gastrointestinal (nausea, vomiting, diarrhea, anorexia, and weight loss, all of which are more common with rivastigmine), and these medications are better tolerated on a full stomach. Side effects of donepezil also include nightmares when taken before bedtime, which can be avoided in most patients if the drug is instead taken in the morning or early in the day.

Bradycardia, usually insignificant, is a side effect that can be dangerous in patients with cardiac conduction deficits, hence supporting the performance of an electrocardiogram prior to treatment. Risk of conduction block and cardiac arrest is compounded by simultaneous administration of multiple cholinesterase inhibitors, which should therefore be avoided. The choice of which acetylcholinesterase inhibitor is most appropriate for each patient is based on titration schedule, dosing regimens, and side effects. Metanalyses and treatment guidelines do not suggest important differences in efficacy but do note differences in the frequency of side effects. For instance, donepezil can be administered once daily and has been suggested to have a lower rate of adverse gastrointestinal effects than rivastigmine.[32] Studies are needed to further assess possible long-term benefits such as delayed institutionalization and economic savings in the cost of patient care.

Although data regarding how long patients should remain on an acetyl-cholinesterase inhibitor is limited,[33] a case could be made to treat patients indefinitely in the hope of slightly delaying the cognitive decline that might have occurred off treatment, unless side effects or other individualized issues arise. In the latter stages of dementia, however, many families elect to discontinue these medications for lack of perceived efficacy.

At this time, the FDA has approved cholinesterase inhibitors for the treatment of mild to moderate stages of AD, and memantine for the moderate to late stages of AD. Some neurologists advocate the use of memantine over the cholinesterase inhibitors in patients with FTD, but there is currently little empirical data to support this practice. There may be some benefit to the addition of one medication class following a full therapeutic trial of the other class. More recently, the issue of cost-benefit has arisen and is controversial, with some claiming therapy reduces long-term costs and others claiming it simply adds to long-term costs,[34] while others suggest serious limitations in those pharmaco-economic studies.

BEHAVIORAL PROBLEMS

There are three categories of behavioral problems that are commonly encountered in patients with AD and related forms of dementia:

1. Psychosis. This includes hallucinations (typically but not exclusively visual), paranoid delusions, and agitation (particularly sundowning). There are no agents that have received FDA approval for the specific treatment of agitated, delirious, psychotic elderly patients with dementia. Anecdotal experience and metanalysis[35] suggest that atypical antipsychotic agents may be the preferred agents especially in patients with Parkinsonism because they can be effective, and because they are less likely to cause or exacerbate extrapyramidal syndromes, although randomized trials have failed to support this clinical impression. They currently lack FDA approval for such an indication; therefore, clinical judgment is essential. In 2005, the FDA issued a warning and has since required a black-box warning label on the use of atyp-

ical antipsychotics in the treatment of elderly patients with dementia because of an increased risk of mortality (http://www.fda.gov/cder/drug/advisory/antipsychotics.htm).[36]

Since then, clinical-trial data has suggested that atypical antipsychotics are ineffective in managing psychotic symptoms in patients with dementia,[37] but a criticism of this study has been that the doses employed were inadequate. Alternate recommendations were not given, although some have advocated the use of anticonvulsant medications.[38] In the absence of a clear alternative, many clinicians continue to feel that these medications remain an important therapeutic option for managing severe behavioral problems. Older agents (the "typical" antipsychotic drugs such as haloperidol) are effective but have a high likelihood of causing or exacerbating Parkinsonism. They also have a much higher risk of tardive dyskinesia, a potentially irreversible drug-induced condition of involuntary, purposeless movements, if used chronically. A more recent analysis suggested mortality associated with neuroleptic use in the older dementia population is more frequent in those treated with conventional neuroleptics compared to the newer atypical neuroleptics.[39]

Therefore, use of atypical neuroleptics will probably continue, provided that the patient's family and other physicians involved in a patient's care feel that the benefits outweigh the risks.

FTD patients frequently exhibit bizarre social behaviors that may be difficult to categorize as specifically psychotic (for example, hoarding food or urinating in public), but which nonetheless create great distress for caregivers and may also place the patient at risk depending on the specific problem the behavior creates. Treatment of such behaviors is particularly difficult. One small study suggested trazodone may be modestly effective,[40] and many have used neuroleptic agents as well for such behaviors with inconsistent success. Whatever psychoactive medication is tried, care must be taken to minimize the dose and duration of use.

2. Depression. Depression is common in patients with AD. Drugs with anticholinergic properties, such as the tricyclic antidepressants, should be avoided because of the risk of exacerbating confusion. Selective serotonin reuptake inhibitors (SSRIs) are preferred[41] and sometimes can also help to ease agitation. However, SSRIs may occasionally precipitate REM sleep behavior disorder (RBD).[42]

In patients with depression who are also having trouble sleeping, some clinicians have advocated the use of a sedating antidepressant, such as trazodone, at bedtime, though randomized controlled trials are lacking and side effects such as orthostatic hypotension should be considered.

3. Anxiety. Dementia patients may become anxious over many things. One common theme is the perceived absence of their caregiver. Some patients will not let their caregiver out of their sight, and this can quickly wear down the caregiver. If other treatments are not effective, a low-dose atypical antipsychotic medication as described above might be considered.[43]

SLEEP DISORDERS

Of the many possible sleep disorders that can affect patients with dementia, the following five are perhaps the most frequently troublesome.

1. Simple insomnia. The patient will not fall asleep, or else gets up very early and will not go back to sleep. A short-acting sedative hypnotic such as zolpidem or zaleplon is often effective and may be given either at bedtime or when the patient wakens in the night.[44]

    Antihistamines are not recommended because of their lack of established efficacy and side-effect profile.

2. REM sleep behavior disorder (RBD). REM sleep is the part of sleep during which dreaming occurs. When we dream we are running down the street, our bodies normally lay motionless in a state of "sleep paralysis" induced by specialized neurons in the brain stem. In RBD, this group of neurons malfunctions and fails to induce a normal state of sleep paralysis. Consequently, patients have dream-enactment behavior. Sleep studies (polysomnograms) monitor muscle tone during sleep and show a loss of muscle paralysis. RBD is associated with several disorders that all share Parkinsonism as a feature, including, in particular, dementia with Lewy bodies (DLB).[45] This can be difficult to treat, but some clinicians have advocated the use of low-dose clonazepam, while monitoring patients carefully for any benzodiazepine-related exacerbation in cognitive impairment or ataxia over the next few weeks.

3. Obstructive sleep apnea (OSA). This should be suspected in any over-weight patient complaining of daytime somnolence. In patients with OSA and mild cognitive difficulties, treating underlying OSA can sometimes improve their cognitive syndrome. OSA is not a cause of dementia but can be a cause of mild cognitive complaints that may be mistaken for early-stage AD. It is also found more commonly in persons with the *apolipoprotein E* (*APOE*) *e4* gene (a common risk factor for AD),[46] which is commonly found in patients with AD. A simple screening test can be overnight oximetry, but if truly suspected, a formal sleep study and continuous positive airway pressure (CPAP) trial should be obtained.

4. Nocturia. This refers to frequent urination at night causing an interruption of sleep. Though not a primary sleep disorder, this is a common reason some patients with dementia are up at night and tired during the day. Treatment options for incontinence are described below.

ASSOCIATED PROBLEMS

These associated problems commonly occur in the dementia population:

1. Parkinsonism. Parkinsonism can occur in some familial forms of FTD and is also an important diagnostic sign of DLB. Intervention with medications for Parkinson's disease can potentially create or worsen psychotic symptoms, particularly visual hallucinations, in vulnerable patients. Treatment should therefore be reserved for those with clinically significant Parkinsonism, especially if balance becomes impaired so that falls become a threat. An arguably related condition, normal pressure hydrocephalus (NPH), has gained recognition by the clinical triad of dementia, gait disorder, and incontinence. This triad is not unique to NPH and occurs eventually in many patients with dementia. Nonetheless NPH remains an important diagnostic consideration since it can sometimes be reversed. NPH usually begins as a predominant gait disorder that is unresponsive to anti-Parkinsonian medications. When correctly diagnosed, it may be treated with brain surgery (ventriculoperitoneal shunting).

2. Urinary incontinence. Two of the more common causes of urinary fre-

quency and incontinence in patients with dementia are flaccid distended bladders that cause overflow incontinence (patients fail to adequately empty their bladders when they void) and spastic bladders (bladders that fail to allow a normal amount of urine to be stored and so are constantly trying to empty). They are easily distinguished by checking a urinary post-void residual, a test in which the amount of urine in the bladder is measured right after the patient voids as completely as possible. The former is treated with intermittent catheterization. The latter can usually be managed with peripherally acting anticholinergic agents such as oxybutinin and tolterodine. These risk exacerbating confusion, and so care must be taken, but if started at low doses, and titrated gradually, they can often be used safely and effectively.

3. Other physical deficits. These may be disease specific, such as apraxia, a form of abnormal movement in which the ability to carry out a familiar movement is lost despite having the physical ability to perform the movement (in patients with corticobasal ganglionic degeneration), difficulty swallowing and choking (dysphagia) in patients with ALS-dementia complex, and impaired vision (cortical visual syndromes) in patients with visual variant AD (or posterior cortical atrophy). These are not generally responsive to medications, but appropriate physical/occupational therapy and safety interventions should be addressed.

ABRUPT DECLINE

Over the protracted course of FTD, many patients have times when they suddenly become much more confused, with slurred speech, somnolence, agitation, tremulousness, unsteadiness, falls, and worsened incontinence. Often, this is due to a superimposed illness, typically an infection (urinary tract and pneumonia most commonly), a medication error, an injury of some type, or some other cause that must be sought with a thorough medical evaluation.

LIFESTYLE CHANGES

Driving

One of the more difficult lifestyle changes for patients with dementia to accept is cessation of driving. The Clinical Dementia Rating (CDR) scale is a widely utilized clinical tool for grading the relative severity of dementia with scores that range from 0 (no impairment) to 3 (severe impairment).[47] Patients with mild cognitive impairment (MCI) typically have a CDR of 0.5 and compose an identifiable subgroup of patients that can be distinguished from those with true dementia.[48] According to the *Practice Parameter of the Quality Standards Subcommittee of the American Academy of Neurology* that was originally issued in 2000 and updated in 2010, patients with MCI and a CDR of 0.5 generally should be cautioned from driving (but those with additional exacerbating factors, such as visual impairment, should be restricted from driving even at the MCI stage). While there is typically no absolute restriction on driving in the absence of overt driving impairment reported either by the patient or a reliable observer, physicians should be aware of reporting requirements in their area. For instance, California requires physicians to report the diagnosis of dementia to the state epidemiologists, who then report the diagnosis to the Department of Motor Vehicles. However, the practice parameter advises that patients be reassessed periodically (every six months) until they have declined to a CDR of 1.0 (or the equivalent), and at that point, the standard changes to no driving. Therefore, according to the practice parameter, a patient with mild AD and a CDR of 1.0 is to be advised he is not to drive.[49]

There are many simple reasons why patients with dementia may not be able to drive. Patients with FTD have severely impaired judgment and may create road hazards, even when their intellectual skills may seem to be relatively intact.[50] Patients with visual-variant AD have disabling visual impairment.[51] Patients with progressive apraxia related to corticobasal ganglionic degeneration have severe motor impairment, and some also have visual impairment. Patients with primary progressive aphasia (PPA) sometimes are capable of driving, but due to the speech disturbance occurring within the context of a dementing degenerative brain disease, they would be ill equipped to explain themselves in the event of a mishap, and legally it would be difficult to defend if challenged. (Hence, it is probably best that they not drive.)

Impaired attention, inability to multitask, and other cognitive disturbances in addition to memory loss all impair driving skills as shown on actual road tests[52] as well as on driving simulation tests[53] resulting in a two- to eightfold increase in rate of collisions in patients with AD who continue driving.[54]

Simply telling a patient with dementia not to drive often is not sufficient, and despite admonitions not to drive, many continue to do so even after they develop evident driving impairment.[55] Patients may take a driving test, and when they do, 40–60 percent fail,[56] but losing their license only makes it illegal for them to drive. The most effective way to stop a patient from driving is to remove his or her access to car keys or to the car itself. This is not always easy to accomplish and has caused some patients to become belligerent, so care must be used in managing this very difficult but important issue.

NOTES

1. M. E. Lytle, B. J. Vander, R. S. Pandav, et al., "Exercise Level and Cognitive Decline: The MoVIES Project," *Alzheimer Disease and Associated Disorders* 18 (2004): 57–64.

2. M. Gatz, "Educating the Brain to Avoid Dementia: Can Mental Exercise Prevent Alzheimer Disease?" *Public Library of Science Medicine* 2 (2005): e7.

3. M. C. Morris, D. A. Evans, J. L. Bienias, et al., "Vitamin E and Cognitive Decline in Older Persons," *Archives of Neurology* 59 (2002): 1125–32.

4. P. P. Zandi, J. C. Anthony, A. S. Khachaturian, et al., "Reduced Risk of Alzheimer Disease in Users of Antioxidant Vitamin Supplements: The Cache County Study," *Archives of Neurology* 61 (2004): 82–88.

5. Ibid.

6. D. Commenges, V. Scotet, S. Renaud, et al., "Intake of Flavonoids and Risk of Dementia," *European Journal of Epidemiology* 16 (2000): 357–63; M. J. Engelhart, M. I. Geerlings, A. Ruitenberg, et al., "Dietary Intake of Antioxidants and Risk of Alzheimer Disease," *Journal of the American Medical Association* 287 (2002): 3223–29.

7. S. Kalmijn, E. J. Feskens, L. J. Launer, et al., "Polyunsaturated Fatty Acids, Antioxidants, and Cognitive Function in Very Old Men," *American Journal of Epidemiology* 145 (1997): 33–41.

8. R. Clarke, A. D. Smith, K. A. Jobst, et al., "Folate, Vitamin B12, and Serum Total Homocysteine Levels in Confirmed Alzheimer Disease," *Archives of Neurology* 55 (1998): 1449–55.

9. Zandi, Anthony, Khachaturian, et al., "Reduced Risk of Alzheimer Disease in Users of Antioxidant Vitamin Supplements."

10. Clarke, Smith, Jobst, et al., "Folate, Vitamin B12, and Serum Total Homocysteine Levels in Confirmed Alzheimer Disease."

11. J. M. Ringman, S. A. Frautschy, G. M. Cole, et al., "A Potential Role of the Curry Spice Curcumin in Alzheimer's Disease," *Current Alzheimer Research* 2 (2005): 131–36.

12. J. A. Luchsinger, M. X. Tang, S. Shea, et al., "Caloric Intake and the Risk of Alzheimer Disease," *Archives of Neurology* 59 (2002): 1258–63.

13. N. Scarmeas, Y. Stern, M. X. Tang, et al., "Mediterranean Diet and Risk for Alzheimer's Disease," *Annals of Neurology* 59 (2006): 912–21.

14. A. Ruitenberg, J. C. van Swieten, J. C. Witteman, et al., "Alcohol Consumption and Risk of Dementia: The Rotterdam Study," *Lancet* 359 (2002): 281–86.

15. D. L. Sparks, M. Sabbagh, D. Connor, et al., "Statin Therapy in Alzheimer's Disease," *Acta Neurologica Scandinavica Suppl.* 185 (2006): 78–86.

16. W. H. Birkenhager and J. A. Staessen, "Antihypertensives for Prevention of Alzheimer's Disease," *Lancet Neurology* 5 (2006): 466–68.

17. M. K. Sun and D. L. Alkon, "Links between Alzheimer's Disease and Diabetes," *Drugs of Today* 42 (2006): 481–89.

18. P. L. McGeer and E. G. McGeer, "Anti-inflammatory Drugs in the Fight against Alzheimer's Disease," *Annals of the New York Academy of Sciences* 777 (1996): 213–20.

19. S. A. Shumaker, C. Legault, S. R. Rapp, et al., "Estrogen Plus Progestin and the Incidence of Dementia and Mild Cognitive Impairment in Postmenopausal Women: The Women's Health Initiative Memory Study: A Randomized Controlled Trial," *Journal of the American Medical Association* 289 (2003): 2651–62; S. A. Shumaker, C. Legault, L. Kuller, et al., "Conjugated Equine Estrogens and Incidence of Probable Dementia and Mild Cognitive Impairment in Postmenopausal Women: Women's Health Initiative Memory Study," *Journal of the American Medical Association* 291 (2004): 2947–58.

20. S. T. DeKosky, J. D. Williamson, A. L. Fitzpatrick, et al., "Gingko Biloba for Prevention of Dementia: A Randomized Controlled Trial," *JAMA* 300 (2008): 2253–2262.

21. P. S. Aisen, K. A. Schafer, M. Grundman, et al., "Effects of Rofecoxib or Naproxen vs. Placebo on Alzheimer Disease Progression: A Randomized Controlled Trial," *JAMA* 289 (2003): 2819–2826.

22. R. C. Petersen, R. G. Thomas, M. Grundman, et al., "Vitamin E and Donepezil for the Treatment of Mild Cognitive Impairment," *New England Journal of Medicine* 352 (2005): 2379–2388.

23. P. S. Aisen, L. S. Schneider, M. Sano, et al., "High-Dose B Vitamin Supplementation and Cognitive Decline in Alzheimer Disease: A Randomized Controlled Trial," *JAMA* 300 (2008): 1774–1783.

24. S. A. Shumaker, C. Legault, L. Thal, et al., "Estrogen Plus Progestin and the Incidence of Dementia and Mild Cognitive Impairment in Postmenopausal Women: The Women's Health Initiative Memory Study—A Randomized Controlled Trial," *JAMA* 289 (2003): 2651–2662.

25. M. Sano, K. L. Bell, D Galasko, J. E. Galvin, R. G. Thomas, C. H. van Dyck, and P. S. Aisen, "A Randomized, Double-Blind, Placebo-Controlled Trial of Simvastatin to Treat Alzheimer Disease," *Neurology* 77 (2011): 556–63.

26. S. L. Rogers, M. R. Farlow, R. S. Doody, et al., "A 24-Week, Double-blind, Placebo-Controlled Trial of Donepezil in Patients with Alzheimer's Disease. Donepezil Study

M. Rosler, R. Anand, A. Cicin-Sain, et al., "Effi-... ...ents with Alzheimer's Disease: International Ran-... ...ical Journal 318 (1999): 633–38; M. A. Raskind, ...amine in AD: A 6-Month Randomized, Placebo-... ...on. The Galantamine USA-1 Study Group," Neu-

...ffler, et al., "Memantine in Moderate-to-Severe ...nal of Medicine 348 (2003): 1333–41.

A 24-Week, Double-Blind, Placebo-controlled ...er's Disease."

Efficacy and Safety of Rivastigmine in Patients with Alzheimer's Disease."

30. Raskind, Peskind, Wessel, et al., Galantamine in AD: A 6-Month Randomized, Placebo-Controlled Trial with a 6-Month Extension."

31. R. S. Doody, J. C. Stevens, C. Beck, et al., "Practice Parameter: Management of Dementia (an Evidence-Based Review). Report of the Quality Standards Subcommittee of the American Academy of Neurology," Neurology 56 (2001): 1154–66.

32. J. Birks, "Cholinesterase Inhibitors for Alzheimer's Disease," Cochrane Database Systems Review (2006): CD005593; A. Lleo, S. M. Greenberg, and J. H. Growdon, "Current Pharmacotherapy for Alzheimer's Disease," Annual Review of Medicine 57 (2006): 513–33.

33. S. L. Rogers, R. S. Doody, R. D. Pratt, et al., "Long-Term Efficacy and Safety of Donepezil in the Treatment of Alzheimer's Disease: Final Analysis of a US Multicentre Open-Label Study," European Neuropsychopharmacology 10 (2000): 195–203; M. A. Raskind, E. R. Peskind, L. Truyen, et al., "The Cognitive Benefits of Galantamine Are Sustained for at Least 36 Months: A Long-term Extension Trial," Archives of Neurology 61 (2004): 252–56.

34. H. Feldman, S. Gauthier, J. Hecker, et al., "Economic Evaluation of Donepezil in Moderate to Severe Alzheimer Disease," Neurology 63 (2004): 644–50.

35. K. M. Sink, K. F. Holden, and K. Yaffe, "Pharmacological treatment of Neuro-psychiatric Symptoms of Dementia: A Review of the Evidence," Journal of the American Medical Association 293 (2005): 596–608.

36. G. Trifiro, K. M. Verhamme, G. Ziere, A. P. Caputi, B. H. Ch. Stricker, and M. C. Sturkenboom, "All-Cause Mortality Associated with Atypical and Typical Antipsychotics in Demented Outpatients," Pharmacoepidemiology and Drug Safety 16, no. 5 (May 2007): 538–44; references in the text refer to the epub, which was available ahead of the print edition, on October 12, 2006.

37. L. S. Schneider, P. N. Tariot, K. S. Dagerman, K. S. Davis, J. K. Hsiao, M. S. Ismail, et al., "Effectiveness of Atypical Antipsychotic Drugs in Patients with Alzheimer's Disease," New England Journal of Medicine 355 (2006): 1525–38.

38. L. A. Profenno, L. Jakimovich, C. J. Holt, A. Porsteinsson, and P. N. Tariot, "A Randomized, Double-Blind, Placebo-Controlled Pilot Trial of Safety and Tolerability of Two Doses of Divalproex Sodium in Outpatients with Probable Alzheimer's Disease," Current Alzheimer Research 2 (2005): 553–58.

39. P. S. Wang, S. Schneeweiss, J. Avorn, et al., "Risk of Death in Elderly Users of Conventional vs. Atypical Antipsychotic Medications," *New England Journal of Medicine* 353 (2005): 2335–41.

40. F. Lebert, W. Stekke, C. Hasenbroekx, and F. Pasquier, "Frontotemporal Dementia: A Randomized, Controlled Trial with Trazodone," *Dementia and Geriatric Cognitive Disorders* 17 (2004): 355–59.

41. L. E. Tune, "Depression and Alzheimer's Disease," *Depression and Anxiety* 8, suppl. 1 (1998): 91–95.

42. C. H. Schenck, M. W. Mahowald, S. W. Kim, et al., "Prominent Eye Movements during NREM Sleep and REM Sleep Behavior Disorder Associated with Fluoxetine Treatment of Depression and Obsessive-Compulsive Disorder," *Sleep* 15 (1992): 226–35.

43. C. Salzman, "Treatment of the Agitation of Late-Life Psychosis and Alzheimer's Disease," *European Psychiatry* 16, suppl. 1 (2001): 25s–28s; D. P. Devanand, "Behavioral Complications and Their Treatment in Alzheimer's Disease," *Geriatrics* 52, suppl. 2 (1997): S37–S39.

44. Devanand, "Behavioral Complications and Their Treatment in Alzheimer's Disease"; P. S. Shelton and L. B. Hocking, "Zolpidem for Dementia-Related Insomnia and Nighttime Wandering," *Annals of Pharmacotherapy* 31 (1997): 319–22.

45. T. J. Ferman, B. F. Boeve, G. E. Smith, et al., "REM Sleep Behavior Disorder and Dementia: Cognitive Differences When Compared with AD," *Neurology* 52 (1999): 951–57.

46. H. Kadotani, T. Kadotani, T. Young, et al., "Association between *apolipoprotein E epsilon4* and Sleep-Disordered Breathing in Adults," *Journal of the American Medical Association* 285 (2001): 2888–90; D. J. Gottlieb, A. L. DeStefano, D. J. Foley, et al., "*APOE epsilon4* Is Associated with Obstructive Sleep Apnea/Hypopnea: The Sleep Heart Health Study," *Neurology* 63 (2004): 664–68.

47. J. C. Morris, "The Clinical Dementia Rating (CDR): Current Version and Scoring Rules," *Neurology* 43 (1993): 2412–14.

48. R. C. Petersen, J. C. Stevens, M. Ganguli, et al., "Practice Parameter: Early Detection of Dementia: Mild Cognitive Impairment (an Evidence-Based Review). Report of the Quality Standards Subcommittee of the American Academy of Neurology," *Neurology* 56 (2001): 1133–42; R. C. Petersen, R. Doody, A. Kurz, et al., "Current Concepts in Mild Cognitive Impairment," *Archives of Neurology* 58 (2001): 1985–92; B. Winblad, K. Palmer, M. Kivipelto, et al., "Mild Cognitive Impairment—beyond Controversies, towards a Consensus: Report of the International Working Group on Mild Cognitive Impairment," *Journal of Internal Medicine* 256 (2004): 240–46.

49. R. M. Dubinsky, A. C. Stein, and K. Lyons, "Practice Parameter: Risk of Driving and Alzheimer's Disease (an Evidence-Based Review): Report of the Quality Standards Subcommittee of the American Academy of Neurology," *Neurology* 54 (2000): 2205–11; Iverson DJ, Gronseth GS, Reger MA, Classen S, Dubinsky RM, Rizzo M, and the Quality Standards Subcommittee of the American Academy of Neurology, "Practice Parameter Update: Evaluation and Management of Driving Risk in Dementia: Report of the Quality Standards Subcommittee of the American Academy of Neurology," *Neurology* 74, no. 16 (April 20, 2010): 1316-24.

50. B. L. Miller, A. Darby, D. F. Benson, J. L. Cummings, and M. H. Miller, "Aggressive, Socially Disruptive and Antisocial Behavior Associated with Fronto-Temporal Dementia," *British Journal of Psychiatry* 170 (1997): 150–54; V. de Simone, L. Kaplan, N. Patronas, E. M. Wasserman, and J. Grafman, "Driving Abilities in Frontotemporal Dementia Patients," *Dementia and Geriatric Cognitive Disorders* 23 (2006): 1–7.

51. R. J. Caselli, "Visual Syndromes as the Presenting Feature of Degenerative Brain Disease," *Seminars in Neurology* 20 (2000): 139–44.

52. D. A. Drachman and J. M. Swearer, "Driving and Alzheimer's disease: The risk of crashes," Neurology 43 (1993): 2448–56; R. G. Logsdon, L. Teri, and E. B. Larson, "Driving and Alzheimer's Disease," *Journal of General Internal Medicine* 7 (1992): 583–88; L. J. Fitten, K. M. Perryman, C. J. Wilkinson, et al., "Alzheimer and Vascular Dementias and Driving. A Prospective Road and Laboratory Study," *Journal of the American Medical Association* 273 (1995): 1360–65; L. A. Hunt, C. F. Murphy, D. Carr, et al., "Reliability of the Washington University Road Test. A Performance-Based Assessment for Drivers with Dementia of the Alzheimer Type," *Archives of Neurology* 54 (1997): 707–12.

53. J. M. Duchek, L. Hunt, K. Ball, et al., "Attention and Driving Performance in Alzheimer's Disease," *Journal of Gerontology*, ser. B, *Psychological Sciences and Social Sciences* 53 (1998): 130–41; G. W. Rebok, P. M. Keyl, F. W. Bylsma, et al., "The Effects of Alzheimer Disease on Driving-Related Abilities," *Alzheimer Disease and Associated Disorders* 8 (1994): 228–40; M. Rizzo, S. Reinach, D. McGehee, et al., "Simulated Car Crashes and Crash Predictors in Drivers with Alzheimer Disease," *Archives of Neurology* 54 (1997): 545–51; D. J. Cox, W. C. Quillian, F. P. Thorndike, et al., "Evaluating Driving Performance of Outpatients with Alzheimer Disease," *Journal of the American Board of Family Practice* 11 (1998): 264–71.

54. Dubinsky, Stein, and Lyons, "Practice Parameter: Risk of Driving and Alzheimer's Disease."

55. Drachman and Swearer, "Driving and Alzheimer's Disease: The Risk of Crashes"; Logsdon, Teri, and Larson, "Driving and Alzheimer's Disease."

56. Hunt, Murphy, Carr, et al., "Reliability of the Washington University Road Test"; G. K. Fox, S. C. Bowden, G. M. Bashford, et al., "Alzheimer's Disease and Driving: Prediction and Assessment of Driving Performance," *Journal of the American Geriatrics Society* 45 (1997): 949–53.

CHAPTER 6

REHABILITATION INTERVENTIONS

Uses and Benefits of Speech, Occupational, and Physical Therapies

Keith M. Robinson, MD;
and Amy P. Lustig, PhD, MPH, CCC-SLP

THE IDEA BEHIND REHABILITATION

Rehabilitation is a holistic, comprehensive treatment approach that incorporates the physical, cognitive, behavioral, emotional, and social dimensions of care. It, thus, has something to offer all major presentations of frontotemporal degeneration (FTD), that is, the behavioral variants characterized by changes in personality; primary progressive aphasia and its subtypes characterized by changes in language; and the motor variants characterized by changes in movement. It operates as a physician-directed team effort that is multidisciplinary in membership and interdisciplinary in process. Rehabilitation treatments focus on everyday-life functions that need to be restored or modified for an individual to maintain an optimal level of control within his or her meaningful environment. For the individual with frontotemporal degeneration, the goal of rehabilitation is to maintain the highest level of empowerment that is realistically and safely possible through skilled and/or preventative/maintenance treatments performed collaboratively by rehabilitation therapists, the individual, and his or her caregivers.

Skilled treatments are those that require specialized interventions by rehabilitation therapists to re-achieve a previously established functional level that has become compromised by acute illness and/or by frontotemporal degeneration. For example, the recovery from an aspiration pneumonia in an individual with frontotemporal dementia inevitably will require a period of inactivity. The physiologic impact of this event may cause the loss of ability to walk, care for oneself, and interact meaningfully with others. Skilled physical therapy would support this individual to re-achieve his or her pre-pneumonia mobility status; skilled occupational therapy would support this individual to support his or her pre-pneumonia abilities to feed, bathe, and dress him- or herself; and skilled speech therapy would support the optimal oral intake of food with the use of safe swallowing strategies to prevent another aspiration event, as well as support this individual to communicate in the most meaningful way in order to express his or her basic needs to caregivers and others.

Preventive/maintenance treatments are those that are performed by the individual autonomously or with the supervision and assistance of caregivers, often as the product of having been treated with skilled therapies, to maintain the highest level of functioning possible for the individual. Preventive/maintenance treatments are viewed as at least as important as treatments because they define, in part, the daily routines of the individual.

Rehabilitation treatments do not separate the individual from his or her caregivers, nor from the environment in which he or she lives. Rehabilitation defines caregivers broadly to include family members, friends, neighbors, church community members, volunteers, and skilled/semiskilled personnel (for example, home health aides, homemakers), as those who supervise or assist the individual with frontotemporal degeneration in his community-based or institutional place of residence. Rehabilitation views the social-support system/caregivers as the interpersonal environment, and the place of residence as the physical environment.

Therapeutic interventions are directed toward the individual and these environments concurrently. For example, in those individuals who have progressed in their frontotemporal degeneration to the point where learning is finite, rehabilitation directs treatments toward these environments to educate caregivers in rational care of the individual (for example, cueing a dysphagic and impulsive individual with amyotrophic lateral sclerosis–associated frontotemporal degeneration who has aspiration risk to tuck his/her chin during swallowing, to take smaller portions or bites with each mouthful, and to slow down the pace of eating), and to create a physically safe environment to reduce risks of physical injury to an individual or caregiver (for example, training the spouse of an individual who has frontotemporal degeneration with Parkinsonism with excessive motor rigidity and slow movements how to properly transfer and walk with this individual).

Rehabilitation emphasizes the mundane in everyday life, that is, those activities in which everyone must participate, (for example, eating and toileting) to negotiate through the day. When considering frontotemporal degeneration, control of one's rituals during everyday life is dynamically defined by how far an individual has progressed in his or her disease trajectory. Loss of function is inevitable. Redefining optimal control as loss occurs is operationalized by rehabilitation strategies. Optimal control, regardless of functional status, can invoke a less negative perception of one's declining situation and a higher sense of quality of life.

Despite loss of cognitive functions, learning new or alternative ways of participating in everyday-life rituals is possible for the individual with frontotemporal degeneration, particularly in the early and middle stages of the disease. As remembering names, places, and events becomes difficult and less important, remembering and learning skills that are grounded in motor control can remain relatively spared. The former type of remembering requires conscious learning, known as declarative or explicit—or the "learning what" memory system; this disproportionately becomes impaired in frontotemporal degeneration. The latter type of remembering requires unconscious learning, known as procedural or implicit—or the "learning how" memory system; this can remain relatively available for learning alternative motor skills to negotiate safely through everyday life, for example, learning to use a rolling walker to walk safely at home, and managing the control mechanism on a stair glide to negotiate on stairs safely.

Rehabilitation views inactivity as harmful to health and well-being. There are well-documented negative anatomic, physiological, and psychological effects of inactivity, summarized in table 6.1. Bed rest, although sometimes a necessary treatment to recover from an acute episode of illness, has negative side effects that can be as disastrous as the side effects of medications. Much of the effort of rehabilitation is directed toward reversing and minimizing these negative effects.

THE ESSENTIAL TOOLS OF REHABILITATION

Functional assessment is the basic method of clinical evaluation to define rehabilitation treatments and to determine the utility or outcome from treatments. The multidisciplinary team operationalizes treatment approaches based on functional assessment. Mutually agreed upon goals of treatment are then negotiated and set among members of the treatment team, the individual with frontotemporal degeneration, and his or her caregiver.

Functional Assessment

Rehabilitation defines function at the level of individual performance in relation to the caregivers' requirements to provide supervision and assistance within a meaningful environment where one lives. Function in these terms does not view the individual as the deconstructed collection of cells, neurotransmitters, and organ systems that composes his or her anatomic and physiologic protoplasm, but rather as how this protoplasm integratively performs basic survival skills to negotiate through everyday life vis-à-vis the burden on caregivers to perform these skills successfully. Functional assessment observes and measures performance in three broad areas of living: communication, self-care, and mobility. Each of these three areas can be categorized into those that are necessary to survive within one's home or place of residence, and those that are necessary to survive in the larger community. These functional survival skills are summarized in table 6.2.

The Rehabilitation Team

The core rehabilitation team includes a rehabilitation medical specialist, that is, a physiatrist, and three nonmedical specialists: a speech therapist, a physical therapist, and an occupational therapist. Each of these specialists traditionally has been considered an expert in treating deficits in each of the three broad areas of functioning: speech therapists treat communication deficits; occupational therapists treat self-care deficits; and physical therapists treat mobility deficits. Over time, their respective areas of expertise have evolved to include treating functional deficits that require overlapping and complementary approaches. For example, as speech therapists also assess and treat swallowing deficits, occupational therapists concurrently assess and treat fine motor strategies that control eating/feeding. These therapy disciplines are more thoroughly defined and discussed in chapters 10 through 14.

The rehabilitation team also includes a larger array of nonmedical specialists who operationalize clinical assessments and treatment interventions collaboratively, based on either a prescription or a referral from a physician (who is typically a neurologist, a primary-care doctor, a physiatrist, or a psychiatrist), or by cross-referral from another nonmedical member of the team. Table 6.3 summarizes the division of labor among the rehabilitation specialists. Rehabilitation includes the individual's caregivers as an essential component of the team.

While any physician can prescribe rehabilitation treatments, the physiatrist understands best the skills of the various team members, and in doing so, often functions as the gatekeeper of rehabilitation services. The physiatrist plays a major role in defining precautions for rehabilitation interventions for therapists, particularly exercise, which can be performed even by severely debilitated individuals. The physiatrist forms a partnership with the primary-care physician or neurologist to manage the rehabilitation aspects of treatment in coordination with the medical treatment. The physiatrist typically will manage the following:

1. Prescribe, monitor, and revise rehabilitation services.
2. Decide which nonmedical specialists are appropriate to intervene at specific points in time.
3. Reinforce the execution of preventive/maintenance treatments by the caregivers.
4. Decide on the best site for rehabilitation services to occur (inpatient, outpatient, home).
5. Prescribe durable medical equipment (DME) such as walkers, wheelchairs, and commodes.

SPECIFIC TREATMENT APPROACHES

Minimizing Deconditioning

Deconditioning is a syndrome that is comprised of the reversible and preventable negative anatomic and physiologic effects of bed rest, inactivity, and sedentary lifestyles. Those with frontotemporal degeneration who have poor initiation and/or apathy (for example, those with Parkinsonism-predominant, and with these behavioral variants), and who have loss of motor control (for example, all variants with motor decline predominant) are particularly at risk. Deconditioning affects multiple organ systems and is cumulative, superimposing the effects of the underlying neurodegenerative process and its complications. There are commonsense interventions that rehabilitation therapists can teach caregivers to manage the effects of deconditioning. Some of these treatments include: daily muscle and joint range-of-motion to minimize the effects of spasticity and rigidity in forming soft-tissue contractures, regular walking programs and upper-limb repetitive activities to prevent loss of stamina and endurance, and the use of wheelchair cushions and mattresses made of specialized materials to decompress bony weight-bearing sites to prevent pressure sores. These are summarized in table 6.1.

Contractures occur when joints and their associated soft tissues (tendons, ligaments, muscles) are immobilized for sustained periods of time. They worsen as the period of immobility lengthens. What occurs is a progressive shortening and remolding of musculoskeletal tissues into positions that can interfere with performing basic survival skills (for example, mobilizing the shoulder for eating and reaching; lifting up the foot and ankle for walking; cleaning skin folds of the armpit, in between the fingers and wrists, and between the legs). Contractures can be minimized with range-of-motion and gentle muscle flexibility programs taught to caregivers by physical and occupational therapists.

Loss of muscle strength and loss of the endurance of muscles to perform repetitive activities without excessive fatigue can start to occur within a few days of bed rest and worsen as the period of immobilization is prolonged. Immobilization can augment aging-related bone demineralization (osteopenia), increasing the risk of a bone fracture during minor trauma. Muscle weakness, loss of muscle endurance, and osteopenia can be minimized with conservative strengthening and muscle-endurance exercises, such as bedside strengthening; sustained sitting at the bedside or upright in a supportive chair; "pre-walking" activities such as repetitive sitting to standing; weight shifting during sustained standing and walking in place; and gait training with an assistive device such as a walker. The physical therapist takes the lead in teaching the individual and caregivers these mobility skills.

Important risk factors for pressure sores in individuals with frontotemporal degeneration include involuntary movement disorders such as those frequently seen in the variants that have motor decline as predominant, that is, spasticity in progressive supranuclear palsy, corticobasilar syndrome, and amyotrophic lateral sclerosis; and rigidity in Parkinsonism. These involuntary disorders of motor control disallow initiation and continuation of fluid movements, resulting in inactivity as a major risk factor. Other risk factors for pressure sores include incontinence with frequent moistening of the skin, poor nutrition, apathy (behavioral variant), and sensory deficits at weight-bearing sites over bony prominences such as the shoulder blades and the buttocks. Prevention of pressure sores is a multidisciplinary effort including bed mobility and transfer training to avoid shearing or friction during movement (physical therapy); repositioning schedules during sustained sitting and when in bed (physical therapy, occupational therapy, and nurses in hospital or home care); specialized cushions and mattresses to decompress weight-bearing sites (physical therapy and nursing); and specialized foot and ankle bracing, such as with Multi Podus™ boots, to unload the heels when in bed (physical therapy, nursing, and orthotics).

The effects of immobilization on the heart, lungs, and blood vessels include an increase in resting heart rate, an abrupt increase in heart rate with minimal activity, and a decrease in cardiac reserve to perform sustained everyday life activities, resulting in easy fatiguabilty. The output of blood from the heart during each contraction to supply vital organs decreases. The integrity of the muscles inside of veins and arteries that controls their diameter becomes compromised; thus, resting blood pressure becomes lower and drops with changes in position from lying to sitting to standing, resulting in dizziness and passing out (orthostatic hypotension). The efficiency of breathing becomes compromised because of loss of strength of the ventilatory muscles (particularly in amyotrophic lateral sclerosis) and collapse of the more dependent segments of the lung (particularly in Parkinsonism when there is chest wall rigidity creating a stiff and inflexible rib cage), resulting in inconsistent and irregular oxygen exchange from the airways into the blood stream. The protective cough reflex weakens, and clearance of secretions becomes less effective, increasing the risk of food, mucus, and gastric contents entering the lungs (aspiration). Vascular blood flow in the leg veins slows down, predisposing the individual to blood-clot formation in the deeper large veins (deep venous thrombosis). If these clots break into small pieces, they can travel to the lungs and interfere with blood flow and air exchange. This is life threatening and known as a pulmonary embolism. Both a deep venous thrombosis and a pulmonary embolism require treatment with a blood thinner such as Coumadin®, which has its own risk of easier bleeding with minor trauma, particularly in people who fall frequently. These cardiovascular and pulmonary consequences of inactivity can be minimized with several therapeutic interventions: graduated sitting, standing, and walking programs (physical therapy); no/low-resistance, high-repetition strengthening exercises such as ankle pumps (physical therapy); ventilatory muscle training; and swallowing assessment and individualized strategies such as modifying food consistencies and adopting behaviors to minimize the risk of aspiration (speech therapy).

Cognitive Remediation of Intellectual Deficits

Frontotemporal degeneration is defined by progressive cognitive and intellectual losses. Neuroscientific investigations have made promising headway into understanding the underlying cellular and neurochemical mechanisms that underpin cognitive functions. Treatment of the cognitive deficits that occur with frontotemporal degeneration is limited by what we know about fundamental neural mechanisms in the brain. A more sophisticated appreciation of cognition, intelligence, and learning is evolving. New models of cognition, intelligence, and learning are being developed and tested through scientific pursuit in a variety of brain disorders. The models that have been developed from studying other diagnoses, such as head injury, multiple sclerosis, and stroke, can be applied to treating frontotemporal degeneration, particularly in the early and middle stages of the disease trajectory. With these thoughts in mind, several principles can be articulated about rehabilitation of cognitive and intellectual deficits, that is, cognitive remediation:

1. A hierarchy of cognitive functions is assumed. Attentional functions and short-term memory can be viewed as infrastructure that support

more complex cognitive processes. Treating attention and short-term memory deficits with a combination of neuromodulating medications and behaviorally based treatments may enhance performance of more complex cognitive functions. A fundamental approach used to treat behavioral impairments in cognitive infrastructure includes repetition and guided forced usage. However, in treating individuals with frontotemporal degeneration, practice will not make perfect, but it may improve function and safety by enhancing attentional systems.

2. Despite common deficits that define frontotemporal degeneration, every individual has his/her own idiosyncratic profile of intellectual strengths and deficits. Detailed behavioral, neurological, and neuropsychological assessment is the best approach to define an individual's profile of cognitive strengths and weaknesses. This profile then can be translated by various members of the rehabilitation team (neuropsychologist, speech therapist, occupational therapist) into behaviorally based cognitive-remediation strategies that are task and goal specific.

3. Learning theory has distinguished the two different systems of learning mentioned above: the conscious/explicit/declarative/"learning what" system, and the unconscious/implicit/procedural/"learning how" system. The former system has a more specific localization of neural networks in the brain, connecting the medial temporal lobes with specific areas of the thalamus, the base of the frontal lobes, and the amygdala. The medial temporal lobes sustain particular damage in frontotemporal degeneration resulting in deficits in the "learning what" system. The latter "learning how" system has a more diffuse representation in the brain and is certainly subject to damage in frontotemporal degeneration yet theoretically may be relatively spared as a learning system until the later stages of disease. Much of what underpins rehabilitation treatments, including cognitive remediation, is dependent on the "learning how" system in that what occurs is teaching cognitive and motor skills and procedures that are task and goal specific, through behaviorally based strategies that either accommodate or compensate for neurological deficits.

4. Cognitive remediation involves two fundamental approaches: utilizing cognitive strengths to bypass cognitive weaknesses, and replacing "lost" information and procedures with external aids. Common examples of a bypass strategy is the procedural motor learning that occurs

when an individual who has Parkinsonism is required to use rolling walker to reduce falling risk during walking as learned in physical therapy. Another example is when an individual who has the behavioral variant of frontotemporal degeneration with impulsivity predominant is taught in speech therapy not to "shovel in" food but to use a slower rate of intake and double swallow maneuvers to minimize aspiration risk during eating. A common example of the use of external aids is procedurally learning the use of daily planners and memory logs to cue the retrieval of critical information necessary for negotiating through everyday life, such as types and times of medication usage, appointments, and safe meal-preparation procedures.

5. Cognitive remediation often links the use of physician-prescribed neuromodulating medications with behaviorally based treatments that are driven by procedural learning, and with structured and nonpunitive behavioral management. It is of fundamental importance that the treating rehabilitation team be made aware when such medications are initiated, modified, and discontinued, so that the therapists can closely observe with caregivers any beneficial/detrimental effects of medication interventions by using behavior trackers that monitor precipitants of undesired behaviors and instances and quality of desired targeted behaviors. See chapter 5 for a more in-depth discussion of neuromodulating medications.

Procedural learning in the context of rehabilitation is task and goal specific. More complex tasks are deconstructed into a logical sequence of steps that are reconstructed during treatment. The learning that occurs tends to become hyperspecific for the targeted task; this means that learning one task does not generalize to master a related task; for example, learning the use of a remote-control device to control cable television channels should not presume that this learning will generalize to apply to successful use of a cell phone.

Treatment of Difficult or Unruly Behaviors

While progressive cognitive deficits define the presence of frontotemporal degeneration, these are often associated with difficult behaviors, particularly in the behavioral variant in which there is a range of problematic behaviors across the spectrum, from apathy and emotional flatness to impulsivity and inappropriate social interactions and displays. These types of undesired behaviors result in compromised safety during everyday-life activities, and can interfere with meaningful participation in rehabilitation therapies and other types of treatment. Within this spectrum, further undesired behaviors include poor initiation, easy distractibility, agitation, wandering, disinhibition, anger, aggression, poor insight or self-monitoring of one's abilities and inabilities, inappropriate communication of basic needs, perseveration or "getting stuck" in the middle of an activity, emotional lability, obsessiveness-compulsivity, and rumination. Often, these behaviors require neuromodulating agents to suppress them. See chapter 5 for a more in-depth discussion of these neuromodulating agents.

Knowledge of some basic principles of behavioral management that are incorporated into rehabilitation treatments can provide caregivers with strategies that support exercising more control in creating a safe interpersonal environment. These include:

1. The environment in which the individual with dementia lives should be structured, consistent, and have minimally distracting influences. This will at least encourage appropriate activity participation to support a normal sleep-wake cycle.
2. Every effort should be made to ensure that the individual's hearing and vision are optimized since they control the primary entry of sensory information from the environment into the brain.
3. Many disturbing behaviors have specific precipitants that can be identified, then modified or eliminated. When a pattern cannot be realized, fatigue from environmental overload should be entertained as an explanation, and "down time" and short naps should be included in the structured daily schedule.
4. Desirable and adaptive behaviors should be rewarded with positive feedback. Undesirable behaviors should be responded to as neutrally and as safely as possible. Providing positive feedback is an easier and more enjoyable response and usually involves displaying a simple positive emotional message such as a smile, verbal encouragement, or touch. Providing neutral responses to problematic behaviors is counterintuitive and effortful; however, automatic negative feedback in response to undesired behaviors may simply reinforce them by bringing more attention to them. Neutral responses in these situations

can be difficult to adopt by family members intimately involved with the individual with frontotemporal degeneration because this requires modifying long-standing patterns of behavioral responses that have fueled close relationships. Furthermore, eliciting a neutral response to unruly behaviors is not always safe in situations in which an individual is threatening to be injurious to self and others. The use of "time out" or removing the individual from an environment to disengage him or her from possible precipitants may be useful in this situation.

Treatment of Involuntary Movement Disorders: Rigidity and Spasticity

Rigidity, tremor, and spasticity are involuntary movement disorders seen in individuals during the middle and later stages of frontotemporal degeneration, particularly in the variants that have progressive motor decline predominating. Rigidity and tremor are associated with Parkinsonism, and spasticity is commonly observed with progressive supranuclear palsy, corticobasilar syndrome, and amyotrophic lateral sclerosis. In many individuals, rigidity and spasticity can be difficult to distinguish clinically. Rigidity is one of several Parkinsonian signs that disallows smooth and fluid motor control during daily-life activities. The individual subjectively experiences stiffness and expends more energy to perform basic survival skills such as eating and walking, which results in easy fatigability. It can also increase falling risk. Tremor is another Parkinsonian sign involving repeated and patterned "oscillations" of specific body parts that can result in clumsy and dangerous participation in such activities as drinking from a cup in the event of finger/hand/wrist tremors, and/or taking food by mouth in the event of a lower facial or neck tremor.

Spasticity can be distinguished clinically from rigidity by an involuntary resistance to an external stretch to a specific muscle group that is "velocity dependent." The more rapidly that one provides an external stretch, the more resistance by the muscle is observed. When there is demonstrated functional interference, spasticity should be treated with antispasticity medications (for example, dantrolene sodium, tizanidine, baclofen) cautiously because these medications are often sedating even in low doses. When specific patterns of spasticity involve particular regions of the body, and when there is associated functional interference (for example, a "frozen shoulder" that interferes with eating; the wrist and finger flexor contractures that interfere with holding utensils or using a computer keyboard; the ankle extension or "equinovarus" contracture that interferes with adequate foot and ankle placement during the stance phase of the gait cycle), treatment with "chemoneurolysis" or injection of botulinum toxin into specific muscle groups by a neurologist or a physiatrist trained to do this procedure should be pursued.

Both rigidity and spasticity can cause shortening of muscles and other musculoskeletal tissues resulting in the formation of contractures. When severe (e.g., a frozen shoulder), they can disallow functional and controlled movement (e.g., eating, brushing teeth) and encourage poor hygiene in skin-folds (e.g., the armpits, between the legs) because of lack of access during bathing. Fundamentally, what will reverse and prevent contracture is daily range-of-motion and flexibility programs that can be taught to caregivers by physical and occupational therapists and incorporated into the daily schedule of the individual with frontotemporal dementia.

CREATING A SAFE ENVIRONMENT

As frontotemporal degeneration progresses, the learning ability of the individual will become finite. The rehabilitation interventions, then, are best directed toward the interpersonal and physical environments. These efforts hopefully improve the sense of control that the caregivers have in an interpersonal situation that can be viewed as relentlessly frustrating and asymmetric.

Creating a safe physical environment can be accomplished inexpensively and with input from home physical therapists, occupational therapists, speech therapists (swallowing and communication; for example, maximizing access to emergency assistance), and nurses, and with the purchase of several pieces of durable medical equipment. Any physician can prescribe a home environmental evaluation by the rehabilitation team with the goal of providing the caregiver advice for creating a safe environment. See chapter 14 for a more in-depth discussion of home modifications to increase safety.

MOBILITY (GAIT AND BALANCE) TRAINING AND DURABLE MEDICAL EQUIPMENT (DME)

Mobility training by physical therapy is fundamental to minimize falling risk and preventing falling episodes resulting in major injuries such as hip fractures and subdural hematomas of the brain. Frontotemporal degeneration is itself a risk factor for falling. For example, for those with the behavioral variant, their limited ability to maintain attention in combination with impulsivity of movement may disallow them to appreciate changes in contours on walking surfaces that demand adjustments in balance in order stay upright when walking on nonlevel surfaces; a fall can result. In those who have the progressive motor decline variant, rigidity associated with Parkinsonism and spasticity associated with the other three subtypes can interfere with smooth and fluid motor sequencing during the cycle of walking; a fall can result.

The large muscles situated in the lower back and abdomen, deep in the pelvis (core muscles), and at the hips and buttocks control one's ability to sit and stand upright during transfers, and to sustain standing and walking. When these large muscle groups become deconditioned, fall risk increases.

Fluid, goal-directed movement during walking is dependent on the integrity of an array of cognitive and sensorimotor factors or "intrinsic" factors that interpret the physical environment and then direct safe movement. These "intrinsic" factors must appreciate and pay attention to "extrinsic" factors in the physical environment, for example, cracks in the pavement, curb cuts, stairs, thresholds through doorways, and slippery surfaces, in order to prevent falling.

As presented in more detail in chapter 11, mobility training focuses on optimizing the intrinsic factors by deconstructing movement into a series of basic and sequential motor tasks that an individual must execute for safe movement: rolling, lying to sitting and vice versa, unsupported sitting balance, sitting to standing and vice versa, transfers or changes in sitting/standing surfaces (for example, onto and off of toilet, into and out of bed), weight shifting once upright, walking on level surfaces and on nonlevel surfaces (for example, stairs, outdoors), and integrative balance reactions to anticipate and react to environmental challenges (for example, getting pushed). During mobility training, all sensory systems are being optimized. It is observed that impaired proprioception or position sense ("knowing where your body is in space") and impaired vision that cues an individual when environmental challenges occur will particularly compromise movement by disallowing optimal sensory direction of movement. This principle, in rehabilitation, is known as sensory-motor integration. Additionally, during mobility training, the focus of strengthening is directed toward improving the core (abdominal, lower back, and deep pelvic muscles), buttocks, hip, and knee group muscles, that is, the large muscle groups of the pelvis and legs, as the power sources that are fundamental for maintaining an upright position during sitting, transfers, standing, and walking.

In many situations when mobility is impaired and falling risk is high, an assistive device may be necessary to allow safe walking. From least restrictive to more restrictive, these include straight canes, quad canes, axillary/forearm crutches, hemi-walkers, rolling walkers, and standard walkers. Successful use of the lesser restrictive devices presumes better balance. All of these assistive devices serve two main purposes: to provide enhanced sensory feedback to the brain to improve motor control; and to decrease energy consumption during walking to conserve strength and endurance. For individuals with frontotemporal degeneration, it is essential that they learn the use of an assistive device under the direction of a physical therapist. Most individuals with frontotemporal degeneration can procedurally learn to use these devices safely. As frontotemporal degeneration progresses, some individuals will be unable to initiate and sequence these devices correctly, thus increasing their falling risk.

In addition to assistive devices to support walking, there are other kinds of durable medical equipment (DME) that can optimize mobility when walking is no longer possible:

1. Wheelchairs—These should be considered when walking at home and longer distances outdoors is no longer possible. Their use in individuals with frontotemporal degeneration presumes that caregivers are available to propel them and that the individual is not self-propelling. For insurance reimbursement, a physician's prescription is necessary. This can be taken to a DME vendor who can supply, deliver, and set up the wheelchair. The DME vendor will send a certificate of medical necessity (CMN) to the prescribing physician for sign-off after documenting the wheelchair's necessity for household use. For the individual with frontotemporal degeneration, foldable, manually controlled, lightweight wheelchairs with swing-away or flip-back desk arms, removable/elevating leg rests, and a firm gel/foam combination cushion are

recommended. This combination of wheelchair components will allow the caregiver to fold/lift the wheelchair up/down stairs or into/out of the car; the individual to be seated comfortably at a table or desk; the individual's legs to be elevated to facilitate venous return; and a firm base of support to be provided to decompress bony weight-bearing sites in the buttocks, to support good sitting posture and prevent pressure sores. Many caregivers find lightweight wheelchairs, weighing between thirty and forty pounds, too heavy to lift. A less supportive, lower cost, and lighter option is a lightweight "travel" or "companion" wheelchair weighing twenty to twenty-five pounds.

Motorized scooters or power wheelchairs are not recommended for individuals with frontotemporal degeneration. Their cognitive deficits will likely interfere with safe driving. Health-insurance plans commonly will not pay for "companion control," that is, when a caregiver drives the power wheelchair.

2. Hospital beds—These should be considered when movement in bed and transferring into and out of bed becomes difficult. Health-insurance plans commonly reimburse semiautomatic hospital beds, that is, when there is remote control of elevating/lowering the head and foot of the bed and manual control of the height of the bed, with a physician's prescription and sign-off on a CMN arranged through a DME vendor. Fully automatic hospital beds provide remote control of the height of the bed and can be reimbursed with an additional letter of medical necessity (LMN) from a physician that documents its need for facilitating safe transfers into and out of bed and when a caregiver is unable to control the height of the bed with manual control.

3. Patient lifts (e.g., Hoyer® lifts)—These should be considered when transfers require at least 50 percent assistance of a caregiver, or less, when the caregiver has health problems. They are manually controlled mobile devices that can be manipulated in the bedroom and bathroom, and include a sling type of lift. A Hoyer "partner" is an accessory sling made of mesh material that dries quickly if exposed to water in the shower or tub and can be removed from underneath the dependent individual so that he or she does not have to sit on the sling for a prolonged period of time. These items are insurance reimbursable with a physician's prescription and sign-off on a CMN arranged through a DME vendor.

4. Commode and raised toilet seats—These are necessary for a one-floor living arrangement when toileting facilities are not available on the same floor where one chooses to live or that necessity dictates that one lives. Even if toileting facilities are available on the same floor, mobility may be impaired, particularly at nighttime, necessitating the use of a bedside commode. The best option is a "three-in-one" commode that can be used at the bedside with its collection pan, or the frame and seat can be used as a raised toilet seat without the collection pan when placed over the permanent toilet. These items are not always insurance reimbursable with a physician's prescription and sign-off on a CMN as arranged through a DME vendor.

5. Stair glides/lifts—These should be considered when walking on stairs is no longer safe, and one chooses to continue to live on two floors. Health-insurance plans will not reimburse them. They can be rented or purchased from specific vendors who will assess the home environment for their feasibility since they do not fit in all stairways. When installed, an individual will usually require a wheelchair or assistive device for each floor between the stair glide. Purchase or rental of the second set of wheelchairs and assistive devices will require payment out of pocket since health-insurance plans will usually not pay for duplicate sets.

Several other caveats about DME are worth mentioning:

1. Many physicians do not know what they are ordering when prescribing DME, and thus depend on the knowledge of a DME vendor. Seek advice from someone on the rehabilitation team who has more experience ordering this equipment—the physiatrist, physical therapist, occupational therapist, or nurse.

2. Select a DME vendor who is known to your rehabilitation providers. If the wrong equipment is ordered, or if ongoing service is needed, a good relationship with a vendor will facilitate equipment return/ exchange and/or reimbursement, and repair.

3. The physiatrist has the most experience writing letters of medical necessity with appropriate clinical justification. Information from rehabilitation therapists and DME vendors, based on their own assessments of the individual/environment, can be incorporated into these letters.

ACTIVITIES OF DAILY LIVING (ADL) TRAINING

As summarized in table 6.2, ADLs can be categorized as those activities that one needs to survive inside the household (eating, grooming, bathing, toileting, etc.), and those that are needed to survive in the larger community (shopping, banking, etc.). Supporting optimal control of these skills is the focus of occupational therapy and nursing treatments and is discussed in more detail in chapters 12 and 13. Occupational therapy is essential for teaching individuals with frontotemporal degeneration and their caregivers the commonsense use of adaptive equipment, such as reachers, leg lifters, and built-up utensils that will serve to conserve energy during the performance of ADL. They can provide practical and resourceful advice on the purchasing of low-cost DME and making changes in the physical environment at home to enhance safety and energy conservation. Occupational therapists have specific training in cognitive functions, particularly memory and visuoperception, and can teach the use of procedural strategies to compensate for deficits. They can help caregivers set up structure and consistency in daily-life schedules as a fundamental behavioral intervention. They work collaboratively with physical therapists and home nurses on ordering and teaching the proper use of DME and the proper techniques of assisting individuals with basic mobility so that caregivers can prevent injuries to themselves. They are experts in fine motor functioning of the hands to facilitate optimal control when performing/assisting ADLs.

Occupational therapists also work collaboratively with speech therapists to assist individuals in the setup and positioning of computerized or other assistive communication devices/tools, such as those sometimes used by individuals with primary progressive aphasia (PPA) and with severe slurring of words that can be seen in amyotrophic lateral sclerosis, to aid in execution of more complex ADLs, for example, generating a shopping list, and in expressing one's basic needs. Alternative and augmentative communication (AAC) devices (along with strategies described in more detail in chapter 10) can help individuals with difficulty in verbal communication to express themselves through use of gestures, visual information, and computer-aided voicing to compensate for difficulties with verbal communication. AAC devices range from very "low-tech" to very "high-tech." Low-tech AAC approaches include use of visual materials such as written alphabets to cue word recall; written words or phrases that can be pointed to for expression of needs or thoughts; and pictures of items, actions, concepts, and important people, places, and events (including familiar photographs), with or without paired written words, that can also be pointed to for self-expression purposes. For individuals unable to point by themselves, communication boards and books can be created and personalized to represent the individual's specific needs, interests, and concerns. The caregiver will be trained by the speech therapist to assist the individual with communication, usually accomplished by teaching them how to point at or direct their loved one's attention to written words or pictures, and to train the individual in a small set of responses that the caregiver will recognize for accurate communication purposes. Sometimes when the individual's physical and/or cognitive limitations prevent use of a typical paper-based communication board/book, a transparent communication board is created where relevant words and pictures are strategically positioned such that the caregiver and their family member can communicate by meeting one another's eye gaze at a certain letter, word, or picture. In cases of very severe disability, sometimes it can be a challenge—albeit a critical one—to establish a reliable strategy for communication of even "yes" and "no" responses. The speech therapist will make every effort to tailor communication strategies to the individual's and caregiver's particular situation and functional contingencies.

High-tech AAC applications typically employ some type of computerized or mechanical device that contains the information to be communicated, along with an electronically based method of getting the message out. Some devices are designed to be relatively small, hand-held units with a limited number of "buttons"; a single message is programmed into each button, and the message is expressed when the button is activated. Sometimes the message is communicated visually through words appearing on a screen, but more frequently it is produced in an audible format through the use of digitized voicing; this is often referred to as a "speech-generating" device or communication solution. For example, a device can have six buttons, each programmed with a different message, such as "I need help" or "Please turn me over." When the button is pressed, it will generate the message in a spoken format so that it may be heard by the caregiver. The quality of the digitized speech used by these devices has improved greatly over the past several years, and often the user will have several options to choose from, such as gender and age, to tailor the digitized speech output most closely to their personal preference.

There are also very high-tech speech-generating devices available that provide a variety of complex and sophisticated solutions to communication impairment associated with loss of speech competence. Usually these devices are too heavy to carry and require some form of mounting solution; they can be placed on a wheelchair, a bedframe, or a freestanding support unit. They are designed with a prominent screen that varies in size, usually from ten to twenty inches in diameter, and they have a lot of electronic "memory" within which a considerable amount of information can be programmed to facilitate communication of needs, thoughts, ideas, and conversation. Individuals can access the information in these devices through a variety of mechanisms, including through use of a computer mouse, an electronic "switch," touch-screen activation, and most recently through technology that allows them to select targets on the computer screen by using their eyes. Such "eye-gaze" technology is typically offered to individuals who have limited cognitive involvement with good attention skills and the ability to learn new tasks, as it can be somewhat challenging to learn, though the material to be communicated can be organized to be as simple and accessible as possible. These devices also offer a variety of other communication modalities, including e-mail, cell-phone texting, and instant messaging, and many have built-in infrared receptivity such that any infrared-compatible device (for example, televisions, radios, doorbells, lights, etc.) can be remotely manipulated by the individual through the communication unit. In addition, a multitude of personal information and recreational activities, such as music, ebooks, movies, games, photograph albums—virtually anything that can be put in digital form—can be easily installed on these devices, allowing the individual and his or her caregivers and companions to share entertaining and meaningful activities along with communication opportunities. Some of the software used by these devices is also available on portable devices, such as cell phones and electronic tablets, and can be used through touchscreen or other interfaces (including, to a limited extent, eye-gaze technologies that are currently on the market for Android[SM] tablets) to select communication targets and generate digitized speech output for communication purposes. Many, if not most, of these software programs are designed to be very flexible and can be specifically tailored to meet the needs of the individual and caregiver with the assistance of the speech therapist.

ASPIRATION PREVENTION DURING EATING AND SWALLOWING

Aspiration occurs when food, saliva, or gastric contents pass through the larynx and enter the upper airways of the lungs. Aspiration can be life threatening, causing airway obstruction and pneumonia. Swallowing dysfunction, or dysphagia, is the major reason that aspiration occurs. Dysphagia can be observed in frontotemporal degeneration for a number of reasons that demonstrate the complexity and elegance of normal swallowing. Swallowing has three major phases: an oral (mouth) phase; a pharyngeal (throat) phase; and an esophageal phase (where food is transported through the esophagus from the throat to the stomach).

The oral phase requires voluntary, conscious, and active attention directed toward the pacing of eating, the size of the food/liquid bolus to be ingested, and the coordination of the mouth, facial muscles, and tongue to chew food and propel food toward the throat. Any problems with focusing and sustaining attention toward these components of the oral phase will increase the risk of aspiration—this can be problematic across all three variants of frontotemporal degeneration. Moreover, those with the behavioral variant who are easily distracted and impulsive will not be able to self-monitor their pace of eating, nor will they consistently select smaller food and liquid portions. Consequently, they will require cueing during meals from caregivers to slow the pace of eating and limit the size of the bites. On the other hand, those with the behavioral variant who are apathetic are at risk for not supporting themselves nutritionally with food because they function slowly and with poor self-initiation during meals, and are indifferent to their sensation of hunger. Furthermore, delayed movement of food/liquid across the mouth toward the throat that may be particularly observed in Parkinsonism will increase aspiration risk.

The pharyngeal phase is a coordinated, involuntary series of reflexes during which muscles of the throat alternately contract and relax to allow passage of food/liquid into the esophagus, which anatomically is behind the larynx. The cricopharyngeus muscle, which sits at the top of the esophagus, relaxes and opens to accept the food/liquid being swallowed, which then travels through the esophagus into the stomach. Otherwise, the cricopharyngeus muscle remains in a contracted, closed position to protect the pharynx from acidic stomach contents that may have entered the esophagus. Sensory receptors at the opening to the larynx work to trigger a cough to clear food or liquid debris from getting into the airway. An effective and protective cough reflex can propel materials from the upper airways at speeds of up to two hundred miles per hour. These reflexes may be slow to respond and poorly coordinated, particularly in the variants of frontotemporal degeneration with progressive motor decline.

Common symptoms that indicate swallowing difficulties and aspiration include coughing during or after eating/drinking, and a "wet" or gurgling voice during or after eating. Speech therapists have emerged as diagnostic and therapeutic swallowing experts. They can perform a clinical swallowing exam in almost any setting with simple tools, and they also work with radiologists to perform more detailed studies of swallowing function. Based on their assessment, they can give practical advice to individuals and their caregivers about operationalizing behavioral strategies during meals to lower aspiration risk and optimize nutritional intake.

When any sort of oral food/liquid ingestion results in aspiration, alternative forms of eating, such as enteral nutritional support (tube feeding), can be considered. This offer of alternative feeding strategies is particularly common in amyotrophic lateral sclerosis when there is disproportionate loss of motor control of the facial and throat muscles that control swallowing, speech production, and handling of secretions (drooling). The choice for enteral nutrition is complicated and does not preclude tasting orally ingested foods with the goal of addressing quality-of-life purposes. The work of the speech therapist is discussed in more depth in chapter 10. A discussion about enteral feeding choices is included in chapters 10 and 17.

THE DECISION TO STOP DRIVING

The decision to stop driving is a difficult one. Chapters 5 and 12 address some of the issues about making this decision. It is important to note that physicians are legally obligated to report unsafe drivers to the state registries of motor vehicles. This is best done with open and informed consent of the individual with frontotemporal degeneration, and with family support and reassurance, whether or not the individual agrees. When the state registry of motor vehicles is informed that someone is no longer medically able to drive, the burden of responsibility is placed on the individual and the family to prove that he or she is a safe driver by passing certified drivers' training and/or a driving test. Occupational therapists are knowledgeable about such training and testing and can refer to regional subspecialists who manage driving programs. Payment for such driving programs is not reimbursable by health-insurance plans.

TABLE 6.1. The Deconditioning Syndrome and Its Preventive Treatments

PRIMARY EFFECTS ON ORGAN SYSTEM	RELATED COMPLICATIONS	PREVENTION AND TREATMENT INTERVENTIONS

Musculoskeletal

Joint contractures	Impedes self-care and ambulation	Proper positioning of limb, sometimes with static splinting; passive and active range-of-motion exercises with terminal stretch at least twice daily
Muscle weakness and atrophy	Decreased strength, coordination, and balance	Conservative isometric and isotonic strengthening
Osteoporosis	Pathologic fractures	Graduated sitting and standing protocol

Dermatological

Subcutaneous tissue ischemia	Pressure sores	Optimize nutritional intake
Skin atrophy		Frequent repositioning; specialized mattresses that distribute pressure away from bony prominences; avoiding shear stress or skin friction when moving patient

Cardiovascular/Pulmonary

Decreased vascular smooth muscle tone	Postural hypotension	Graduated sitting and standing protocols
Tachycardia at rest and during submaximal exercise with reduced cardiac output	Poor endurance	Graduated ambulation
Hypercoagulable blood	Deep venous thrombosis (DVT); pulmonary embolism	Strengthening exercises (low resistance, high repetition) of the legs; frequent ankle pumps
Basilar lung collapse	Poor ventilation	Incentive spirometry
Compromised secretion clearance	Aspiration pneumonia	Aspiration prevention strategies while drinking/eating

Genitourinary

Increased calcium clearance	Kidney stones	Graduated sitting protocols
Incomplete bladder emptying	Urinary-tract infections	Use of bedside commode; regularly scheduled voiding

TABLE 6.2. Everyday-Life Functional Survival Skills

SELF-CARE	MOBILITY	COMMUNICATION

Household

SELF-CARE	MOBILITY	COMMUNICATION

Eating/drinking
Bathing/grooming
Dressing
Toileting
Bowel/bladder
  control
Sexuality
Cooking
Laundry
Housekeeping
Taking
  medications
	Bed mobility
	Transfers (bed to chair,
	  chair to toilet, chair to
	  shower seat)
	Ambulation with or
	  without an assistive
	  device, level versus
	  nonlevel surfaces
	  (stairs)
	Balance
	Wheelchair ambu-
	  lation and parts
	  management
		Hearing
		Vision
		Orientation
		Attention
		Memory
		Language (talking/reading/
		  writing/gesturing)
		Spatial perception
		Organization
		Problem solving

Community

SELF-CARE	MOBILITY	COMMUNICATION

Shopping
Banking
Managing finan-
  cial and legal
  affairs
	Nonlevel surface ambulation with
	  or without an assistive device
	  (curbs, ramps, uneven terrain)
	Community wheelchair ambulation
	  (manual vs. motorized)
	Driving
	Using public transportation (bus,
	  taxi, wheelchair, van)
		Using telephones
		Writing, typing, use
		  of low- or high-tech
		  assistive communi-
		  cation devices
		Supervising others
		  in self-care and
		  mobility needs

TABLE 6.3. The Division of Labor among Rehabilitation Providers

Physiatrist

Medical specialist in rehabilitation; gatekeeper of rehabilitation services; prescribes and monitors therapies and durable medical equipment (DME); coordinates rehabilitation team.

Nurse

Nurses, particularly those employed by home-care agencies, will support the caregivers in many ways, including proper administration of all medications; supervision of home health aides and homemakers employed by the same agency; and frontline follow-through of rehabilitation-generated skilled treatment strategies that must be integrated into the daily routines of the individuals who have FTD during preventive/maintenance programs. A nurse also assists and supervises the patient in using cognitive and functional skills learned in therapies; educates the patient in medication schedule and self-monitoring of medical problems such as diabetes; trains the patient to follow bowel and bladder programs; provides direct wound care and pressure-sore prevention.

Physical therapist

Assists in basic mobility skills, including bed mobility, transfers, wheelchair mobility, and ambulation; selects appropriate assistive devices for ambulation, including canes, walkers, and wheelchairs; manages spasticity with therapeutic exercises; facilitates sensorimotor control, gait training, lower limb bracing (orthotics), and balance training.

Occupational therapist

Involved with daily-living skills, including feeding, grooming, toileting, dressing, and homemaking; develops fine motor skills of the hand and upper limbs, including splinting (orthotics) and wheelchair accessories; assists with cognitive remediation, especially in the areas of memory and visuoperception.

Speech/swallowing therapist

Provides cognitive remediation as it relates to meaningful communication, especially in the areas of attention, memory, language comprehension, conceptual organization, language production (including nonverbal technologies), and oral-motor articulation; performs swallowing evaluation and treatments, specifically regarding oral-motor and pharyngeal function, aspiration precautions, and oral feeding with different food consistencies.

Nutritionist

Collaborates with physicians and therapists to establish caloric and nutritional requirements; makes recommendations for nutritional-support options, depending on the most reliable means of food entry (oral, enteral), and dietary advancement.

Psychologist

Counseling psychologists provide psychotherapeutic treatment of emotional-loss reactions, depression, and other mood disorders for the individual with frontotemporal degeneration and the caregivers.

Behavioral psychologists design and manage behavior strategies and programs (often in concert with medications) aimed at optimizing communication with patients having difficulty with self-monitoring, aggression, poor initiation, and other behaviors that disrupt rehabilitation treatments and social interactions.

Neuropsychologists provide formal assessment of cognitive and intellectual functions and translate cognitive strengths and weaknesses into behaviorally based cognitive remediation strategies.

Orthotist

Fabricates devices that enable motor control and conserve energy consumption during mobility (orthotics or bracing), especially of lower limbs.

DME vendor

Supplies and services durable medical equipment based on physician/therapist prescription/recommendation with health-insurance plan reimbursement or through private payment.

Recreation therapist

Evaluates and remediates motor and cognitive dysfunction in a setting that focuses on leisure activities.

Social worker/case manager

Clarifies social-support system and supports caregivers and their ability to provide safe and stable emotional support, residential sites, personal care, and transportation; clarifies eligibility and coverage of health and welfare services and health-insurance plans; mobilizes resources for coverage of essential health and rehabilitation services with informal and formal care providers acting in complementary roles; provides emotional support for patients and their caregivers; orchestrates appropriate medical, surgical, rehabilitation, and social services, depending on disease trajectory and during recovery from acute illnesses, treatment priorities, and health-insurance/financial resources.

Caregiver

Supervises and assists in personal care at home; performs preventive/maintenance rehabilitation interventions at home; includes family members, friends, volunteers, neighbors, church community members, and anyone willing to act as an unpaid or informal care provider.

BIBLIOGRAPHY

Gitlin, L. N., and T. V. Earland. "Dementia (Improving Quality of Life in Individuals with Dementia: The Role of Nonpharmacologic Approaches in Rehabilitation)." In J. H. Stone and M. Blouin, eds. *International Encyclopedia of Rehabilitation*. 2010. Center for International Rehabilitation Research Information and Exchange (CIRRIE), http://cirrie.buffalo.edu/encyclopedia/en/article/28/.

Robinson, K. M. "Assessing Function." In M. A. Forciea, R. Lavizzo-Mourey, and E. P. Schwab. *Geriatrics Secrets*, 2nd ed. Philadelphia: Hanley and Belfus, 2000, pp. 121–28.

Robinson, K. M. "Rehabilitation Applications in Caring for Patients with Pick's Disease and Frontotemporal Dementias." *Neurology* 56, suppl. 4 (2001): S56–S58.

Robinson, K. M., and M. Grossman. "Rehabilitation of Dementia." In M. E. Selzer, S. Clarke, L. G. Cohen, P. W. Duncan, and F. H. Gage. *Textbook of Neural Repair and Rehabilitation*. New York: Cambridge University Press, 2006, pp. 488–501.

Sandel, E. M., K. M. Robinson, G. Goldberg, and V. Graziani. "Neurorehabilitation." In J. Gruz, ed. *Neurologic and Neurosurgical Emergencies*. Philadelphia: W. B. Saunders, 1998, pp. 503–46.

Zorowitz, R. D., and K. M. Robinson. "Pathophysiology of Dysphagia and Aspiration." *Topics in Stroke Rehabilitation* 6, no. 3 (1999): 1–16.

CHAPTER 7

AS THE SYMPTOMS PROGRESS

Understanding the Stages of the Disease

Carol F. Lippa, MD; and Kate J. Bowen

While caring for someone who is ill, family members and other caregivers often wish to have information regarding the progression of an individual's disease. After the diagnosis, this type of inquiry is the most frequent, and the common concerns typically involve three main areas. First, caregivers want information about the rate of disease progression. Second, they want to know what symptoms to expect as the disease progresses. Third, families and other caregivers are interested in ways to slow the rate of disease progression and manage the symptoms.

RATE OF DISEASE PROGRESSION

After diagnosis, questions regarding the rate of disease progression inevitably arise. Accurate progression-rate estimates are helpful for the patient, family, and physician because treatment decisions are based, in part, on this information. However, there is inherent variability in the rate of progression from one patient to another. In some cases, progression is over the course of months. At the other extreme, cases with a duration of more than twenty-five years have been reported. Generally, people live two to ten years from the time of diagnosis, with a mean of eight years.[1]

A number of variables complicate determining an exact estimate of progression, including psychosocial risk factors, genetics, comorbidities, and identification of disease onset. Each of these variables has differing implications dependent on the frontotemporal degeneration (FTD) subtype.

Controllable psychosocial factors may influence the amount of time that an individual can remain at home and may also influence the survival time. For example, FTD patients with behavioral features commonly partake in risky behaviors due to their lack of inhibition and increased impulsivity, such as overeating, alcoholism, and inappropriate sexual behavior. These unsafe behaviors may decrease life expectancy by increasing the likelihood of developing other health concerns, such as obesity, liver disease, and sexually transmitted diseases, respectively. It is necessary for the caregiver to provide supervision in order to prevent or decrease the frequency of these risky behaviors to increase lifespan.

When genetic factors are present, they can provide prognostic information. Genetics are not only key to FTD diagnosis (and subtype classification in some cases), but they also play a role in the rate of disease progression. It is established that several genetic abnormalities may lead to FTD, including the progranulin, chromosome 9 open reading frame 72 (*C9orf72*), and microtubule-associated protein tau genes. By some reports, *APOE* genotype and vascular endothelial growth factor gene variations are also associated. Of these, abnormalities in the progranulin and tau genes may impact the rate of disease progression.[2] In particular, progranulin mutations are associated with poor prognosis, likely due to biological processes that lead to accelerated brain atrophy. Carrying the H2 allele within the tau gene is also associated with poor prognosis, although the exact mechanism for this is unknown.[3] Ask your physician about genetic testing to determine if these genetic risk tests are appropriate in your situation; often consultations are needed with cognitive specialists or genetic counselors to help make this determination. (For additional information regarding genetics, see chapter 3.)

Certain comorbidities also have the ability to influence the rate of progression of the disease. FTD may occur in association with motor neuron disease, such as amyotrophic lateral sclerosis (ALS). FTD plus motor neuron disease decreases life expectancy compared to those with only FTD, with an overall survival of less than three years.[4] In a study that compared the dominant subtypes of FTD, the researchers found that FTD patients with motor neuron disease had a longer mean survival time than those with language variant FTD plus motor neuron disease. These results indicate that language variant FTD in conjunction with motor neuron disease progresses at a comparatively faster rate.

Another complicating factor in assessing the rate of disease progression is that the disease onset in FTD can often be difficult to date with certainty.

Symptoms are caused by a progressive loss of brain cells and brain-cell processes in the frontal and temporal lobes. Biologically, the disease process starts years before the individual shows any symptoms. Symptoms are typically insidious at onset. Furthermore, many of the symptoms that patients with FTD experience are initially exaggerations of previous behaviors, which are sometimes confused with signs of a midlife crisis. With an unclear onset, the rate of progression is difficult to determine. Identification of the FTD subtype may help pinpoint disease onset. For example, behavioral variant FTD and semantic FTD patients tend to have an earlier age at onset, while progressive nonfluent aphasia FTD patients tend to have a later age at onset.[5]

When trying to determine whether an individual will progress quickly, the presence or absence of other neurological symptoms is helpful. Patients with problems involving chewing and/or swallowing, or with reduced voice volume tend to do poorly. However, before deciding that the prognosis is poor, you will want to assess the reasons for these symptoms. If the patient doesn't eat because he is inattentive or because she lacks the initiative to feed herself, prognosis is more favorable if strategies can be developed to circumvent the problem. Patients with movement problems, such as stiffness, slowness, tremors, and a gait disorder may progress at a more rapid rate than those who show no problems with movement. Alternately, loss of ability to control the mouth, throat, and tongue suggests that the disease has involved deep brain regions that are important for survival.

If there are early problems with movement, it is important to first rule out other medical conditions that have features that mimic FTD. These disorders include progressive supranuclear palsy and corticobasal degeneration. A neurologist can help with these diagnoses, particularly early or in the importation of the disease course. It is important to make this distinction because the symptoms these patients develop may differ from pure FTD. Also, there may be medications available to help treat the motor symptoms of progressive supranuclear palsy and corticobasal degeneration. Once the disease has advanced and the patient becomes mute or immobile, it is more difficult for the physician to determine the diagnosis since many dementia subtypes look similar in the end stages.

As yet, we can only estimate how rapidly a patient with FTD will progress. One general rule is that individuals with dementia often maintain their disease tempo. Those with a slow onset are likely to continue to progress slowly. Those with a more rapid change in behavior or cognition may be more likely to progress quickly. Obtaining annual MRI scans and neuropsychological testing may help objectify how rapidly the disease is progressing and the current state of the disease. Neuropsychological testing involves administering scales to monitor a patient's cognition. The Folstein Minimental State Examination (MMSE),[6] is probably the most commonly administered cognitive scale; however, it is not particularly sensitive in FTD because it does not accurately assess key FTD symptoms. The changes that are common in FTD (i.e., personality, energy, and behavior) are not evaluated, and cognitive losses due to aphasic symptoms may overestimate a patient's severity.

There is an inherent bias in the time the diagnosis is officially made and the rate of progression. This time frame will influence where you fall on the continuum of progression. If symptoms have been present for many years before a diagnosis is made, the disease will have progressed further and there will be less time left. If symptoms are new and subtle, the person with FTD is likely to have a longer life expectancy.

WHAT SYMPTOMS TO EXPECT OVER TIME

The second question about progression is what symptoms to expect as the disease progresses. Patients with FTD are more complicated than those with other dementing diseases due to the wide variety of symptoms they experience, their tendency to go through different phases during the disease process, and the number of FTD variants. FTD patients typically experience changes in cognition, behavior, language, and the ability to complete activities of daily living.

When compared with Alzheimer's disease (AD), those with FTD have different initial symptoms and may also develop symptoms at an earlier age. FTD subjects are more likely to experience language problems or personality changes as initial symptoms, while AD patients usually present to the physician with memory problems, specifically in short-term memory and orientation.[7] Patients with FTD often do worse on cognitive tests (except for visuospatial tests) and scales of activities of daily functioning than AD patients at the time they are initially assessed by a physician. They show a more rapid progression of language problems and a more rapid decline on global measures of dementia than do AD patients. FTD patients also exhibit a greater difficulty in executive functions (i.e., planning, organizing, problem solving) when completing cognitive tests.

Generally, there are certain symptoms that can be anticipated as FTD progresses. Classifying FTD into two subgroups, language or behavioral, can aid in predicting which symptoms will occur, especially during the initial stages of the disease. Patients with the language variant of FTD will experience difficulty with language-based tasks. When the left side of the brain is involved, the affected individual has trouble with speech fluency, word finding, sentence length, writing, object identification, and understanding language. Those affected with the behavioral FTD variant will experience changes in personality and mood. Apathy, lack of motivation, compulsive and inappropriate behavior, dietary changes (especially carbohydrate cravings), and poor judgment are common symptoms.

Overlap of symptoms between the subtypes is likely to occur as the disease progresses; over time, symptoms will emerge that were not initially present. Most FTD patients develop language problems, especially speech-expression problems, at some point during their clinical course. If language difficulties are not yet a presenting symptom, they should be expected. Many individuals with FTD become mute as the disease advances.

Energy and initiative are common problems in FTD and may be anticipated at some point in the disease. Apathy, inertia, and an overall flat mood can be major problems in FTD patients as the disease progresses. Restlessness is not uncommon, especially in the earlier disease stages. Restlessness combined with impulsiveness is occasionally exhibited through "roaming" behavior, such as pacing from room to room or visiting the same location repeatedly. Roaming behavior is not the same as wandering, which is typically seen in AD patients, because the roamer is fully oriented to his or her location. FTD patients, regardless of the subtype, also tend to experience a decline in function as it relates to completion of activities of daily living.[8]

INFLUENCING DISEASE PROGRESSION

There is not a cure for FTD, nor is there a definitive way to slow the rate of disease progression. Few clinical drug trials have occurred due to the perceived rarity of the disease, the small subject pool at each site, and the variation in symptoms and progression among those affected. Medications developed for AD, such as cholinesterase inhibitors, including donepezil, rivastigmine, and galantamine, are sometimes used empirically to help stabilize cognitive symptoms. These agents may provide a degree of symptomatic benefit, but they have not been shown to slow the rate of progression. Their use should be discussed with the individual's physician; there are differing opinions about the effectiveness and safety of these agents, and it is not clear that cholinergic losses occur in FTD. If prescribed, these medications should be monitored carefully since FTD patients may experience side effects. (See chapter 5 for more information.)

Medications are available to target the behavioral problems of energy extremes, aggression, agitation, extreme/unjust emotions, and depressive symptoms. These medications are not specifically approved for use in FTD, but rather are prescribed for those suffering from psychiatric conditions. Selective serotonin reuptake inhibitors (SSRIs) are the most widely studied group of medications in FTD. These agents may decrease disinhibition, repetition, and inappropriate behavior in FTD patients.[9] They may enable affected individuals to remain in a less restrictive environment for extended periods of time. Behavioral interventions are also effective for many of the behavioral symptoms these individuals experience. No medication provides a major benefit to language problems in this population.

Although there are not any studies proving the effect of physical and mental activity on the symptoms of FTD, there are studies in AD subjects (and dementia in general) indicating that those who remain physically and mentally active fare better over time. As such, it's reasonable to encourage regular physical, social, and intellectual activity. The specific physical/mental activities do not matter as much as the regularity of practice. However, to prevent frustrating the individual, care should be taken to avoid complex and advanced mental or physical challenges. It is best to select and encourage increased involvement in activities that the individual enjoys and in which he or she can still actively participate.

In most cases, FTD does not directly cause death. The brain areas most severely affected by FTD are those involved with cognition, language, and personality, rather than those that regulate the heart and breathing muscles. FTD patients are likely to die as a result of their deteriorating health. For example, as the disease advances, individuals become less mobile, which can result in falls. Once dementia patients stop walking, they are susceptible to developing infections, particularly pneumonia and urinary-tract infections, and their body is less able to clear these infections. Overall, infection is the most common cause of death among those with FTD. FTD patients are also less likely to express pain and medical concerns. The language variant patients may feel ill but are unable to correctly communicate the discomfort, while patients with behavioral variants may be indifferent and not acknowledge the problem. Elderly individuals with FTD may also die from age-associated diseases, such as cancer and heart attacks.

SUMMARY

Overall, there is marked variability in symptom progression in FTD. Estimation of the rate of progression is dependent on a number of factors, including psychosocial risk factors, genetic makeup, comorbidities, and the clarity of the exact time of disease onset. If disease duration can be estimated, the rate of progression typically remains stable during the early years. Patients often first present with either language, behavior, or cognitive complaints, and the initial symptom may progress over several years before other FTD symptoms arise. FTD patients may develop a variety of language and behavioral symptoms, or they may experience phases in which different symptoms predominate. Problems with high-order thinking (organization, problem solving, and maintaining goal-directed behavior) can be severe. Those with difficulty moving or swallowing often have a more rapid clinical course. Medications and behavioral strategies may be used to influence an individual's symptoms and maintain his or her ability to remain in an optimal environment.

NOTES

1. The Association for Frontotemporal Dementia, "FTD Fast Facts," http://www.theaftd.org/frontotemporal-degeneration/ftd-fast-facts.

2. B. Borroni et al., "Genetic Background Predicts Poor Prognosis in Frontotemporal Lobar Degeneration," *Neurodegenerative Diseases* 8 (2011): 289–95.

3. Ibid.; B. Borroni et al., "Establishing Short-Term Prognosis in Frontotemporal Lobar Degeneration Spectrum: Role of Genetic Background and Clinical Phenotype," *Neurobiology of Aging* 31 (2010): 270–79.

4. J. K. Johnson et al., "Frontotemporal Lobar Degeneration: Demographic Characteristics of 353 Patients," *Archives of Neurology* 62 (2005): 925–30; E. A. Coon et al., "Predicting Survival in Frontotemporal Dementia with Motor Neuron Disease," *Neurology* 76 (2011): 1886–93; E. D. Robertson et al., "Frontotemporal Dementia Progresses to Death Faster Than Alzheimer Disease," *Neurology* 65 (2005): 719–25.

5. Johnson et al., "Frontotemporal Lobar Degeneration."

6. M. F. Folstein, S. E. Folstein, and P. R. McHugh, "Mini-Mental State—A Practical Method for Grading the Cognitive State of Patients for the Clinician," *Journal of Psychiatric Research* 12 (1975): 189–98.

7. G. Binetti et al., "Differences between Pick Disease and Alzheimer Disease in Clinical Appearance and Rate of Cognitive Decline," *Archives of Neurology* 57 (2000): 225–32.

8. E. Mioshi and J. R. Hodges, "Rate of Change of Functional Abilities in Frontotemporal Dementia," *Dementia and Geriatric Cognitive Disorders* 28 (2009): 419–26.

9. M. Manoochehri and E. D. Huey, "Diagnosis and Management of Behavioral Issues in Frontotemporal Dementia," *Current Neurology and Neuroscience Reports* 12, no. 5 (2012): 528–36.

CHAPTER 8

AN IMMORTAL LEGACY

How Donation of Human Tissues Impacts Research and Drives Advances in Diagnosis and Therapy

David J. Irwin, MD; Elisabeth McCarty Wood, MS;
Virginia M.-Y. Lee, PhD;
and John Q. Trojanowski, MD, PhD

THE IMPORTANCE OF AN AUTOPSY

For patients and families with frontotemporal degeneration (FTD) and other rare neurodegenerative diseases as well as more common brain disorders such as Alzheimer's disease (AD), autopsy has been the "ultimate medical consultation" as clinical diagnosis has been challenged by the lack of confirmatory testing. Since FTDs are a heterogeneous group of complex disorders, but, as a group, are the second most common cause of dementia after AD in individuals under age sixty-five, autopsy has provided families with the additional information about their loved one's disease that they were not able to ascertain during life. This chapter will provide information on the following:

- background information on autopsy
- autopsy process
- research on human tissue and bodily fluids
- impact of autopsy research on FTD in addition to AD and related nervous-system disorders
- disease classification of FTD based on autopsy

A rigorously conducted autopsy or postmortem investigation will establish a proximal (actual) cause of death and identify other disorders that contributed to the failure and compromised health status of an individual afflicted by disease. Also, it serves important roles in the oversight or monitoring of the quality and adequacy of the medical care a patient has received during life by confirming, clarifying, and correcting clinical diagnoses. Therefore, autopsies often provide unique and critical information on the relative effectiveness of novel versus established medications, operative procedures, and other disease interventions. Autopsy studies further serve to document disease rates and provide data for local and national population registries concerning changing trends in mortality, infection, and other healthcare concerns. Epidemiological autopsy data also are essential for accurate estimates of the true occurrence rates of existing and well-known—as well as underdiagnosed and newly emerging—diseases. Autopsy data can also provide important information leading to the identification of new or unsuspected diseases. Examples of disorders that are better understood now compared to a few decades ago, as a result of autopsy studies, include Legionnaires' disease, AD, and sudden infant death, toxic shock, and acquired immunodeficiency syndromes. Indeed, a growing body of data from an increasing number of postmortem studies of FTDs, the focus of this chapter, is providing a much clearer picture of these relentlessly progressive and ultimately fatal neurodegenerative disorders. This surge in data on FTDs suggests that they may be more common than has been previously reported.

Other socially beneficial purposes served by autopsies include (1) biomedical research to discover causes and better treatments for disease, (2) detecting the health-related consequences of a wide variety of occupational exposures, and (3) delivery of lifesaving treatments for living individuals by playing a key role in the acquisition, preservation, and donation of human skin, bone, cornea, and other organs for transplantation therapy. In medicolegal cases, autopsy establishes the means and manner of death. For instance, autopsies have helped link fatal poisoning to product tampering in several over-the-counter drug preparations. Autopsy once played a major role in medical-school education, but because of declining autopsy rates in hospitals, use of this important teaching medium for medical students is dwindling throughout the United States.

A BRIEF HISTORY OF AUTOPSY

The Greek word *autopsia* means "to see with one's own eyes." Ancient Greeks focused their attention on an imbalance of fluids and vapors or humors, rather than organs and anatomic structures, as causes of disease. Egyptian embalmers of the Early, Middle, and Late Kingdoms had knowledge of human anatomy. They routinely removed organs in their work to mummify or preserve the bodies of deceased pharaohs and other members of the ruling elite for the after-life. But these highly skilled anatomists did not convey many of their observations in writing to the scientific community. Prompted by new autopsy-derived data, Erasistratus abandoned the popular humoral theory of disease developed earlier by Hippocrates, and Erasistratus is generally credited for making the association of organ change and disease by carrying out dissections of the human body as long ago as 300 BCE.

In the European Middle Ages, the church did not generally accept post-mortem dissections, although popes did direct autopsies to be performed to search for a cause of the plague, which decimated large populations at that time. It was not until the Renaissance in the fifteenth century that the autopsy became an established investigative method and began to play a significant role in advancing medical science. Subsequently, by the eighteenth century, scientists and clinicians were carrying out comprehensive studies to corre-late clinical and autopsy data at leading medical centers throughout Europe. By the mid-nineteenth century, the social and medical benefits of the autopsy were widely appreciated. Following informed consent of authorized family members, individuals dying in academic health centers as recently as the mid-twentieth century in the United States had approximately a 50 percent chance of being autopsied to determine the cause of death.

Today in the United States, the autopsy rate in most academic health centers hovers around 10 percent, and is still falling. Autopsies are rarely per-formed in for-profit hospitals, and this has occurred for several reasons. First, in 1971, after the Joint Commission for the Accreditation of Health Organiza-tions dropped the recommended 20 percent autopsy rate for hospitals, there was a diminished emphasis on autopsy as part of the medical-school curric-ulum at many universities. Also, the growing success and emphasis on tech-nical advances (e.g., medical imaging) and many advances in experimental research led to a decreasing reliance on postmortem examination as a means of gaining new knowledge. This was despite the fact that the clinical or ante-mortem diagnostic error rates determined through autopsy examinations has remained constant at around 12 percent for the past several decades.

Since autopsies are not revenue-producing activities but cost approximately $3,000 to $5,000 per case, they have been subject to cutbacks in an era of health-care-cost containment. If the death of a patient occurs outside a facility where he or she had been monitored by clinicians, there are charges for the transportation of the body to the clinicians' facility for postmortem examination. This charge (which can range from a few to several hundred dollars) may be an overwhelming financial burden for families that influences their decision to decline an autopsy on their loved one. In addition, physician attitudes have changed such that they may be less inclined to request an autopsy out of a fear of increased risk of medical liability. Despite the lack of concrete evidence for this, these factors have led to inadequate numbers of pathologists (physicians specializing in laboratory medicine) to perform autopsies. Finally, recent trends in scientific research have focused less on innovative findings from postmortem studies. This also has contributed to a declining interest of the biomedical-research community in autopsy studies and data derived from them.

Religious beliefs and philosophical views of different ethnic groups have profoundly influenced the extent to which diverse cultures in the United States as well as in regions throughout the world value the social and medical benefits of autopsy studies, as well. However, many religions (e.g., Christianity, Hinduism, Buddhism, Taoism, Confucianism, Shintoism) have no specific religious tenets that prohibit the postmortem examination of deceased members of their faith. Jewish religious authorities have permitted autopsies since the eighteenth century, although Orthodox Judaism forbids its followers from consenting to an autopsy. This also is the view of Muslims.

THE AUTOPSY PROCESS

Currently, in the United States, a family member of the deceased must give written or verbal permission for an autopsy of his or her loved one, except in certain medicolegal cases that fall under the jurisdiction of the municipal medical examiner's office. The spouse of the deceased individual usually has the overriding right to give consent for an autopsy, but state laws vary regarding which family member can exercise this right if there is no surviving spouse. Consent for complete postmortem examination is obtained in approximately 75 percent of autopsies. Family members may limit their consent for autopsy to specified organs or body parts (such as the trunk or brain only). These "problem-targeted" (diagnosis-oriented) autopsies can answer specific questions regarding one or more of the patient's clinical diagnoses. In contrast to a complete autopsy, in which all major organs are removed and examined, a limited autopsy may include inspection of the organs without removal of any of them. It also may permit the microscopic examination of small biopsy samples from selected organs. Many spouses or family members of an individual with FTD, AD, Parkinson's disease (PD), amyotrophic lateral sclerosis (ALS), or related neurodegenerative disorders who have consented for autopsy have specified "brain-only" or "brain and spinal cord–only."

While the foregoing applies to most autopsies, the ground rules are different for forensic autopsies that are conducted for medicolegal reasons. Briefly, forensic medicine refers to the scientific application of medical knowledge to resolve legal problems. Medicolegal deaths refer to deaths that must be investigated in accordance with state and federal laws, such as unexpected or violent deaths, suspicious deaths, and so on. In a forensic autopsy, which refers to postmortem studies focused on determining the cause of death for legal reasons, several distinctions need to be made to fully explain the death. For example, the cause of death in a forensic autopsy report refers to the disease or injury that is responsible for the death. The proximate cause of death is the event or disease that started the sequence of events ending in the death of the individual, and the immediate cause of death includes complications and terminal events that result from the proximate cause of death.

Although similar issues are addressed in academic or nonforensic autopsies, the emphasis in autopsies conducted for research studies is on determining not only the key diagnoses but also the disease mechanisms that led to the death of the patient—including the underlying physiological or pathological process. However, since there are many poorly understood diseases that remain to be investigated, as exemplified by FTDs, it may not be possible to specify this in all cases. Thus, in the case of an individual afflicted with a neurodegenerative disease such as FTD that is associated with progressive cognitive impairments, the patient may be determined to have FTD as a proximate cause of death, pneumonia as the immediate cause, and infection as the mechanism of the individual's death. When autopsy is limited to a specific organ such as the brain, information is learned only about the direct pathology observed in the particular organ. In the case of FTDs, a brain and spinal cord–only autopsy is sufficient for providing diagnostic information and also allows researchers access to important tissue for further studies of the causes and mechanisms of the underlying condition.

A complete postmortem examination begins with careful evaluation of the exterior of the body and includes notations of wounds, scars, and any other skin abnormalities. Dissection begins with a small abdominal incision to enable inspection of the chest and abdominal organs, which the pathologist removes and further dissects to examine organ parenchyma, ducts, blood vessels, and lumens. In most autopsies, the pathologist dissects all organs and samples small portions of each organ for microscopic analysis of evident abnormalities. The pathologist examines the brain in a similar manner, following removal through an incision made at the back of the head, but the face and limbs are never dissected in an academic or nonforensic autopsy. Hence, even a sophisticated pathologist cannot surmise whether an autopsy has or has not been performed on someone viewed at a traditional open-casket funeral service.

After overall examination, the pathologist studies each organ and records its weight and measurements as well as other salient normal or abnormal features. Following fixation to preserve the tissue samples for subsequent investigations, the pathologist uses a microscope to study samples selected for histological analysis. Additionally, as the case dictates, the most critical diagnostic information may come from biochemical or microbiological analysis of small tissue samples or fluids. In selected cases, toxicology studies may be performed to rule out drug- or toxin-induced medical disorders. At academic institutions, once the diagnostic studies are complete, the remaining tissue can be carefully stored for research studies. This has been incredibly important for the advancement in knowledge in rare or new diseases, such as FTDs. It is such research that allows scientists to further understand what has occurred biologically to cause the disease and work toward improve treatments.

Finally, all of the pertinent data from the autopsy studies are summarized into a coherent technical report of the patient's illness. This is correlated with the autopsy findings to reconcile both data sets into a lucid account of how all of the pathological findings contributed to the clinical manifestations of the patient and led to his or her demise. An autopsy and the formal report have several benefits to the family, including:

- clarification of the relevant diagnoses
- reassurance from knowing the cause of death and relief of any guilt when a patient dies unexpectedly or from poorly understood diseases
- knowledge that the appropriate care has been provided for the patient during his or her illness
- identification of genetic conditions that might have contributed to disease onset or progression
- knowledge about any contagious diseases the patient might have had so that appropriate measures can be taken to protect the family members
- advancement of medical research to develop better or new therapies for diseases

Common concerns about giving consent for an autopsy are:

- body disfigurement, mutilation, and delaying of funeral
- lack of information about the reasons for autopsy and the benefits it provides to families and society
- objection from other family members, based on religious background, family dynamics, or lack of understanding
- cost and logistics

These issues should be discussed with your healthcare providers and researchers, family members, and support resources (e.g., clergy) to help make a decision that is good for you and your family. One common misconception is that the clinical diagnoses of a deceased loved one are correct, therefore an autopsy is not necessary. But it is known through autopsies conducted at academic health centers over many decades that clinical diagnoses are incorrect approximately 12 percent of the time, and for FTDs and all other neurodegenerative dementias or movement disorders, the only certain diagnosis is through an autopsy.

Oftentimes, another concern is that family members may feel the deceased or family has suffered enough and that an autopsy will only serve to prolong the suffering. However, information gleaned from an autopsy often promotes closure among family members. Furthermore, families should be reassured that a pathologist is a highly skilled member of the healthcare team who will perform the autopsy with respect and concern for the dignity of the deceased. Organs will be removed for study through the incisions mentioned above and will be hidden by clothing, thus allowing for an open-casket funeral service. Additionally, concerns about interference with funeral arrangements are unwarranted, since the removal and inspection of organs at autopsy takes only one to two hours and arrangements can be made to facilitate timely examination.

The complete analysis of samples removed at autopsy may require the expertise of several pathologists with special knowledge of diseases involving the heart, brain, kidneys, and other relevant organ systems. It may take several weeks for all of the relevant studies to be completed and for the final autopsy report to be compiled, but the family can request a copy of this technical document. Although an autopsy report may be challenging for the nonspecialist to understand, the family can seek consultation with the patient's doctor and/or the pathologists involved in the postmortem studies.

RESEARCH ON HUMAN TISSUES AND BODILY FLUIDS

While the previous considerations about autopsy do not apply in exactly the same manner to biological samples (e.g., blood, tissue biopsies, bodily fluids) from living patients, many considerations do. Some of these considerations are:

- the need for informed consent from the individual or family member for obtaining and conducting studies on the samples
- the critical importance of such samples for determining an accurate diagnosis of the patient's condition
- the benefit to furthering biomedical research and learning more about the underlying causes of disease and developing therapies

The myths or misunderstandings about what is involved when patients and family members provide biological samples to medical researchers need to be addressed. With increased understanding of the issues, patients and families have provided biological samples from living and deceased individuals, contributing substantially to basic and clinical studies of FTDs and related disorders. This is driving biomedical progress in neurodegenerative dementias with breathtaking speed.

IMPACT OF BIOMEDICAL AND AUTOPSY RESEARCH ON FTD

Translating biological research studies into clinical care that impacts the quality of medical care and treatment received by an individual is the ultimate goal and challenge. Knowledge that has been gained through autopsy-based research has advanced biomedical research in neuropathology (the study of brain, spinal cord, and nerve cells) and our understanding of FTDs. This has most dramatically been proven in the ability to identify unique clinical and diagnostic features, syndromes, and subtypes among FTDs, as reviewed in chapter 2.

Brain-tissue studies of neurodegenerative conditions have led to the realization that most of these conditions have unique or hallmark brain findings, such as abnormal accumulations of specific proteins in defined regions and/or loss or shrinkage of brain tissue in defined regions of the brain. Table 8.1 provides a listing of neurodegenerative conditions and the specific proteins found to be abnormal in the brain. For example, in PD it was shown that the protein alphasynuclein is the building block of the Lewy bodies in neurons (nerve cells or brain cells).

Common neurodegenerative diseases like AD, which have been the focus of intense research for many years, have paved the way for the more recent work on FTDs. Enormous progress has been made to improve the reliability and accuracy of methods and procedures for the antemortem and postmortem diagnosis of AD and other dementias. This has led to the recognition that AD is a disorder caused by multiple genetic and environmental influences and with a set of distinct clinical and postmortem features that distinguish AD from other dementias.

Insights into the composition of the neurofibrillary tangles of AD have directly advanced our knowledge of FTDs. These tangles contain abnormal forms of a protein called tau. Normal tau has an important function in the brain cell: it is the crosspiece between microtubules. One can think of microtubules as train tracks and tau as the railroad ties used to hold the tracks together properly. The microtubules and tau are important for sending information through the cell. Nerve cells can be very long; therefore, a secure transmitting structure is important. When tau is abnormal, it forms paired and twisted filamentous structures that take on a helical shape, thus the term "paired helical filaments" is used, as it describes the appearance of the abnormal tau proteins under the microscope. Abnormal tau is like having a broken rail tie that causes the track to be insecure. Just as a train cannot travel down an insecure track, information in the cell cannot travel down a microtubule that is twisted or comes apart. When information cannot travel through a cell, that cell is more likely to die than the surrounding unaffected cells. Abnormal tau in the brain has been documented in many neurodegenerative conditions, including FTDs. As a group, these conditions are commonly referred to as "tauopathies." Table 8.2 contains a list of some of the conditions characterized by abnormal tau in the brain. Mutations in the gene that encodes tau (*MAPT* gene) have been shown to cause rare hereditary forms of FTD. This is discussed in chapter 3 in more detail.

Based on these studies of tau and additional autopsy studies of patients thought to have FTD during life, it is now appreciated that several proteins and pathological profiles define the spectrum and neuropathological classification of FTDs (see figure 8.1). The family of neuropathological entities diagnosed at autopsy are collectively referred to as frontotemporal lobar degeneration (FTLD); the term *frontotemporal degeneration* (FTD) and its variants are now reserved for the clinical diagnosis obtained during life. This distinction is important, due to the significant heterogeneity of FTLD diagnoses at autopsy associated with FTD clinical syndromes. A major direction of current research in FTD is to develop biomarkers, or clinical tests, that help determine what type of FTLD a patient has during life. Autopsy studies are crucial in this effort.

FTLDs are characterized by brain degeneration, primarily in the frontal and temporal lobes. Some types of FTLDs have accumulations of tau-containing neurofibrillary tangles. As in AD, these tangles are caused by the abnormal tau protein that aggregates in the neurons. Research has further defined the abnormal forms of tau (based on length and additional chemical tags, or phosphorylation). The presence of specific forms of tau in different variants of FTLDs has recently been documented and used for diagnostic purposes. These forms of FTLD are delineated on the left-hand side of the chart in figure 8.1. Other types of FTLDs do not have tau accumulations in the neurons but rather other characteristic features and proteins.

The other main type of FTLD is characterized by inclusions of the DNA/RNA-binding protein, TDP-43 (i.e. FTLD-TDP). This discovery in 2006 provided evidence for the clinical link between FTLD and ALS, as inclusions of TDP-43 are found in both disorders.

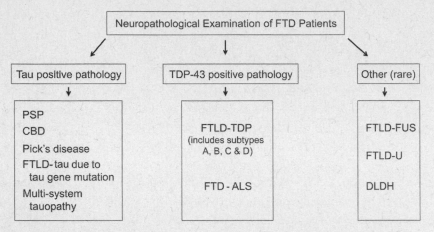

Figure 8. 1. This figure shows how the presence of specific proteins known to cause FTD are evaluated to help provide a neuropathological diagnosis of FTD. Abbreviations for the neuropathological diagnoses are provided. PSP = Progressive supranuclear palsy; CBD = Corticobasal degeneration; FTLD-tau = frontotemporal lobar degeneration with tau due to tau gene mutations (previously known at FTDP-17); FTLD-TDP = frontotemporal lobar degeneration with TDP-43 pathology; FTD-ALS = frontotemporal degeneration with amyotrophic lateral sclerosis; FTLD-FUS = frontotemporal lobar degeneration with FUS pathology; FTLD-U = frontotemporal lobar degeneration with ubiquitin positive inclusions; and DLDH = dementia lacking distinctive histopathology.

FTLD-TDP pathology is found in a significant proportion of all FTLD cases at autopsy. Studies that correlate clinical characteristics with the autopsy result have found FTLD-TDP to be the cause of the majority of semantic variant of primary progressive aphasia cases and those cases with comorbid ALS. Conversely, the nonfluent-agrammatic form of primary progressive aphasia most often corresponds to FTLD-tau. Finally, the behavioral variant of FTD is found to have roughly equal proportions of FTLD-tau and FTLD-TDP; thus, the relationships of clinical syndrome to underlying neuropathological diagnosis in FTLD is not absolute and current research efforts are aimed at correctly diagnosing FTLD-tau and FTLD-TDP during life. This is important because future clinical trials would benefit from being able to accurately predict the type of protein causing the disease. FTLD-TDP can be subdivided based on the appearance and location of the inclusions (i.e., subtypes A–D). Of note, these subtypes correspond reasonably well to specific genetic etiologies of FTLD-TDP but are not predictive of a particular FTD clinical syndrome.

Very recently, the link between ALS and FTD was further defined with the discovery of a hexanucleotide expansion in the non-coding region of the gene *C9orf72* on chromosome 9 as a pathogenic mutation resulting in ALS and/or FTLD-TDP. This mutation is an expansion of a repeated sequence of genetic material in the *C9orf72* gene (see chapter 3). The function of this protein is currently unknown, as is its link to TDP-43. This is the most common genetic form of both ALS and FTD. Furthermore, this expansion is found in a small subset of apparent sporadic cases, or patients without a known family history of ALS or FTD. Future studies are aimed at understanding the variable cognitive and motor deficits in patients with *C9orf72* expansion and how this relates to TDP-43 accumulation and resultant neurodegeneration.

Prior to the discovery of TDP-43 as a key pathologic inclusion in FTLD, FTLD-TDP was previously called dementia lacking distinct histopathological features (DLDH) and frontotemporal lobar degeneration with ubiquitin positive inclusions (FTLD-U). These terms are now reserved for a small minority of cases with no clear signs of neurodegeneration (DLDH) or those who have inclusions containing ubiquitin that are negative for tau and TDP-43 (FTLD-U), and most likely are composed of a currently unknown protein. FTLD-U can be caused by rare mutations in the *CHMP2B* gene on chromosome 2. Finally aggregations of a similar RNA-binding protein to TDP-43, fused in sarcoma (FUS), are found in a small subset of FTLD (i.e., FTLD-FUS) and ALS.

The importance of identifying these neuropathological diagnoses during life is highlighted by breakthrough experiments that recently have shown that synthetic tau fibrils (tau filaments that make up tangles) alone can transmit disease between neurons in mouse and cultured cell models of FTLD-tau. Further, pathological tau obtained from human tissue can be transmitted to transgenic mice, or animals that genetically are altered to express high levels of pathological tau in the nervous system, to cause a spread of pathology and neurodegeneration in this these animals. Interestingly, the pathology seen in these animals occurs much earlier and has a different form and structure, as it resembles human disease, from the tau accumulations that eventually develop in these genetically altered mice. Animal studies of transmission of TDP-43 are yet to be developed, but autopsy examination of ALS and FTLD-TDP cases finds TDP-43 deposits in the brain that mirror these animal transmission studies. That is, examination of many patients with TDP-43 disease at autopsy suggests that these inclusions may spread from neuron to neuron through the brain as disease progresses. A similar approach examining autopsy tissue in

AD and PD has resulted in a system that allows for staging of the pathology based on the location and severity of tau and alpha-synuclein deposits. These findings are similar to properties of prion disease, or human spongiform encephalopathy, where the pathogenic prion protein is misfolded and spreads throughout the nervous system to cause neurodegeneration. A major distinction is that prions are infectious particles that can spread disease between individuals if they are exposed to the pathogenic protein from an affected individual. There is no definitive data to suggest FTD, AD , PD, or other neurodegenerative diseases can be spread between individuals through casual contact or extreme circumstances such as exposure to brain tissue. Thus, it is highly unlikely that these disorders are infectious or have the potential to be infectious in humans, in sharp contrast to prion diseases. The properties of transmission from neuron to neuron of these protein aggregates within an individual is a major discovery in neurodegenerative-disease research and provides a potential therapeutic target to treat disease; therapeutics that can stop or slow the aggregation and spread of tau and/or TDP-43 could potentially make a meaningful impact in FTD and help preserve patient independence.

Recent developments in the genetics of FTLD include genome-wide association studies (i.e., GWAS) of patients with autopsy confirmed FTLD-TDP and FTLD-tau (progressive supranuclear palsy). These studies compare the rates of single-nucleotide polymorphisms (i.e., SNPs), between patients and controls to discover which SNPs associate with disease at a rate greater than would be expected by chance. Although the human genome is 99.9 percent similar between individuals, there is variation (i.e., SNPs and other polymorphisms) that may influence disease. SNPs are variations in a single unit of DNA, some of which may influence how a gene or protein is processed or how it functions. SNPs that significantly associate with FTLD-TDP or FTLD-tau are promising candidates for therapeutic targets and diagnostic or prognostic markers of disease. Further, research targeting these SNPs and/or the gene(s) in which they are contained could provide insights into the underlying biology of the disease. Further studies of GWAS-identified SNPs and future GWAS studies with other types of FTLD hold promise to identify useful markers to improve diagnostics and advance the goal of developing disease-modifying treatments that target tau and/or TDP-43.

Finally, since the neuropathological diagnoses and traditional clinical diagnoses do not always agree, this is a cause of confusion for many healthcare providers and patient families. For example, as illustrated in figure 8.1, the term

Pick's disease is now used only to define/diagnose individuals with a specific type of tau-positive inclusions. This is because not all patients with clinical "Pick's disease" (now referred to as bvFTD) have underlying tau inclusions at autopsy. Therefore, when individuals with a clinical diagnosis of Pick's disease pass away and undergo autopsy study and a diagnosis is later communicated back to the family, this diagnosis might be FTLD-TDP or another FTLD-tau disease based on the specific findings in the brain. Conversely, not all patients with findings of Pick's disease at autopsy had the classic clinical presentation of progressive cognitive and behavioral symptoms, now referred to as bvFTD. While this can be frustrating and confusing to families, the next of kin of a deceased patient are encouraged to meet with the neurologist as well as the neuropathologist or other healthcare professionals on the research team to discuss the results and to help them understand the significance of the final neuropathological diagnosis. At most academic medical centers where such autopsy investigations are performed, the neuropathologists, neurologists, and other research staff are willing to talk to families. This disagreement about terminology will continue until we have better diagnostic tests to use in the clinic, regardless of how many pathologists, researchers, and clinicians are working together to try to improve and agree on terminology. Indeed, as more is learned about the relationships between FTLD neuropathology and clinical FTD, physicians will be better equipped to diagnose patients and have markers that can track disease. Investigations of cerebrospinal fluid (CSF) or blood highlight many potential markers that could be useful, not only to differentiate FTD from AD, but also FTLD-tau from FTLD-TDP in living patients. Other modalities, such a imaging of the brain using traditional magnetic resonance imaging (MRI) or nuclear scans that can detect tau inclusions are currently under intense research. A combination of these different tests may improve accuracy of one test alone and help physicians more accurately diagnose FTD.

CONCLUSION

The FTLD research field is experiencing a sense of optimism as key breakthroughs in understanding these complex nervous-system disorders have been recently announced. Many of these breakthroughs have been realized based on pathological and research studies that have been possible due to an increased number of autopsy requests and brain and spinal-cord donations from deceased patients, along with continued access to human biological samples from living FTD patient families.

Indeed, academic centers that pursue studies of FTLDs and other neuro-degenerative disorders are obligated to adhere to strict protocols to retain their funding from granting agencies. Thus, for these reasons, it is recommended that families seek out institutions that have followed the protocols when they are contemplating plans for brain donation.

In summary, donation of biological samples through autopsy of deceased patients, or by other means from living subjects, satisfies altruistic needs and the personal interests of individuals. These magnanimous acts of patients and their families leave an immortal legacy to future generations of human beings, since knowledge obtained from research on these samples will have lasting benefits far into the future.

TABLE 8.1. Neurodegenerative Diseases Characterized by Lesions in the Brain That Are Formed by Abnormal Aggregate Proteins

DISEASE	LESIONS	PROTEIN
Alzheimer's disease	Senile plaques Neuro-fibrillary tangles Lewy bodies	Beta-amyloid Tau Alpha-synuclein
Amyotrophic lateral sclerosis	Motor neuron inclusions	TDP-43
Lewy body dementia with Lewy bodies	Lewy bodies	Alpha-synuclein
Multiple system atrophy	Glial cytoplasmic inclusions	Alpha-synuclein
Parkinson's disease	Lewy bodies	Alpha-synuclein
Prion diseases (Creutzfeldt-Jakob disease)	Plaques	Prions
FTLD-tau	Neurofibrillary inclu-sions in glial neurons	Tau
FTLD-TDP	Neuronal and glial cyto-plasmic inclusions and threads	TDP-43

TABLE 8.2. Neurodegenerative Conditions That Have Tau or TDP-43 Pathology

Diseases with Tau inclusions

Primary Tauopathies:

Progressive supranuclear palsy
Tangle-predominant senile dementia
Pick's disease
Corticobasal degeneration
FTLD-tau due to tau gene mutations (previously known as FTDP-17)
Argyophilic grain dementia

Secondary Tauopathies:

Chronic traumatic encephalopathy
Alzheimer's disease
Down's syndrome
Neurodegeneration with brain iron accumulation type 1 (formally known
    as Hallervorden-Spatz disease)
Multiple system atrophy
Nieman-Pick disease type C
Prion diseases (Creutzfeldt-Jakob disease)
Guam amyotrophic lateral sclerosis/Parkinsonism-dementia complex

Diseases with TDP-43 inclusions

Primary TDP-43 proteinopathies:

Frontotemporal lobar degeneration (FTLD) with TDP-43 inclusions
    (FTLD-TDP)
Amyotrophic lateral sclerosis (ALS)

Secondary TDP-43 proteinopathies:

Hippocampal sclerosis of aging
Alzheimer's disease
Schizophrenia
Alexander's disease
Pathological aging
Parkinson's disease
Guam amyotrophic lateral sclerosis/Parkinsonism-dementia complex

Note: This is not a complete listing. The notation of a disease as "primary" means that the disease has either tau or TDP-43 as the predominant or exclusive disease protein, whereas "secondary" means that tau or TDP-43 is present, but not the predominant protein for that diagnosis.

AUTHORS' NOTE

Virginia M.-Y. Lee is the John H. Ware 3rd Chair of Alzheimer's disease research, and John Q. Trojanowski is the William Maul Measey-Truman G. Schnabel Jr., MD, Professor of Geriatric Medicine and Gerontology at the University of Pennsylvania. Work done in the laboratories of the authors is supported by grants from the National Institute of Aging of the National Institutes of Health (AG10124, AG17586, AG32953 and T32-AG000255) and the Alzheimer's Association. We thank our many collaborators and past as well as current members of the Center for Neurodegenerative Disease Research (CNDR) for contributions to the research from CNDR summarized here. Finally, the support of the families of our patients has made this research possible.

The University of Pennsylvania Alzheimer's Disease Center (ADC) was funded by the NIA in 1991, and it is the first and only NIA–funded ADC in the Delaware Valley (for more information on AD and details on the Penn ADCC, see www.med.upenn.edu/cndr/ and http://pennadc.org/).

BIBLIOGRAPHY

Brettschneider, J., K. Del Tredici, D. J. Irwin, et al. "Sequential Distribution of pTDP-43 Pathology in Behavioral Variant Frontotemporal Dementia (bvFTD)." *Acta Neuropathologica* (2014): in press. doi 10.1007/s00401-013-1238-y.

Brettschneider, J., K. Del Tredici, J. B. Toledo, et al. "Stages of pTDP-43 Pathology in Amyotrophic Lateral Sclerosis." *Annals of Neurology* (2013): 20–38.

Clark, C. M., and J. Q. Trojanowski, eds. *Neurodegenerative Dementias: Clinical Features and Pathological Mechanisms.* New York: McGraw-Hill, 2000.

Forman, M. S., J. Farmer, J. K. Johnson, et al. "Frontotemporal Dementia: Clinicopathological Correlations." *Annals of Neurology* (2006): 952–62.

Grossman, M. "Primary Progressive Aphasia: Clinicopathological Correlations." *Nature Reviews Neurology* (2010): 88–97.

Hu, W. T., J. Q. Trojanowski, and L. M. Shaw. "Biomarkers in Frontotemporal Lobar Degenerations—Progress and Challenges." *Progress in Neurobiology* (2011): 636–48.

Hughes, M. E., J. Peeler, J. B. Hogenesch, and J. Q. Trojanowski. "The Growth and Impact of Alzheimer's Disease Centers as Measured by Social Network Analysis." *JAMA Neurology* (2014): in press. doi:10.1001/jamaneurol.2013.6225.

Mackenzie, I. R. A., M. Neumann, E. H. Bigio, et al. "Nomenclature and Nosology for Neuropathologic Subtypes of Frontotemporal Lobar Degeneration: An Update." *Acta Neuropathologica* (2010): 1–4.

Mackenzie, I. R. A., P. Frick, and M. Neumann. "The Neuropathology Associated with Repeat Expansions in the *C9ORF72* gene." *Acta Neuropathologica* (2014): in press. doi: 10.1007/s00401-013-1232-4.

McKhann, G. M., D. S. Knopman, H. Chertkow, et al. "The Diagnosis of Dementia Due to Alzheimer's Disease: Recommendations from the National Institute on Aging–Alzheimer's Association Workgroups on Diagnostic Guidelines for Alzheimer's Disease." *Alzheimer's & Dementia: The Journal of the Alzheimer's Association* (2011): 263–69.

Montine, T. J., C. H. Phelps, T. G. Beach, et al. "National Institute on Aging-Alzheimer's Association Guidelines for the Neuropathologic Assessment of Alzheimer's Disease: A Practical Approach." *Acta Neuropathologica* (2012): 1–11.

Neumann, M. "Frontotemporal Lobar Degeneration and Amyotrophic Lateral Sclerosis: Molecular Similarities and Differences." *Revue Neurologique* (2013): 793–98.

Neumann, M., D. M. Sampathu, L. K. Kwong, et al., "Ubiquitinated TDP-43 in Frontotemporal Lobar Degeneration and Amyotrophic Lateral Sclerosis." *Science* (2006): 130–33.

Polymenidou, M., and D. W. Cleveland. "Prion-like Spread of Protein Aggregates in Neurodegeneration." *Journal of Experimental Medicine* (2012): 889–93.

Souder, E., and J. Q. Trojanowski. "Autopsy: Cutting away the Myths." *Journal of Neuroscience Nursing* (1992): 134–39.

Svoronsky, D. M., V. M. Lee, and J. Q. Trojanowski. "Neurodegenerative Diseases: New Concepts of Pathogenesis and Their Therapeutic Implications." *Annual Review of Pathology* (2006): 151–70.

Weiner, M. W., D. P. Veitch, P. S. Aisen, et al. "The Alzheimer's Disease Neuroimaging Initiative: A Review of Papers Published since Its Inception." *Alzheimer's & Dementia: The Journal of the Alzheimer's Association*, suppl. 1 (2012): S1–S68.

CHAPTER 9

SEARCHING FOR THE ANSWERS

The Future of Research and Clinical Care

David S. Knopman, MD

Since the first edition of this book was published over ten years ago, the scientific understanding of frontotemporal degenerations (FTDs) has grown enormously. It is now becoming possible to link the symptoms of a particular patient to ever more sophisticated models of FTD biology. The next step, for a future edition of this book, is to be able to prescribe therapies for specific underlying diseases for all of our FTD patients. As you read this chapter, you may want to reference the abbreviations and glossary provided at the end of the chapter.

THE PROGRESS OF GENETIC AND PATHOLOGICAL SUBTYPES OF FTD

In the early part of the twentieth century, Pick's disease was the first FTD to be identified. Yet eighty years later, very little progress had occurred. Pick's disease was thought to be diagnosable only with a brain autopsy. While neurologists had known of other disorders that resembled Pick's disease, there was no common understanding of how Pick's disease was related to any other brain disease. By the 1990s, things began to change. Special microscopic staining procedures were devised that allowed researchers to identify specific proteins in brain tissue obtained at autopsy. These new techniques, called "immunohistochemical stains," were used to detect specific proteinaceous materials on microscopic sections. Discoveries in other areas of neuroscience research had, by then, established that the microtubule-associated protein tau, which we will refer to simply as *tau* was part of the inner skeleton of nerve cells (neurons). Tau protein turned out to be the main constituent of the Pick body, the abnormal structure originally identified microscopically in 1911 that signifies Pick's disease. A stain for a second protein called ubiquitin had also been developed by the 1990s and applied to research in brain diseases. Ubiquitin is frequently found in brain regions damaged by many different diseases. Around the same time, there were advances like the introduction of magnetic resonance imaging and the improved recognition the symptoms that occurred in Pick's disease. Coupled with a push for more brain autopsies, it became clear that some of the cases that clinically were diagnosed as frontotemporal dementia showed abnormal tau staining and some showed only ubiquitin staining under the microscope. Thus, by the mid-1990s, neuroscientists suspected that Pick's disease was just the tip of the iceberg of a larger group of disorders that had a particular predilection for the frontal and temporal lobes of the brain of middle-aged and older adults.

In 1998, studies of families with symptoms of frontal and temporal lobe dysfunction demonstrated several distinct genetic abnormalities ("mutations") in the gene that contained the code for the tau protein (the gene is known as microtubule associated protein tau or *MAPT*). The tau proteins that were produced by the mutated gene affected their structure. The abnormal changes in the tau protein ultimately led to damage to neurons in the frontal and temporal lobes. These genetic studies definitively established that the disorder that came to be known as the frontotemporal lobar degenerations, or frontotemporal degenerations (FTD) for short, was due to abnormalities in the chemistry of the tau protein. To make the story richer but more complicated, two other disorders that had been described as disorders of mobility or Parkinson-like syndromes, progressive supranuclear palsy (PSP) and corticobasal degeneration (CBD) were also due to abnormalities in the chemistry of the tau protein.

Although it is a certainty that mutations in the gene that codes for tau called the *MAPT* gene that alter the tau protein's structure produce FTD, the exact mechanism(s) by which that occurs is still being worked out. Neuroscientists have identified at least half a dozen or more mechanisms where the damaged tau protein begins to damage neurons. Knowing the critical abnormality is not a trivial matter, because finding a successful treatment depends on interrupting the process before damage has occurred. As of 2014, prevention of aggregation (glomming together of many individual proteins) of tau protein is a therapeutic strategy being pursued by several laboratories.

There remained a large number of cases of FTD that occurred in families that was not due to mutations in the *MAPT* gene. In 2006, a second gene involved in FTD was found. The discovery of this second gene, progranulin (and abbreviated *GRN*), answered some questions about the genetic nature of the disease in a large number of families, but its discovery raised many more new questions. The nature of the mutations in *GRN* led to much lower levels of the progranulin protein in persons who carried the mutation. How lower levels of progranulin cause damage to neurons in the frontal and temporal lobes is not understood as of 2014. Intensive work on the many possibilities is beginning to yield some clues. Once again, the goal of research is to identify the earliest mechanism where progranulin deficiency causes disease in order to devise treatments. Alternatively, because FTD in persons carrying mutations in the *GRN* gene appears to be caused by deficiency of the progranulin protein, a novel therapeutic strategy being pursued is aimed at enhancing production of progranulin using the existing cellular machinery.

In 2011, a third major gene causing FTD was discovered. For the second time, the discovery provided great insight into the familial nature of the illness in a large number of families, but the new gene for FTD has functions or roles that have yet to be understood. The gene is called *C9orf72* (chromosome 9 open reading frame number 72). The abnormality in the gene is a repeating of a series of six nucleic acids (called a hexanucleotide repeat expansion) hundreds or thousands of times within the gene. As of 2014, what this genetic abnormality does to the neuronal mechanics is unclear. Some unusual proteinlike structures might be produced, or alternatively, the abnormal DNA could interfere with production of other proteins. Remarkably, the mutation in *C9orf72* is the most common cause of familial amyotrophic lateral sclerosis (ALS, also widely known as Lou Gehrig's disease). Although neuroscientists had been aware of the overlap of ALS and FTD, the linkage of the two to a genetic cause was a major step toward understanding their causes.

Another biochemistry advance showed how the genetic cases of FTD due to mutations in *GRN* and *C9orf72* genes shared a common disease mechanism and also shared a common microscopic abnormality with the many persons with FTD not due to genetic causes. In patients with FTD who did not have tau-protein abnormalities, neuroscientists found that a protein called "transactive response DNA binding protein of 43 kilodalton molecular weight" (TDP-43) occurred in the neurons of FTD cases. About two-thirds of all FTD involves abnormal accumulation of TDP-43 in nerve cells. (The other third is due to tau-protein accumulation.) TDP-43 abnormalities are seen in selective regions of the brains and spinal-cord nerve cells in both ALS and FTD. Its role in FTD and ALS is poorly understood.

We now know that 30–40 percent of FTD is genetic, meaning that the majority of cases of FTD are apparently not genetic. The cause of the disorder in the not-genetic cases (called "sporadic" disease) of FTD is still poorly understood. There are a few more rare genetic causes of FTD, but so far their contribution to the big picture is limited.

LINKING PATHOLOGY OF FTD TO CLINICAL DIAGNOSIS

Let us now consider how FTD biology, pathology, and genetics are being applied to clinical diagnosis. There are two principal syndromes (a syndrome is a collection of symptoms that tend to co-occur) that are almost always caused by FTDs. They were the disorder of personality and the control of interpersonal relationships that is now known as behavior variant FTD (bvFTD) and the disorders of language called primary progressive aphasia (PPA). There are two types of PPA that are invariably due to FTD. One is called semantic variant PPA, and the other is called nonfluent/agrammatic variant PPA. There is a third type of PPA whose clinical features are more variable and whose underlying cause sometimes includes FTD but often is due to Alzheimer's disease.

A solid knowledge of clinical neurology is required for optimal diagnosis of bvFTD or PPA. Many physicians, including neurologists, don't encounter these syndromes often enough to develop familiarity with them. Brain imaging with MRI and positron emission tomography (PET) have proved to be excellent though not infallible in helping to confirm a physician's diagnosis of FTD.

Virtually all cases of semantic variant of PPA are linked to abnormal accumulation of TDP-43 in the temporal lobes. Semantic variant PPA almost never occurs in families. Virtually all of progressive supranuclear palsy (PSP) is due to abnormal accumulation of tau protein in several locations in the cerebral hemispheres and the brainstem. It too is rarely genetic. In contrast, the most common syndromes of FTD, namely bvFTD and nonfluent agrammatic variant PPA, may be caused by any of the genetic or nongenetic varieties of FTD.

Brain MRIs have greatly improved the ability to diagnose FTD because in about two thirds of cases, distinctive abnormal shrinkage of the frontal or temporal lobes is evident. Unfortunately, the pattern of brain shrinkage on an MRI does not usually reveal the type of underlying chemistry. Similarly, FDG PET scans also show a pattern of abnormality (reduced glucose uptake) in the frontal and temporal lobes. Sometimes FDG PET scans can detect abnormalities in those regions when the MRI scan still looks normal. Newer types of PET scans are being developed that can detect the tau protein and are just beginning to be tested as of January 2014. Tau PET imaging, if successful, might have a major impact on diagnosis of FTD.

For the majority of patients with FTD, neither the MRI-scan results nor the clinical symptoms allow determination of the biochemical and neuropathological subtype. That is true now, but in the future, prospects are more favorable.

TAKING PROMISING COMPOUNDS AND MAKING THEM DRUGS

The prospects for finding treatments for FTD may be greater than they are for AD. That may sound patently irrational, given the differences in resources that are devoted to FTD compared to AD. But there is a reason for optimism. Each of the major different causes of FTD—tau-protein abnormalities, progranulin deficiency, abnormal TD-P43 aggregation—seem solvable. Therefore, with the help of animal models of FTD, as well as investigations in patients with the FTDs, the hope is that one or more critical biochemical processes can be discovered, where interruption of the disease process could be stopped or slowed down. Even though the funding for FTD research is small compared to AD, research in FTD may be facilitated by efforts that go on under the rubric of AD research because the two diseases share many common processes. For example, funding and effort that is directed at tau pathology in AD is directly applicable to FTD. Many AD researchers are now focusing on how the brain normally rids itself of damaged proteins. The mechanisms by which the brain gets rid of damaged proteins related to AD are almost certainly similar to those involved in FTD. Thus, there is considerable cross-fertilization of ideas between the AD and FTD research worlds, and that will benefit FTD. And the extent to which FTD research helps AD is a tremendous inducement and opportunity for promoting increased research (and research funding) into FTD.

For all of the optimism about improved diagnosis, it is another matter to make genuine progress in treatment. The path from a very promising drug target to successful therapy is arduous, uncertain, and full of pitfalls. Unfortunately, finding therapies is not simple. There are some major questions that need to be addressed before a substance that is claimed to work in animal models of FTD can be certified as a therapy for the human disease. And let's be very clear, the hurdles that stand in the way are not mere bureaucratic ones imposed by the US Food and Drug Administration. Safety of a drug in humans and efficacy of the drug in the human disease can never be ensured on the basis of laboratory-animal data alone. Careful clinical trials in humans are a necessity. As a consequence, it is appropriate to be skeptical about claims that a drug worked beautifully in mice and therefore "just has to" be successful in humans. It is also appropriate to be very skeptical of claims of benefits of a therapy based on results from small numbers of individuals with no control group.

The standard approach to clinical trials and the proof of efficacy and safety of drugs has evolved over the past fifty years. In the parlance of the US FDA, there are three defined phases to drug development in humans. Phase 1 involves an initial determination of safety in healthy young volunteers. Issues about how the drug is absorbed after oral administration, how long the drug remains in the blood, how the body disposes of the drug, and other matters are worked out in phase 1 studies. These technical pharmacological issues are crucial to understanding how to administer the medication. They are also crucial to understanding the potential for side effects. Phase 2 studies involve administration of the drug to patients with the disease in question—for us here, FTD. Phase 2 studies are typically used to find the highest dose that can be administered safely. Phase 2 studies cannot be relied on to determine if the drug is effective, nor can phase 2 studies guarantee that no serious side effects will emerge later. Phase 2 studies are typically modest in size, involving perhaps fifty to one hundred patients.

Problems with the pharmacology could prevent a practical way of administering the drug. It could turn out that the new drug cannot be taken by mouth. That might occur if it so happens that stomach acids destroy the drug's potency. Unexpected side effects are probably the biggest "wild card" in drug development. It is very difficult to predict what kinds of side effects will occur with a drug. It could turn out that the drug caused kidney or liver failure. It could turn out that the drug causes epilepsy or even worsens mental functioning.

Finally, once an optimal dose is determined, and the side-effect profile of the drug is proved to be acceptable or manageable, a phase 3 study can be conducted. Phase 3 studies are called "pivotal" because if they show that the drug is effective and safe, the drug can be put forward for approval by the FDA. In the case of all neurological-disease clinical trials, phase 3 trials (a) are placebo-controlled, meaning that some participants will receive an inactive substance that looks and tastes like the drug being tested; (b) are randomized, meaning that treatment—active drug or placebo—is assigned by a process that is equivalent to tossing a coin for each participant; (c) are double-blinded, meaning that neither the participant nor the investigator is aware of the assignment of drug or placebo to participants; and (d) require all participants meet all inclusion and exclusion criteria. Most often in neurological diseases like FTD, phase 3 trials (a) have a parallel design, meaning that participants, once assigned to the drug being tested or the placebo, remain on that treatment throughout the double-blinded portion of the study; (b) are at least six months in duration and often longer, though not usually longer than eighteen months, and (c) usually include an "open-label long-term extension," meaning that once the double-blind portion of the trial is completed, participants will be placed on the active drug for an extended period of time. For the foreseeable future, a "control" group that receives an inactive substance will be an invariable part of clinical trials in FTD.

Conducting phase 3 studies in FTD will be very challenging because such studies typically require hundreds of participants who are (a) willing and able to come to a research center for six to twelve visits over the course of the trial, (b) neither too early-stage nor too impaired by the illness to match the participation criteria, and (c) free of other medical or neurological conditions that could put the patient at higher risk due to the side effects of the drug or require the use of prescribed medications that could interfere with the study procedures. It is likely that extensive imaging studies will be required to measure the effects of the treatment, as may repeated lumbar punctures to test spinal-fluid chemistries. As symptoms progress over time, maintaining compliance with medication-taking and completing scans and other trial procedures becomes more difficult. On the other hand, some future clinical trials may be conducted in asymptomatic persons who are known to be at risk for FTD because of their family history. In those individuals, safety of the drug becomes even more crucial. Any trial, whether it be with persons who already have symptoms or with those who do not, will involve much effort on the part of participants. It is understandable that many caregivers and families of FTD patients may have a hard time accepting the scientific necessity of participating in a twelve- or eighteen-month placebo-controlled trial in which there is a chance that their loved one is not receiving the active drug. Yet clinical trials with a control group are an absolute necessity in FTD. Clinical trials are not easy to design, are time-consuming for participants and their families, and are typically very expensive for those conducting the trial. Progress will require high levels of participation by patients with FTD. Clinical trials are the only way for us to find effective treatments for our patients with FTD.

There are two avenues for therapeutics in FTD that should both be explored: treatment of persons who are symptomatic and treatment of persons who are asymptomatic but at risk. The first is treating those who already have symptoms. Tailoring the treatment to the specific biochemistry is going to be necessary, and that means that very accurate diagnoses for every patient will be required. Treating people once they already have symptoms may not always be satisfying to the patient or the family, if the symptoms are distressing enough. In fact, maintaining a person with FTD who has distressing symptoms of one type or another, some of which may last for a longer period of time, may not be acceptable to many. Therefore, if we are going to have to treat people with FTD once they have symptoms, we need to find treatments that actually improve symptoms. Bringing about improvement is a much higher bar for therapeutics than is delaying decline. But improving symptoms must be the goal of FTD therapeutics in the next decade.

The second therapeutic approach is that of prevention. Identifying persons at risk for FTD on the basis of their family history might be feasible in a small number of persons who come from families with known genetic abnormalities. But, for the majority of patients with FTD who have no family history, detection of the disease before symptoms appear currently seems out of reach. Preventing FTD should be another goal for research, but perhaps that is one for the future.

THE FUTURE OF RESEARCH IN FTD

Researchers in the FTD field have learned to develop strong feelings of optimism and skepticism simultaneously. It is not easy to maintain the belief that we can find effective treatments, while at the same time recognizing the daunting challenges we face.

Optimism is certainly justified by improvements in diagnosis. Over the past ten years, the FTD research community has reached consensus on many of the key elements of the clinical diagnoses of FTD subtypes. Two techniques have become available to enable physicians to diagnose AD biochemical changes. One method is with spinal-fluid measurement of beta-amyloid protein, and the other is with a PET scanning technique called "amyloid imaging." These tools now give the field of FTD the capability of being able to determine whether a patient with an FTD-like set of symptoms, such as a prominent language disorder or a major change in personality and behavior, actually has underlying Alzheimer's as the primary cause.

In the next few years, it will be possible to distinguish between FTD subtypes. The new PET imaging for tau protein that first began testing in 2013 is an example of a new imaging technique that might dramatically improve our abilities in diagnosis of FTD. Performing tau imaging in an FTD patient would allow doctors to say whether or not the FTD was due to a tauopathy. It is possible that new imaging techniques will also become available to detect abnormal levels of TDP-43 in the brain. Or, alternatively, perhaps a spinal-fluid test will be developed to diagnose TDP-43 abnormalities. It is also possible that new genetic tools will become available that will aid in diagnosing specific FTD subtypes. Accurate diagnosis of the precise chemical basis of FTDs seems like a reasonable possibility in the next decade.

ABBREVIATIONS

AD: Alzheimer's disease

ALS: amyotrophic lateral sclerosis

bvFTD: behavioral variant FTD, the behavioral/personality disorder almost always due to FTD

C9orf72: gene that, when carrying a repeated sequence of DNA ("hexanucleotide repeat expansion), causes FTD or ALS or a combination of the two syndromes

FDG: fludeoxyglucose, a radioactive diagnostic agent used in imaging

FTD: frontotemporal degeneration

FTD-ALS or FTD-MND (MND = motor neuron disease): a combination of FTD and ALS

GRN: gene that encodes progranulin

MAPT: gene that encodes microtubule associated protein tau

MRI: magnetic resonance imaging

PET: positron emission tomography

PPA: primary progressive aphasia, the language variant of FTD

TDP43: transactive response DNA binding protein of 43 kilodalton molecular weight that is abnormally located in several forms of FTD

GLOSSARY

DNA: deoxyribonucleic acid, a substance found in the center ("nucleus") of cells that contains the genetic code. DNA consists of a series of four nucleic acids ("nucleotides") assembled in long chains called chromosomes

neurons: brain cells that transmit, store, and process information through chemical connections ("synapses") with other neurons

protein: a substance found in all living cells consisting of a particular sequence of any of 20+ amino acids

syndrome versus disease: a collection of symptoms that tend to co-occur; for example, behavior variant frontotemporal dementia or primary progressive aphasia are syndromes that are often caused by the disease frontotemporal degeneration

PART 2
MANAGING DAILY CARE

INTRODUCTION

A FRAMEWORK FOR QUALITY OF LIFE WITH FTD

Sharon S. Denny, MA

Part 1 of this book provides information that is critical to understanding frontotemporal degeneration (FTD) from the perspective of science and medicine. Part 2 focuses on day-to-day life after diagnosis. You will find wonderful information on how nonmedical interventions and rehabilitation therapies can help you to manage symptoms and preserve quality of life. Information is critical and necessary, but information alone is not sufficient. Especially with FTD, to be most valuable the facts and figures must be enriched by lived experience. A growing number of professionals have worked with people diagnosed with FTD, and seasoned caregivers and FTD-support-group leaders generously share their hard-earned wisdom. Theirs is the guidance that creates a framework for managing care in daily life.

Navigating the day-to-day challenges of FTD is truly more art than science. It requires skill, creativity, and inspiration. If science is about testing hypotheses and verifying results, caregiving at its best is about operationalizing personal values through daily decisions and changing circumstances. It has been described beautifully as a close dance with your partner. The dance may be a slow, flowing waltz or a fast, frenetic tango. The partners may be spouses or family members, friends, or professionals. The caregiving dance is less about the defined relationship between the person with FTD and his or her partner than it is about a commitment to persevering together for dignity and quality care. You can learn skills and techniques and hone your own style. When this flows from a strategy for decision making that is grounded in your hierarchy of values, you can shape the experience in invaluable ways.

THE IMPACT OF FTD ON THE PERSON DIAGNOSED AND IMMEDIATE FAMILY

For most people, the road to a diagnosis of FTD is long, winding, and difficult. Symptoms develop gradually and are often mistaken for signs of situational stress, depression, or other psychiatric disorders, sometimes for several years, before an FTD disorder is identified. Daily life is affected before the changes are adequately explained. Relationships experience strain, employment is disrupted or lost, and financial stability is shaken. There can be relief in learning that a disease is responsible for these changes, but that relief evaporates as the prospect of living with FTD settles in. The role of "caregiver" is not one embraced eagerly by all family members or necessarily welcomed by the person with dementia. It takes time to incorporate the new knowledge, recalibrate expectations, and find a path forward.

The particular effect of FTD is on the "social brain"; those complex emotional, behavioral, and communication skills controlled by the frontal and temporal lobes that determine how we interact with others. Changes to these cognitive skills are not easy to see or understand. The gradual decline in language and activities is insidious, often becoming firmly established and causing damage before being noticed. People with FTD experience a mix of areas of significant impairment and areas of enduring strength and capability. The typically younger age of onset means that people are physically robust and active. They are closer to the height of their work and family lives than they are settled into retirement. While awareness of FTD is growing, the number of people affected by FTD remains small and is far fewer than other types of dementia such as Alzheimer's and Lewy body dementia. The rare nature of the disease combined with poorly understood symptoms and a person's younger age and family developmental stage make the impact of FTD especially challenging.

There are many faces of FTD. People may be diagnosed when they are married with young children at home, in college, or just starting out on their own. Others are divorced as a result of behavior and personality changes that developed before disease was suspected. And many people diagnosed with FTD are single and manage care on their own. Parents solidly past retirement may take on care for their adult child who is ill. Each scenario affects the context in which decisions about care are made.

The diversity of family arrangements is matched by diversity in the subtypes and range of possible symptoms of FTD. Some people speak hesitantly because they are losing the grammatical structure that holds sentences together. Others speak fluently but lose the meaning of words and concepts. Someone diagnosed with behavioral FTD may show declining interest in hobbies, activities, and socializing. Another person may talk excessively to strangers or make rude comments or off-color jokes that are out of character. The most prominent symptoms in the first two years indicate where the disease started in the brain and determine the clinical diagnosis. What happens next—what brain circuits are affected next, how quickly, and what symptoms develop—is impossible to predict.

A strategic approach to the disease that addresses these challenges—younger onset, rare disease, with poorly understood symptoms—will promote confidence in managing care.

A FRAMEWORK FOR DAILY LIFE

> *"I didn't cause it. I can't change it, and I can't control it. But I do have choices about how to live each moment. . . . I will make life as enjoyable, dignified, and meaningful as possible for as long as I can."*
> —Eleanor, caregiver for her husband

Not too long ago, people receiving a diagnosis of dementia were advised to get their affairs in order and prepare for the end. Public awareness of Alzheimer's disease and other dementias and advocacy by people who are themselves diagnosed is starting to reduce past stigma and put more focus on living with the disease. Someone with FTD did nothing to cause the disease, and in the absence of much-needed treatment, cannot control its eventual outcome. But countless large and small choices will help you live as well as possible for as long as possible.

Consider How You Want to Live

While there are many things about FTD and changing care needs that cannot be predicted or controlled, you can control your approach to the disease. Discuss your goals with as much input as possible from the person diagnosed. Are there ways to position yourself to be near supports and resources before you need to access them? What can you do to lower the stress and stimulation around you? Are there things you want to do together or trips you want to take? You will need to do some things differently, but you can still pursue shared goals and interests and create memories together.

Adjust Expectations

Someone with FTD will have more trouble focusing and interacting when they are tired or in an overly stimulating environment. Look for new ways to do things you enjoy and value. Adjusting expectations and planning activities and commitments accordingly will make it possible to stay engaged more effectively with fewer difficulties.

Develop a Positive Daily Routine

No lifestyle change will stop the progression or reverse the disease. However, items that promote overall physical health and mental and emotional well-being are positive practices for all, including those with FTD. Predictable routines provide an important outline for the day for both the person with FTD and the caregiver. Create an engaging and balanced routine of daily-living activities such as meals, household tasks, and errands with physical activity; mental stimulation; hobbies; social interaction and spiritual development. Be consistent yet flexible to accommodate your day-to-day reality.

Try It and See

Clinicians are beginning to study the effectiveness of pharmacological and non-pharmacological interventions in FTD, but evidence-based practices are lacking. The principles of general dementia care must be adapted to fit the particular needs of people with behavioral variant FTD and primary progressive aphasia. Each intervention must be tailored creatively to the individual, based on knowledge of the person and his or her situation. Nothing will work optimally from the start. When you routinely observe and adjust each intervention, it becomes an experiment that will provide ideas to build on in the next situation.

Be Prepared to Advocate and Educate

Awareness is improving, but there are far too few services that are experienced in serving people with FTD. Do not be surprised that friends, family, and service providers are not familiar with FTD. The main caregiver knows best the affected person's background, preferences, abilities, and needs. Your advocacy is the most effective way to access care. Develop a folder of relevant articles, booklets, and resources for more information that you can take to new providers. Being prepared to educate can help to temper the frustrations you encounter.

Do Not Go It Alone

The emotional, physical, and logistical challenges of managing daily care are impossible for anyone to handle alone. Those who choose to accept assistance will be more effective and satisfied caregivers. People grow in confidence gradually as they begin to speak with closest family or friends about the disease. Identify specific tasks that are needed and people who can help. Most people want to help and appreciate suggestions for how they can.

Remember, the goal is to make each day as good as it can be.

*   *   *

CREATING YOUR MASTERPIECE OF CARE

Frontotemporal degeneration disorders are complex; they bring daunting challenges and devastating losses to the individuals and families affected. Just as advances in research offer hope for future cures, advances in our tools for care provide hope to those living with FTD now. There is a rich trove of expertise in the chapters that follow that can inform the daily care of persons with FTD. Daily life with the disease requires the flexible and creative application of principles and tools to fit each unique situation. Each individual has strengths to draw on and choices to make about how to approach the challenges ahead. More than ever before, you do not face these challenges alone. Professional expertise and the wisdom of other FTD caregivers can provide guidance and support. The decisions within each day with FTD are numerous and often difficult. When you approach them from a framework that acknowledges the reality and promotes your vision of quality of life, you will create a masterpiece of compassionate care.

CHAPTER 10

GETTING IT DOWN AND GETTING IT OUT

Swallowing and Communication Concerns

Amy P. Lustig, PhD, MPH, CCC-SLP

SWALLOWING ISSUES: DYSPHAGIA

We know that dementia is a progressive illness. As such, people with fronto-temporal degeneration (FTD) will show changes over time in their cognitive and functional abilities. These changes can interfere with activities of daily living, including eating, drinking, and medication compliance, all of which rely on a safe, effective swallowing mechanism.

The clinical term for swallowing problems is *dysphagia*. People with a diagnosis of FTD may or may not develop dysphagia at some point in the course of the illness. It has been reported that swallowing problems in FTD appear to be associated with a more difficult course of illness overall (Langmore et al. 2007).

Believe it or not, we swallow up to two thousand times per day! This is necessary to manage our saliva and other oral secretions we produce throughout the day and night. Swallowing is a complex act involving many muscles, nerves, and structures of the mouth, throat, and respiratory system.

The same areas in the brain that are affected in FTD are some of the same areas responsible for motor coordination and sensory feedback involved in swallowing. Sensory changes can affect an individual's ability to taste and smell foods by altering or eliminating these responses, which can lead to reduced interest in eating, refusal of foods that were previously enjoyed, or trouble managing foods and liquids in a timely and efficient way. Motor changes can affect the strength, range of motion, and precise coordination required when foods, liquids, or medications are introduced into the mouth, chewed, propelled into the throat, and brought down through the throat into the esophagus (the pathway from the throat to the stomach).

The primary health concern when dysphagia is present is the potential for foods, liquids, or medications to accidentally enter the airway while they are passing through the throat. During this phase, the bolus (a term referring to whatever food/liquid/medication is being swallowed) travels through the same part of the pharynx (throat) through which air passes during inhalation and exhalation. When swallowing is impaired, the airway can become highly vulnerable to being breached by bits of food or liquid.

Despite the fact that breathing is essential to our survival, there are remarkably few mechanisms in place to protect the airway during swallowing. Nevertheless, it is crucial that the airway be protected from entry of any bolus material. Should bolus material enter the airway, it can result in coughing, choking with difficulty or inability to breathe, or respiratory infection such as pneumonia, due to aspiration, a term meaning penetration of bolus material into the lungs. Pneumonia associated with aspiration is frequently identified as the cause of death for people with FTD (Grasbeck et al. 2003). Aspiration often occurs silently, meaning that food or liquid debris enters the airway and goes down into the lungs without triggering any coughing, throat clearing, or other obvious response.

Other concerns related to dysphagia include compromised nutritional status, dehydration, chronic respiratory problems, diminished enjoyment of eating and drinking, social embarrassment if noticeable signs such as coughing or drooling are present, and social isolation related to lack of participation at mealtimes. For these reasons and more, it is important to identify dysphagia when it is present and to make efforts to maximize the individual's ability to swallow safely and effectively.

People with primary progressive aphasia and other FTDs may experience swallowing difficulties that they are not able to express clearly to those around them, due to declines in their ability to use language to communicate. People who care for individuals with primary progressive aphasia may need to observe their care recipient during mealtimes and make judgments concerning their ability to safely manage foods, liquids, and medications.

Swallowing can be broken down into three stages: oral, pharyngeal, and esophageal. Dysphagia can occur at any or all of these stages. Aspects of the medical history can also inform the presence of dysphagia. There are some signs and symptoms of swallowing problems that can be observed by people who spend time with individuals with FTD. Here are some things to look for that can signify changes in and potential problems with swallowing.

SIGNS AND SYMPTOMS OF DYSPHAGIA

Oral Signs/Symptoms:

- difficulty taking bites, sips, or medications
- difficulty chewing foods
- delayed swallowing
- drooling
- eating or drinking very rapidly or impulsively
- retention of food particles in the mouth well after meal/snack is over

Pharyngeal Signs/Symptoms:

- frequent throat clearing after swallowing
- coughing (brief or prolonged) after swallowing
- choking on foods, liquids, or medications
- wet, gurgly or strangled-sounding voice after swallowing (this can also be heard in between meals due to difficulty swallowing saliva/secretions)
- regurgitation of bolus debris through the mouth or nose

Esophageal Signs/Symptoms:

- feeling that foods are "sticking" or "not going down" (this can be felt anywhere from the collarbone to the waist)
- increase in acid-reflux symptoms such as heartburn, indigestion, etc.
- pain or discomfort anywhere along the path of the esophagus

Medical History Signs/Symptoms:

- history of pneumonia, especially one or more since diagnosis of fronto-temporal dementia

- chronic low-grade fever
- unexplained weight loss
- change in appetite (decrease or increase) and/or food preferences
- dehydration
- change in mental status; decline in attention and concentration
- difficulty recognizing or organizing familiar objects (can affect how food on the plate is seen)
- speech changes (can signify oral/pharyngeal weakness or discoordination)

WHAT TO DO IF YOU SEE SIGNS OF DYSPHAGIA

If you think your care recipient may be demonstrating difficulties with swallowing, the first thing to do is talk with your medical doctor as soon as possible. Problems with swallowing in frontotemporal degeneration will not usually resolve on their own, and they can have potentially serious consequences if they are not addressed.

Your medical doctor will typically refer you to a speech-language pathologist (SLP) for dysphagia evaluation and treatment. SLPs, also called speech therapists, are considered the primary clinical expert for managing functional swallowing disorders and are usually the next provider consulted after the medical doctor. They will also collaborate as necessary with other health professionals, including nutritionists; occupational therapists; gastrointestinal (GI) specialists; and ear, nose, and throat (ENT) specialists to provide a comprehensive, multidisciplinary approach to dysphagia diagnosis and management.

The speech therapist will typically schedule an office visit to meet with the individual with FTD and concerned caregivers. During this visit, the speech therapist will obtain the patient's history and will discuss the signs and symptoms of dysphagia that triggered the visit. The speech therapist will talk with the patient to obtain his or her direct report of swallowing problems to the extent possible and will evaluate the patient's oral motor strength, range of motion, and coordination for foods, liquids, and medications. Because changes in communication and behavioral status can also affect swallowing, these may also be queried and/or directly evaluated by the speech therapist.

The speech therapist may recommend further evaluation to obtain a more detailed and specific evaluation of the patient's swallowing function, such as a modified barium swallow (MBS) study that uses x-ray films to view the swallowing mechanism using foods and liquids impregnated with a contrast material, or a fiberoptic endoscopic evaluation of swallowing (FEES), which views swallowing activity in the throat using a small camera threaded through the patient's nasal cavity. These studies can provide detailed and specific evidence about the extent to which aspiration is occurring during the swallow, and what food and liquid textures may be more or less safe where airway protection is concerned.

Speech-therapy recommendations for dysphagia management are based on factors including the patient's airway-protection status and what foods and liquids are safest to consume; the efficiency with which bolus items clear the throat into the esophagus and if these could be altered to make them easier to swallow, and whether other behavioral or compensatory strategies would be useful. Following are some suggestions typically provided by speech therapists to address swallowing impairments in FTD:

DIET AND FEEDING STRATEGIES

- Avoid or limit thin liquids, foods, and/or medications if they are entering the airway and/or causing coughing/choking.
- Chop solid foods and add extra moisture to make them easier to chew (in more severe cases it may be necessary to blend or puree all foods); avoid foods that are hard, dry, sticky, crumbly, or are otherwise difficult to chew and swallow; choose foods that are softer, moister, and more cohesive. There are several cookbooks and Internet resources with recipes for soft/pureed foods.
- Thicken all thin liquids, including all drinks, soups, and medications (the terms *nectar* and *honey* are often used to describe the texture of the thickened liquid). Products used to thicken liquids may be obtained from local drugstores or supermarkets and may or may not be eligible for medical-insurance reimbursement. Recommendations for thickening liquids are typically made for two reasons: because they have been determined to be less likely to enter the airway during swallowing; and because they can be easier to manage in the mouth due to their relatively heavier, denser texture. *It is important to consult with a speech therapist before adding a thickening agent to liquids*, as these also have the potential to be aspirated into the lungs.
- Add nutritional supplements to the diet as recommended by your doctor

or nutritionist (liquid supplements may need to be thickened along with other thin liquids).

- For those with advanced dementia, limit visual items during mealtimes to essentials only (plate, utensils, cup); remove unnecessary items from the individual's visual field and eliminate background noise and interruptions to minimize confusion and maximize attention.
- Individuals with advanced dementia may require partial or full assistance with feeding; this should be done with a smooth utensil such as a spoon, alternating foods and liquids (which may also need to be provided by spoon) slowly and carefully, and allowing time for complete swallowing and breathing between mouthfuls. It may be necessary to check the mouth for unswallowed food after meals are completed, and to clear any debris so it is not accidentally aspirated.

MEDICATION STRATEGIES

- Take medications with a heavier/thicker liquid or follow medication doses with a spoonful or two of applesauce, pudding, or another easy-to-swallow item to assist in quickly moving the medication from the mouth to the throat to the esophagus.
- If pills are too difficult to swallow, empty capsules and crush or split medications (as possible; check with your pharmacist first) and mix into pudding, applesauce, or other cohesive and easy-to-swallow food items. Liquid medications can also be mixed with food items or thicker liquids to make them easier to manage.

BEHAVIORAL AND COMPENSATORY STRATEGIES*

- ALWAYS SIT FULLY UPRIGHT whenever eating, drinking, or taking medications! Do NOT recline and eat or drink—this is a big choking risk.
- Take small bites and sips; take only one bite or sip at a time; eat slowly and carefully.
- Alternate bites and sips to make it easier to swallow solid foods.
- Swallow everything from one bite/sip before taking the next one—no guzzling or gobbling.

- Do not talk when there is still unswallowed food in the mouth.
- Rather than eating three large meals, take several smaller meals throughout the day if poor attention or fatiguing during meals is a problem, or if weight loss persists.
- Sometimes changing the position of the head, such as a turn to the side or tucking the chin down, can improve swallowing safety and effectiveness; these recommendations are patient-specific and provided by the speech therapist.

*These recommendations may require ongoing verbal, written, and/or pictorial reminders for individuals with poor memory or attention, or with compromised language skills.

MOUTH CARE

It is very important to maintain good oral hygiene for individuals with FTD, especially if swallowing problems are present. In addition to foods and liquids, individuals with dysphagia can also be at risk of aspirating their own saliva and other oral secretions.

Some people with FTD experience changes in their saliva production that can affect swallowing. For some, saliva production can become excessive (sialorrhea), and for others there may be less saliva produced, leading to xerostomia, a chronically dry oral cavity. Both situations require attention and intervention. Sialorrhea can lead to drooling and skin irritation and can interfere greatly with swallowing as well as speaking. Xerostomia, in addition to interfering with swallowing and speech, is a potential breeding ground for bacteria that could cause respiratory infection if aspirated into the lungs.

There are prescription medications that can potentially help to improve both conditions, an injection medication that can help to reduce saliva production, and some over-the-counter remedies to increase oral-cavity moisture. Your speech therapist or medical doctor may refer you to a neurologist for further evaluation.

Changes in FTD can make it increasingly difficult to maintain good oral hygiene. Sometimes it can be helpful to consider modifying how tasks such as toothbrushing are carried out, especially if the individual has difficulty spitting, struggles with keeping his or her mouth open for extended periods of time, or has other compromised oral motor and/or sensory function. For example, toothbrushes with built-in suctioning can clear toothpaste and saliva, eliminating the need to spit. Dentists and occupational therapists familiar with frontotemporal dementia are good resources for information and strategies to maintain good oral hygiene.

SEVERE DYSPHAGIA

Sometimes dysphagia can be so severe that swallowing becomes extremely difficult or even impossible to accomplish. For people in this situation, the act of trying to eat and drink can be highly distressing and exhausting. The risks of severe dysphagia include unintentional weight loss, dehydration, and failure to obtain important medications. When this situation occurs, it may be necessary to consider an alternative way to take food, liquid, and medication into the body.

When it becomes clear that the person with FTD is unable to maintain adequate intake of calories, fluids, and medicines because of severe swallowing impairment, the typical recommendation is use of a feeding tube to provide sustenance. Though there are tubes that can be temporarily placed through the nose and into the stomach for this purpose, usually consideration is given to use of a percutaneous endoscopic gastrostomy (PEG) tube that is more permanently situated in the upper part of the stomach. The PEG tube can used to obtain calories (in the form of liquid nutrition or pureed foods), fluids, and crushed medications in an efficient and relatively safe manner. Use of the PEG tube will reduce the risk of choking and aspiration that is present when taking foods and liquids by mouth in severe dysphagia. However, aspiration is still possible when calories and fluids are taken through a PEG tube, and it is important to work with your medical provider to understand the necessary safety precautions to take when the tube is in use. Most PEG tube placements are uneventful, but as with every medical procedure there are associated risks; these include injury to skin or underlying organs. Sometimes it is necessary to use a different type of feeding tube that is placed lower in the digestive tract.

For people with frontotemporal degeneration, severe dysphagia can occur at any stage of the disease, though it often presents later in the course of the illness. Sometimes decisions concerning alternative ways of taking calories, fluids, and medications are tied to larger considerations about preferences for end-of-life care. Chapters 18 and 22 discuss approaches for decision making in advance of severe disability; these include creating a living will, appointing a healthcare power of attorney to act in the best interests of the individual, and participating in hospice or palliative care. There is no evidence that use of feeding tubes increases survival rate, quality of life, or overall health and nutritional status for individuals with late-stage dementia (Alagiakrishnan et al. 2013).

COMMUNICATION ISSUES: PRIMARY PROGRESSIVE APHASIA AND SPEECH/LANGUAGE IMPAIRMENT

Many, if not most, people with FTD experience changes in their ability to communicate as their illness progresses. These changes can occur earlier or later in the disease process, and the severity of the problem can range from mild to profound. Declines in communication ability can cause significant difficulty and stress for everyone. Problems can range from not being able to indicate what one wants for breakfast to not being able to say what one is feeling or thinking about critical life events.

Communication is essential to our lives. We create all of our relationships in life, as well as our own personal identity, through communication. Our ability to communicate is directly related to how well we can identify, express, and fulfill our needs and desires. It allows us to follow our hopes and dreams, and to be there for others in their own life pursuits. Losing the ability to communicate can have profound effects on the lives of everyone involved.

Central to communication is our use of language to understand and express what we and those around us are thinking, feeling, and desiring. Think of language as a code of sounds and symbols we use to represent ideas. Right now I am using my knowledge of English to write these words, and you are using your knowledge of English to decode and understand them.

One thing that can happen in FTD is that the ability to use language to express one's self, and to understand what others express, can be progressively lost. This problem is known as *aphasia*, a term that represents problems with using language for communication. Aphasia can take many forms: it can present as difficulty thinking of the words you want to say, problems comprehending what others say, or trouble with reading and/or writing. In more severe cases it can even interfere with understanding typical gestures we use to express ourselves, such as a "thumbs-up" sign to indicate a positive response, or waving at someone to call them over.

DIAGNOSIS OF PRIMARY PROGRESSIVE APHASIA

When language problems appear as the first sign of FTD, the problem is usually referred to as primary progressive aphasia (PPA). The diagnosis of PPA is provided by a neurologist, typically in collaboration with a speech therapist. The neurologist consults with family members and conducts various tests, including taking images of the brain, such as magnetic resonance imaging (MRI), to determine the presence of disease. The speech therapist conducts detailed language testing and also works with family caregivers to better understand their concerns and the changes they are observing in the patient. Often, the speech therapist will establish an ongoing relationship with the family to assist them in developing strategies to compensate, to the extent possible, for the breakdowns in communication caused by the aphasia.

For people with primary progressive aphasia, difficulties with self-expression and with understanding others will most likely be the predominant symptom for the first few years of the illness. Typically, the aphasia will worsen over time; some people end up unable to speak at all. In addition to losing their language skills, some people will also experience declines in other cognitive abilities, such as memory and attention, and some will also demonstrate behavior and personality changes.

There are currently three different types of aphasia that have been identified for individuals with primary progressive aphasia: nonfluent/agrammatic, semantic, and logopenic (Gorno-Tempini 2011). Each of these classifications is associated with a different pattern of language impairment. Describing different types and patterns of language impairment in specific terms can be helpful for suggesting possible interventions and strategies for improving communication, and for better understanding of the underlying disease process.

In the nonfluent/agrammatic variant changes in expressive language can be seen in grammar errors such as omitted words (e.g., "Let's go store") or incorrect word order (e.g., "Let's to the store go"). The act of speaking may require more effort and there may be errors in how speech sounds are produced (e.g., "Let's ko to the sore"). The individual with nonfluent/agrammatic variant may have difficulty understanding sentences that are longer or more complex, though comprehension of single words and object knowledge are generally intact.

In the semantic variant there is a decline in the ability to recall the correct words for objects, persons, and actions, as well as difficulty understanding word meanings. Longer phrases and sentences are often better understood than single words. Reading may also be impaired. Speech production in the semantic variant, including repetition, is typically unchanged and grammar use is generally correct.

In the logopenic variant word-finding problems are seen during naming and conversation, and repetition of longer phrases or sentences is difficult or impossible. Speech production is generally smooth, though there can be occasional sound errors, and comprehension of words and object knowledge are usually stable.

These three classifications represent different patterns of language impairment that are observed at the time the diagnosis of primary progressive aphasia is made. They are general classifications, and many people will not fully conform to one or another category. It is expected for individuals with primary progressive aphasia that language competence will decline and impairment patterns will change as the disease progresses over time.

TREATMENT FOR PRIMARY PROGRESSIVE APHASIA

Because communication is so vital to overall quality of life, speech therapists focus on working with individuals with PPA, along with family members and other caregivers, to maximize the individual's ability to convey his or her thoughts and feelings to others. There are different strategies that can be used to compensate, to some extent, for the difficulties that develop with language expression and comprehension. Because no two people are exactly alike, speech therapists work with each individual to develop a set of strategies tailored to his or her specific situation, taking into account the other important people with whom they interact. In addition to identifying the ways in which language expression and/or comprehension have been impaired, it is crucial to ascertain what the individual's communication strengths are, as they will form the basis upon which any useful strategies will be built.

Generally speaking, there are two broad components to speech therapy for primary progressive aphasia: direct practice with the speech therapist, and establishment of strategies that can be used outside the clinical environment with family, friends, and caregivers. The strategies that are developed for home use are typically identified through the speech therapist's evaluation of the patient's strengths and challenges, and they are practiced, reinforced, and modified during individual treatment sessions. Goals are designed to be functional, meaning they are developed to address the individual's personal needs and the challenges experienced in everyday life. Homework is often given for additional practice outside of therapy. Strategies are regularly reevaluated and modified to account for progressive changes in language competence over time.

Strategy planning takes several factors into account, including the nature and severity of the language impairment; the individual's living situation and important support persons involved in providing care; hobbies, interests, and other meaningful life events in which the individual participates; needs associated with daily life and healthcare status; and other personally relevant material. The speech therapist will attempt to identify what is most important to the individual, and where his or her greatest frustrations are where communication is concerned. The more the individual and family caregivers are motivated to participate in therapy, the better the outcomes will be.

Communication strategies can be "self-cued," meaning initiated and carried out by the patients, who may also use other visual materials to help them get out what they want to say. Strategies can also be initiated by others to assist the patient in eliciting successful communication. Since communication is by definition a two-way street, participation in speech therapy by persons close to the individual with primary progressive aphasia is essential to identifying goals and strategies that will be relevant and successfully employed.

A general effect of aphasia, across all primary progressive aphasia types, is that it takes language-impaired individuals longer to communicate. They need more time to organize their thoughts into words and sentences, and they also need more time to process what they hear and read. As such, one of the most helpful things family members or other caregivers can do is to develop a patient attitude when speaking with people with PPA, and allow them the time they require to speak, listen, and respond. For those used to fast-paced conversations, this can be quite a challenge that requires ongoing practice and self-control when learning not to interrupt or jump in too quickly.

Following are examples of some strategies that may be utilized to enhance communication by individuals with primary progressive aphasia and by their family, friends, and other caregivers. It is strongly recommended that you work with a speech therapist to identify the strategies that will be most appropriate and useful, and to obtain expert training on their use.

Problem: Trouble Recalling Words during Conversation

Self-cueing strategies:

- Circumlocution ("talking around" the missing word)
- Alphabet first-letter search (using written or sound cues)
- Write it down or tap it out (when the word is "stuck")
- Draw a picture
- Use gestures to get the point across

Help provided by others:

- Fill in missing word (with the patient's permission)
- Ask the patient to circumlocute ("tell me about it")
- Provide two to three options ("Is it this . . . or this . . . ?")

Problem: Difficulty Understanding General Conversation

Self-cueing strategies:

- Ask speakers to repeat themselves or to speak more slowly
- Turn off the TV or other interfering background noise
- Take a short rest and then return to the conversation

Help provided by others:

- Ensure only one person is speaking at a time
- Speak moderately slowly
- Eliminate background noise
- Provide written words to keep the patient on topic
- Use pictures to keep the patient on topic

Problem: Difficulty Understanding Specific Questions

Self-cueing strategies:

- Ask speakers to repeat themselves or to speak more slowly

- Eliminate background noise or other distractions
- Ask speakers to write, use pictures, draw, or gesture

Help provided by others:

- Speak slowly
- Eliminate background noise
- Write down the question
- Keep the question short
- Reduce question complexity by providing choices; for example, instead of asking, "What do you want for breakfast?" ask, "Would you like eggs or cereal?"
- Reduce question complexity by asking yes/no questions; for example, "Would you like eggs?"
- Use gestures to communicate; for example, point to an egg while looking at the patient with a questioning expression

WHERE TO GET HELP

If you would like more information about communication or swallowing concerns in frontotemporal degeneration or primary progressive aphasia, or if you are seeking a referral source for a qualified therapist, you can contact the American Speech-Language-Hearing Association (ASHA) at 800-638-8255 or through www.asha.org. ASHA manages oversight for all graduate-level education and certification of speech-language pathologists in the United States.

GLOSSARY

aphasia: difficulty using language for communication purposes; can include problems speaking, understanding what others say, or trouble with reading or writing

aspiration: inhalation of food, liquid, or medication into the airway and lungs

bolus: that which is being swallowed; includes foods, liquids, and medications

dysphagia: difficulty with swallowing; can refer to problems in the oral cavity, pharynx, and/or esophagus

esophagus: structure connecting the pharynx (throat) to the stomach fiberoptic endoscopic evaluation of swallowing (FEES): evaluation of swallowing by viewing the upper part of the airway via a small camera passed through the nasal cavity

honey-thick liquid: liquid thickened to the consistency of honey (very thick and dense; drips very slowly; cannot be drawn through a straw)

magnetic resonance imaging (MRI): a method of studying internal body parts, including the brain, with a noninvasive procedure utilizing magnetic fields

modified barium swallow study (MBS): a method of evaluating swallowing function utilizing x-ray technology

nectar-thick liquid: liquid thickened to the consistency of a nectar-type juice (moderately thick but less dense than a honey-thick liquid; can be drawn through a straw)

oral cavity: the mouth and its contents (tongue, teeth, etc.)

percutaneous endoscopic gastrostomy (PEG) tube: a device placed into the stomach through which calories, fluids, and medications may be obtained

pharynx: more commonly referred to as the throat; a structure connecting the oral cavity to the esophagus

primary progressive aphasia (PPA): a form of frontotemporal dementia in which difficulty using language to communicate is the predominant symptom for the first several years

sialorrhea: excessive production of saliva

speech-language pathologist (SLP): the more formal title for a speech therapist

speech therapist: a rehabilitation therapist who focuses on evaluation and treatment of disorders of communication and swallowing

xerostomia: excessive dryness of the oral cavity

BIBLIOGRAPHY

Alagiakrishnan, K., R. A. Bhanji, and M. Kurian. "Evaluation and Management of Oropharyngeal Dysphagia in Different Types of Dementia: A Systematic Review." *Archives of Gerontology and Geriatrics* 56 (2013): 1–9.

Gorno-Tempini, M. L., A. E. Hillis, S. Weintraub, et al. "Classification of Primary Progressive Aphasia and Its Variants." *Neurology* 76, (2011): 1006–14.

Grasbeck, A., E. Englund, V. Horstmann, U. Passant, and L. Gustafson. "Predictors of Mortality in Frontotemporal Dementia: A Retrospective Study of the Prognostic Influence of Pre-Diagnostic Features." *International Journal of Geriatric Psychiatry* 18 (2003): 594–601.

Langmore, S. E., R. K. Olney, C. Lomen-Hoerth, and B. L. Miller. "Dysphagia in Patients with Frontotemporal Lobar Dementia." *Archives of Neurology* 64 (2007): 58–62.

CHAPTER 11

A STEP AHEAD

Exercise and Mobility

Heather Cianci, PT, MS, GCS

HOW DOES PHYSICAL THERAPY HELP INDIVIDUALS WITH FTD?

The role of rehabilitation in the treatment of frontotemporal degeneration (FTD) is to preserve an individual's functional ability in everyday activities for as long as possible, while also limiting disability. Through the use of the therapies discussed in chapter 6, assistance can be provided to both the individual with FTD and his or her care partner throughout the entire disease. Training and education in mobility and safety can help to lessen challenges faced throughout the disease. This chapter will look at how physical therapy can help those with FTD and their care partners.

Physical therapy is a rehabilitative service provided by physical therapists and physical therapists' assistants. Physical therapists assess individuals' safety and quality of life by evaluating joints, muscles, mobility, balance, and activities of daily living. Treatments can consist of aerobic conditioning, strength and flexibility training, gait and balance training for fall prevention, new mobility technique training, and training with assistive devices such as walkers or wheelchairs.

Individuals with the behavioral and speech variants of FTD generally do not require physical therapy until later in the course of their disease. This is because the areas of the brain affected by these variants are different from those involved in movement control. It is the individuals with progressive motor decline variants of FTD (such as progressive supranuclear palsy [PSP], corticobasal syndrome [CBS], and frontotemporal degeneration with motor neuron disease [FTD-MND]) that need therapy early on due to difficulties with balance, gait, coordination, and strength.

Physical therapy deals with not just the individual's physical limitations but also with the challenges the care partner faces. Therapists can teach care partners how to physically assist their friends or loved ones, as well as help them with new ways to set up the home and use new adaptive equipment to prevent falls and other injuries. Therapists also train care partners in new ways of interacting with the person with FTD and helping the patient to still participate in activities he or she enjoys.

RECEIVING PHYSICAL THERAPY

The majority of states now allow individuals to go directly to a physical therapist without a physician's prescription. However, it is important to remember that your insurance provider does set guidelines for receiving therapy. You may first need to visit your primary-care physician and obtain a referral, or you may even be limited to seeing only therapists within a certain network.

For this reason it is very important that you speak with your insurance provider before making an appointment for physical therapy. Remember, though, if you are not comfortable with the therapy facility your insurance provider recommends, you do have the right to appeal. Reasons for wanting to appeal can include: the specialty training of the therapy staff, a poor prior experience with the facility, travel distance, or the ratio of therapy staff to patients (those with dementia tend to perform better with one-on-one, consistent care from the same person). For more specific information on this, visit the website of the American Physical Therapy Association (APTA) at www.apta.org. There is a link for the public, which provides resources. You may also call them at 800-999-APTA (2782).

It is important to know that you have the right to request physical therapy. It is not just up to the physician. You also do not need to wait until mobility or balance changes occur. A therapy program can start early to help prevent falls and functional decline, and to provide education on fitness and exercise. Early therapy intervention also helps to provide a baseline of function that the therapist can use as changes occur throughout the disease. It is also very helpful to the patient to look for therapy facilities that offer a team approach of physical, occupational, and speech therapy.

FINDING THE RIGHT THERAPIST

It is recommended that individuals with any type of dementia receive treatment by a physical therapist who is able to spend one-on-one time with them during treatment. Outpatient facilities that primarily deal with the neurological or geriatric population are generally best at providing this type of care.

Recommendations to help find the best therapist/facility for your needs:

- Ask others dealing with FTD what therapist/facility they have successfully used.
- Call facilities and inquire about its therapist-to-client ratio, how long each therapy session lasts, and the therapy staff's experience in treating patients with dementia.
- Search for a therapist via the APTA website.

A PHYSICAL-THERAPY PROGRAM

The degeneration of the brain that is seen in FTD can indirectly cause degeneration in functional ability. The following table shows how the two can be related.

FRONTOTEMPORAL DEGENERATION	PHYSICAL/ FUNCTIONAL CHANGES
Loss of initiative and decreased interest in daily activities	Less movement, muscle weakness and atrophy, stiffness, risk of skin breakdown
Impaired judgment	Falls, burns, various injuries
Excessive manual exploration of the environment	Falls, burns, lacerations of hands

Decreased ability to read or write	Injuries from inability to recognize safety hazards
Apraxia—loss of skilled movement abilities	Muscle weakness and atrophy, stiffness, difficulty with self-care and walking, falls
Spatial neglect—inability to properly recognize body or objects to one side	Muscle weakness, stiffness, difficulty with self-care and walking
Increased muscle spasticity or tone	Muscle contractures, impaired mobility and posture, skin breakdown—decubitus ulcers/bed sores

PHYSICAL THERAPY IN THE EARLY STAGES

It is not uncommon for those diagnosed with FTD to show some balance or walking problems early on in the disease. Individuals with FTD may also show changes in the way they normally performs tasks such as getting in and out of bed or getting dressed. Beginning a course of physical therapy early on in the disease can have many benefits. At this stage, individuals are the most likely to be able to learn and incorporate new movement techniques, exercises, and safety instructions into their everyday lives. A therapy program can focus on balance, mobility techniques, and fall prevention. It can also include training in a home program to help prevent functional decline and the loss of muscle strength and joint flexibility.

Although there is currently no specific research on the effects of exercise on FTD, there are studies that show and suggest exercise is beneficial for those with Alzheimer's disease (AD), PSP, and CBD. Two recent studies looked at how a multimodal exercise program affected frontal cognitive function, gait, and balance in those with AD. A multimodal exercise program is one that combines physical and cognitive exercises in a dual task. An example would be trying to stand tall and catch a ball while counting backward or naming items in a group. Both studies showed improvements were made to some degree in all categories.

Exercise should continue after the completion of formal physical therapy for not only the individual with FTD but also the care partner. Care partners need to maintain their strength and endurance, and also manage their stress.

A therapist can teach you how to safely and effectively exercise at home by:

- showing you how to use elastic resistance bands to strengthen muscles
- showing you how to use areas of your home for exercise: the corner of a room can be used to stretch the muscles in the front of the chest for better posture by placing the forearms and hands along each wall of the corner at differing heights, and then leaning the body through the arms (see figure 11.1.)

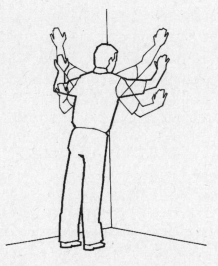

Figure 11.1. *Illustration by Rough Sketch Studio.*

- showing you how to use furniture in your home for exercise: a chair can be used to perform tricep dips to strengthen the muscles located on the back of the upper arms by sitting on the edge of a chair and trying to lift your bottom up off of the chair using only your arms (see figure 11.2.)
- helping you plan an aerobic exercise program (such as walking, biking, or dancing) to help with circulation and endurance

For those exercising out of the home, a physical therapist can help you by:

- making recommendations on what equipment at the gym is best to use
- helping you locate exercise classes that promote fitness and socialization

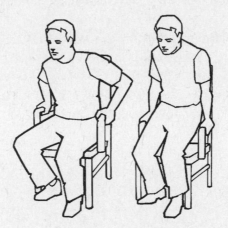

Figure 11.2. *Illustration by Rough Sketch Studio.*

PHYSICAL THERAPY IN THE MIDDLE STAGES

As individuals advance with FTD, they may begin to experience more diffi-culty with walking, balance, and mobility. At this stage, therapists can deter-mine if an assistive device, such as a rollator is needed. This type of walker has four wheels, hand brakes, a basket, and a seat. It is particularly helpful for those who want to walk but may fatigue easily or have poor balance. However, if walking outside or in unfamiliar places is becoming more challenging, a lightweight transport wheelchair can be used to make travel safer and easier. A therapist can help to guide you through the process of how to obtain assis-tive devices.

At this stage in the disease, activities of daily living such as bathing may become more difficult also. This is where care partners often need training in how to safely manage themselves while helping the individual with FTD. Devices such as tub benches, lift chairs, or bed rails may become necessary to ensure safety. Again, a therapist can make recommendations about which devices are best for your needs.

A home exercise program should continue, but now the care partner may need to provide more physical assistance. Exercises should be revamped to address the particular needs of the individual with FTD. Rigidity can become more of a problem now, and exercises that emphasize stretching and rotational movements should be added and emphasized. Heating pads and massage to tight areas may offer relief and work well in conjunction with exercise. Therapy should also work on promoting good posture to help with breathing, swallowing, and communication.

Now may be the time that home modifications become necessary. Relatively simple changes like placing handrails in the bathroom, moving furniture to open up space, and adding lighting can all improve safety. Therapists can come to your home to perform an environmental assessment and make recommendations about necessary changes. They can also help with ways to make the environment less distracting so that individuals with FTD can focus their attention more effectively. A drawer or a closet with too many items can be overwhelming for some people who are afflicted with FTD. Keeping only a few items organized in groups could help simplify a task and reduce stress. Other examples are removing clutter, changing colors or patterns, and reducing noise.

NOTE: If the individual with FTD cannot handle traveling to an outpatient facility at this stage, in-home therapy can be arranged. Issues that are addressed in outpatient therapy can be addressed equally well within the home.

PHYSICAL THERAPY IN THE LATER STAGES

As individuals with FTD become less mobile, it is important to start addressing the prevention of skin breakdown. Sitting or lying in one position for even a few hours at a time can lead to skin breakdown. In addition, moisture from incontinence and/or perspiration can speed this process along. Tissue over bony areas of the body, such as the elbows, heels, ankles, and sacrum, are commonly affected. Pressure to these areas from infrequent position changes leads to an impaired blood supply to those areas. If not relieved, the skin can go from being red and irritated to ultimately being ulcerated.

Those who are spending the majority of their time sitting should be reminded or helped to change their position every twenty minutes. Those who are bedridden should be helped to change position at least every two hours. Home therapists can make recommendations about special beds, lifts, and transfer devices to make positional changes easier and safer. Therapists can also assist with making decisions on specialized cushions, wedges, padding, and braces that promote comfort and prevent contractures and skin breakdown. One example is a foot brace known as a pressure relief, ankle/foot orthosis (PRAFO). This brace helps to keep pressure off of the heel, while keeping the ankle in a position to prevent contractures.

When an individual can no longer safely ambulate, even with the use of an assistive device, a customized wheelchair should be considered. A wheelchair allows the individual to still have some functional independence, and it makes mobility much easier and safer for the care partner. Transport, and off-the-shelf wheelchairs are not recommended for individuals who need to sit in them for long periods of time. A therapist will work with your physician and a durable medical equipment company to ensure that the correct wheelchair is provided. A prescription and a letter of medical necessity from the physician are necessary for insurance coverage. Some insurance providers even help with the cost of ramps for the home. If your insurance provider does not do this, check with your local area agency on aging (AAA) at http://www.n4a .org, a support group, or a social worker recommended by your physician or therapist for suggestions on funding.

An exercise program should continue to be performed; however, now that program may require increased help of a care partner. Physical therapists can provide training in how to properly perform range-of-motion and stretching exercises to help with flexibility, circulation, and the prevention of contractures.

SUMMARY

Physical therapy provides many different treatment options to individuals with FTD and their care partners. Therapy can help with physical fitness, fall prevention, safe mobility, and the prevention of functional decline. For this reason, it is important to get started in therapy sooner rather than later. The progressive nature of FTD often leaves individuals feeling a loss of control. However, by using treatments and equipment that focus on ability rather than disability, physical therapy can give back some control to those affected by FTD.

Remember:

You have the right to request physical therapy.
You have the right to request a therapist who specializes in the areas you are having difficulty with.

Look for therapy facilities that offer a team approach of physical, occupational, and speech therapy.

There are many options for making a home safer and mobility easier.

Exercise should be an everyday occurrence for both the individual with FTD *and* the care partner.

Programs that encourage combined physical and cognitive exercises are best.

BIBLIOGRAPHY

Berkow, R., and A. J. Fletcher, eds. *The Merck Manual*, 16th ed. Rahway, NJ: Merck Research Laboratories, 1992.

Buchanan, J. A., A. Christenson, and D. Houlihan. "The Role of Behavioral Analysis in the Rehabilitation of Persons with Dementia." *Behavioral Therapy* 42 (2011): 9–21.

Coelho, F. G, et al. "Multimodal Exercise Intervention Improves Frontal Cognitive Functions and Gait in Alzheimer's Disease: A Controlled Trial." *Geriatrics & Gerontology International* 13 (2013): 198–203.

de Andrade, L. P, et al. "Benefits of Multimodal Exercise Intervention for Postural Control and Frontal Cognitive Functions in Individuals with Alzheimer's Disease: A Controlled Trial." *JAGS* 61 (2013): 1919–26.

Family Caregiver Alliance Fact Sheet: Frontotemporal Dementia. 2014. Retrieved from http://www.caregiver.org/caregiver/jsp/content_node.jsp?nodeid=573.

FTD Disorders, The. 2014. Retrieved from http://www.theaftd.org/frontotemporal-degeneration/disorders.

Guccione, A. "What Is a Physical Therapist?" *American Physical Therapy Association* (online). October 1999. http://internet.apta.org/pt_magazine/oct99/closer.html. Retrieved January 10, 2002. This URL is no longer active.

Hodges, J. R. "Frontotemporal Dementia (Pick's Disease): Clinical Features and Assessment." *Neurology* 56 (2001): S6–S10.

Hopper, T. L. "'They're Just Going to Get Worse Anyway': Perspectives on Rehabilitation for Nursing Home Residents with Dementia." *Journal of Communication Disorders* 36 (2003): 345–59.

Hutton, T. J. *Preventing Falls*. Amherst, NY: Prometheus Books, 2000.

Kawahira, K., T. Noma, J. Iiyama, S. Etoh, A. Ogata, and M. Shimodozono. "Improvements in Limb Kinetic Apraxia by Repetition of a Newly Designed Facilitation Exercise in a Patient with Corticobasal Degeneration." *International Journal of Rehabilitation Research* 32, no. 2 (June 2009): 178–83.

Mioshi, E., and J. R. Hodges. "Rate of Change of Functional Abilities in Frontotemporal Dementia." *Dementia and Geriatric Cognitive Disorders* 28, no. 5 (2009): 419–26.

Perry, R. J., and B. L. Miller. "Behavior and Treatment in Frontotemporal Dementia." *Neurology* 56 (2000): S46–S51.

Robinson, K. M. "Rehabilitation Applications in Caring for Patients with Pick's Disease and Frontotemporal Dementia." *Neurology* 56 (2001): S56–S58.

Rosen, H. J., et al. "Frontotemporal Dementia." *Neurologic Clinics* 18, no. 4 (November 2000): 979–92.

Steffen, T. M., B. F. Boeve, C. M. Petersen, L. Dvorak, and K. Kantarci. "Long-Term Exercise Training for an Individual with Mixed Corticobasal Degeneration and Progressive Supranuclear Palsy Features: 10-Year Case Report Follow-Up." *Physical Therapy* 94, no. 2 (February 2014): 289–96; references in the text refer to the epub, which was available ahead of the print edition, on October 10, 2013 (accessed December 5, 2013)

Steffen, T. M., B. F. Boeve, L. A. Mollinger-Riemann, and C. M. Petersen. "Long-Term Locomotor Training for Gait and Balance in a Patient with Mixed Progressive Supranuclear Palsy and Corticobasal Degeneration." *Physical Therapy* 87, no. 8 (August 2007): 1078–87.

Warren, J. D., J. D. Rohrer, and M. N. Rosser. "Frontotemporal Dementia." *BMJ* 347 (2013): f4827.

Zampieri, C., and R. P. Di Fabio. "Balance and Eye Movement Training to Improve Gait in People with Progressive Supranuclear Palsy: Quasi-Randomized Clinical Trial." *Physical Therapy* 88, no. 12 (December 2008): 1460–73.

CHAPTER 12

CHALLENGING THE MIND

Activities and Socialization

Lisa Ann Fagan, MS, OTR/L

INTRODUCTION

Engaging in activities, or "doing things," benefits us in many ways. Activities can bring us joy or a sense of purpose. They can shape our identity and help structure our days and nights. Engaging in activities during the day can lead to more restful nights. Without meaningful activities and social roles, we would become so bored that time would seem endless, and we would have difficulty defining ourselves. One of the tragedies of dementia is that it alters a person's ability to participate in activities and relationships long before the body is ready to stop.[1]

Frontotemporal degeneration (FTD) can cause a myriad of symptoms that can alter an individual's ability to engage in activities. Behavioral manifestations, including a decline in interpersonal conduct, poor impulse control, and depression, can cause social isolation and decreased opportunities for interaction.[2] Linguistic deficits common in FTD (word finding, word substitution, progressive nonfluent aphasia, semantic dementia, and other disorders) impact an individual's ability to communicate, thereby limiting social interaction.[3] Cognitive and perceptual changes, such as a decline in memory, inability to plan and sequence activities, and diminished visual-perceptual skills, can cause further limitations in initiating and participating in desired activities.[4]

A decline in active engagement with life (lack of activity participation and interpersonal relationships) has been linked to many negative outcomes, including depression, anxiety, pacing, and agitation.[5] Finding activities that are meaningful and provide successful experiences, and are not viewed as "childish" or "busy work," is a major challenge for caregivers.[6]

INDEPENDENCE ISSUES

Individuals with FTD are, first and foremost, adults. They have led successful lives, simultaneously balancing a variety of roles: spouse, parent, employee, hobbyist, religious participant, community volunteer, and others too varied to mention. Losing the ability to control one's own actions, thoughts, and feelings is distressing, and some individuals valiantly strive to remain autonomous in the early stages of dementia. In some individuals, there is an early loss of insight into their abilities, and the loss of self and abilities appears to cause them less concern than it does their family.

Activities and social interaction should promote maintenance of skills and abilities, compensate for declining capabilities, and incorporate familiar roles and routines of daily life. Allowing for choices in activities fosters a sense a control.[7] Success-oriented tasks allow the individual to feel pride in accomplishments and to sustain self-identity.[8]

THE JUST-RIGHT CHALLENGE— MODIFYING ACTIVITIES FOR SUCCESS

Finding the "just-right challenge" that balances abilities with interests is a daunting task for caregivers. To be able to complete a task independently, sometimes the activity must be simplified. Making cookies from a premeasured mix is easier than making them from scratch. Setting a table is easier if all the needed objects are gathered and put on the table before you ask the individual with FTD for assistance.

We often provide many directions for an activity at one time (e.g., "Finish watering the plants, then come inside and wash your hands before lunch"). Providing one-step directions may be needed to ensure successful task completion and promote continued independence (e.g., "Please water those plants" as you hand the individual a watering can, and point toward the plants that need attention). Many individuals find giving one-step direction to be challenging, but it becomes easier with time and practice.

The environment in which the activity takes place can either promote independence or constrain abilities. Excess noise and excess clutter can cause difficulty in concentration, resulting in distraction from the desired task. An environment that is too hot or too cold can impact performance, as can an environment that is not well lit.

Your mood as a caregiver can influence the activity as well. If you are stressed or irritable, the individual with FTD may perceive your mood and become anxious as well. Anxiety often leads to decreased task performance. Try to remain calm and maintain your sense of humor when possible.

SPECIFIC TYPES OF ACTIVITIES

Activities can be divided into four categories based on various characteristics of the tasks: activities of daily living, work/productive activities, play/leisure, and rest/relaxation. These are the groupings used by occupational therapists to classify the intent of the activity.[9] These categories cover the range of activities and interactions in which an individual participates throughout the day. Individuals need a balance of these tasks to maintain a healthy lifestyle.

Activities of daily living (ADLs) include several tasks discussed in other chapters: grooming, hygiene, bathing, dressing (chapter 13), feeding (chapter 10), and mobility (chapter 11). Other ADLs include socialization, functional communication, and sexual expression. These activities promote physical and psychological health and well-being.

For many individuals with FTD, socialization is challenged by behavioral disinhibition that may not be understood by friends, neighbors, and distant relatives. It would be wise to discuss behavioral changes with visitors before the interaction so that the visitor is not shocked or offended by comments made by the individual with FTD. Small gatherings (one to four individuals) are usually more successful than larger-group activities.

Functional communication refers to the manner in which we express and receive information regarding thoughts, feelings, needs, and desires. Verbal-language abilities, facial expressions, gestures, body language, written language, and use of symbols and pictures are all forms of functional communication. Individuals with FTD often have difficulty with verbal language and many have blunted affects, making it difficult to express emotions.

Occasionally, written language or symbols and pictures may provide a more accurate method of communicating than relying on verbal language and facial expression. For individuals with prior knowledge or experience with keyboards, typing may be more successful than oral communication. Picture boards (graphic depictions of commonly needed items, such as a glass of water, toilet, sweater, book, etc.) can be useful when an individual is unable to verbally request a specific item.

Sexual expression or engaging in intimacy is often severely altered by FTD. Individuals may make inappropriate comments or violate other social norms of conduct. Some may become apathetic to their partner's wants and needs and seek only their own fulfillment. Others may become depressed and withdrawn and will not initiate any forms of intimacy.

Work/productive activities include household tasks (meal preparation, cleaning, clothing care, money management, household maintenance, and other tasks), care of others (grandchildren, pets, etc.), and vocational and volunteer activities. These tasks can often be divided into chunks that can be easily managed by the individual with FTD, if the activity is meaningful and interests the person. These activities promote self-identity and self-esteem.

A gentleman who considers himself to be a good home maintainer might take pride in changing light bulbs, raking leaves, or balancing a checkbook. A woman who went to great lengths to keep the home neat might enjoy dusting or folding laundry. Meal preparation can be broken into many smaller activities: making a salad, setting the table, frosting a cake. Many individuals with dementia enjoy the unconditional love of pets. Feeding, grooming, petting, or walking an animal may be very rewarding activities.

The kitchen can present many safety hazards for individuals with dementia. If an individual is likely to attempt a cooking task involving the stove, an electrician can install a range cut-off switch. Chapter 14 provides more home safety recommendations.

Care must be exercised when deciding whether or not to let an individual with FTD babysit young children. Due to the difficulties with cognitive language and social skills that many individuals with FTD experience, another adult should always be present when young children are in the home.

Play/leisure activities are another source of meaningful engagement for many individuals. Amusement, spontaneous enjoyment, and self-expression are possible outcomes of play and leisure activities.[10] Although some previous pursuits may become too challenging as the disease progresses, many individuals are able to participate in former pastimes in some manner.

Games with complex rules (e.g., chess, Scrabble®), may need to be played as a team, or in a simplified manner. Card games may need to be simplified from games with complicated rules (such as pinochle or poker) to simpler games (blackjack or matching games) to games of chance (such as war).

Physical activities (such as dancing or taking a walk) can provide exercise as well as recreation, as can playing catch with a grandchild.

Music is a terrific activity. For those who played the piano or other musical instruments, that ability often remains unaffected until the late stages of dementia. Although they might not be able to read music or learn a new piece, many individuals have memorized musical pieces that they frequently played, and can still recall them. Others may simply enjoy listening.

Gardening is the most popular leisure activity in the United States. Many individuals enjoy puttering in the garden, pulling an occasional weed, cutting a few flowers, or picking a ripe tomato. Others enjoy tending to indoor plants (e.g., watering, removing dead leaves, repotting larger plants that have out-grown the present container). Gardening activities can provide links to the former self and promote self-esteem.

Art can provide an outlet for many who are unable to express themselves verbally. Some individuals with dementia who previously thought of them-selves as "unartistic" can produce beautiful, expressive works. Creating small pieces from modeling clay can be enjoyable for some. There are many colored plastic clay products available in arts-and-crafts stores. Others enjoy painting or coloring activities. Some individuals enjoy creating art from a blank canvas or paper; others benefit from the structure of adult-appropriate patterns books that they fill in with color. Pattern books cover a wide array of interests, from flowers and butterflies to trains, cars, and sport scenes. Patterns may be printed on translucent paper (creating a stained-glass effect) or on paper that accepts watercolors. One series of pattern books features outlines of famous works of art that you color or paint.

Reading is an activity enjoyed by many individuals. In the early stages of FTD, an individual might be able to read a large-print short story or poem aloud with a friend, family member, or caregiver, and discuss the story after-ward. Others may enjoy hearing familiar poems or stories being read to them. Some people enjoy looking at or reading magazines. The photographs and shorter article length in most magazines are more easily understood than those in bigger or longer publications.

Reminiscence activities, such as looking through photo albums or watching old family movies, may be a meaningful activity to some individ-uals. For others, it may cause confusion or sadness.

Family celebrations might be overwhelming for some individuals. Family members may not understand the behavior of the individual with FTD and the individual with FTD might not recognize friends and family or be able to verbalize names. Smaller groups tend to be easier to tolerate. Familiar traditions and rituals may need to be modified in response to the individual's capabilities (e.g., someone else might need to carve the Thanksgiving turkey or make the birthday cake).

Rest/relaxation includes passive activities (e.g., watching TV, listening to music) that require little participation, and spiritual activities that renew the soul. Some individuals have difficulty discriminating between TV and reality, and may become anxious when watching the news or action programs. Movies may be too long in duration for the individual to follow, but familiar movies might be enjoyed for brief periods. Avoid using children's programs as entertainment. There are several companies that make adult-appropriate videos (e.g., nature, animals, travelogs through foreign countries that the individual has visited). Some may be available at the local library.

Many individuals may not be able to tolerate attending religious services, but they might enjoy televised or taped services and familiar songs and hymns. Prayers learned in youth might be recalled and provide a source of comfort for some.

Some individuals benefit from stress reduction and relaxation techniques when anxious. A hand massage with scented lotion, some deep-breathing exercises (with simple verbal cues, such as "Breathe in" and "Breathe out"), or reciting a favorite poem can assist a person to become calmer. Petting a cat or a soft-textured fabric (e.g., chenille or velvet) may work for other people. Finding an effective stress-reduction or relaxation technique is an individualized process, but a very important one, if you are caring for a person who frequently becomes anxious. If the individual is unable to be calmed after several alternatives are attempted, the physician should be contacted.

EXERCISE

Daily physical activity is important for everyone, regardless of current fitness level.[11] Walking, dancing, swimming, riding a stationary bike, or engaging in other forms of physical movement is recommended to maintain muscle mass, promote cardiovascular health, maintain flexibility and balance, decrease depression, enhance cognitive functioning, and promote general psychological well-being. For optimal cardiovascular benefit, aerobic activity is usually recommended for at least twenty minutes per session, with three to five sessions per week, after approval from your physician. This topic is covered in more detail in chapter 11.

For some individuals, exercise can be made more enjoyable with music, videos, or games. Dancing or marching to favorite music, participating along with a video, playing basketball or golf, or imitating movements done by a caregiver are all forms of exercise.

Some individuals prefer a more regimented exercise program that includes hand-held weights, exercise bands, or pulleys. There are many styles of hand-held weights and cuff-style ankle/wrist weights available at sporting-goods stores and mass-merchandise stores. Exercise bands are available at some sporting-goods stores as well as through therapy-supply vendors listed in the "Resources" section at the end of this chapter. Over-the-door pulleys encourage full arm movement. They can be used as needed, then removed from the doorframe; and they are available through the therapy-supply vendors listed in the "Resources" section.

FREEDOM AND SAFETY

Some individuals with dementia are at a high risk for wandering and/or getting lost, due to decreased topographical orientation (the ability to find one's way). Even familiar routes may become confusing at some point during the disease process. An individual may not be able to state where she lives or be able to give her name. Such an individual should wear an identification bracelet or necklace so that police and rescue authorities could return a lost individual to his home. The MedicAlert® + Alzheimer's Association Safe Return® program offers such an identification bracelet or necklace, along with a communications network to alert authorities of a missing person. There are also safety services that use GPS and cellular technology to manage a person's location.

Home-safety modifications are a vital part of a safety program. If possible, an enclosed yard offers a safe area to enjoy nature without the risks of wandering. See chapter 14 for more information.

DRIVING

For many individuals (with or without dementia), surrendering a driver's license is one of the most emotionally upsetting times in their life. Many individuals in the United States fear losing their driver's license more than they fear going to a nursing home or dying.[12] In the United States, being able to drive a car fosters independence and freedom.

In some states, a person cannot hold a driver's license once a diagnosis of dementia is made. In other states, there is no such restriction. A driving evaluation may be recommended by the neurologist or physician to determine if the individual is still capable of driving.[13] The evaluation is usually completed by an occupational therapist, and the results are sent to the referring physician and (if required by state law) to the Department of Motor Vehicles.

Individuals may still attempt to drive after a driver's license has been surrendered; therefore, in some cases, car keys need to be hidden or cars need to be sold, so that the individual with dementia will not drive.

SUMMARY

Activities are the everyday tasks that provide our lives with meaning, shape our identity, and allow us to accomplish our daily routines. Dementia can rob a person of the ability to initiate a task or complete a complex activity. Tasks can be simplified, or given in one-step directions, to promote continued independence and success.

There are many types of activities, including daily living, work/productive, play/leisure, and rest/relaxation activities. Those that require special consideration include driving, babysitting, and other safety-related issues. Maintaining a balance of activities that are success-oriented and meaningful to the individual helps promote physical and psychological well-being.

TABLE 12.1. The Dos and Don'ts of Activities Planning for Individuals with FTD

(adapted from *Activity Programming for Persons with Dementia: A Sourcebook*)

DO	DON'T
Treat the person as an adult	Speak to the person as if he/she is a child
Provide a calm environment	Yell at or scold the person
Simplify instructions	Give up
Establish a familiar routine	
Provide encouragement	
Be patient and flexible	
Help the person remain as independent as possible	

TABLE 12.2. Suggested Activities

Exercise/Physical Activities	taking a walk
	dancing
	raking leaves/gardening
	vacuuming
	exercising (may need to follow demonstrated exercises)
Creative Activities	doing art projects (clay, painting, coloring, etc.)
	playing musical instruments
Relaxation Activities	listening to music
	watching TV or movies
	getting a hand massage
	singing religious hymns or saying prayers
	petting a cat or dog
Cognitive-Stimulation Activities	listening to stories/poems
	playing simplified word or card games
	reminiscing (recalling family events)

Purposeful Activities

assisting with household chores (setting
the table, folding laundry, etc.)
assisting with meal preparation
providing self-care (bathing, dressing,
grooming)
giving pet care

RESOURCES

Exercise equipment is available from several vendors. An Internet search using the keywords *TheraBand*™ or *over door pulleys* will yield several results. Here is a sample of vendor sites:

TheraBand, The Hygenic Corporation, 800-321-2135 (toll-free), www .thera-band.com

Over the Door Pulleys, PrePak Products, Inc., 800-544-7527 (toll-free), www.prepakproducts.com

NOTES

1. J. M. Zgola, *Doing Things: A Guide to Programming Activities for Persons with Alzheimer's Disease and Related Disorders* (Baltimore: Johns Hopkins University Press, 1987);1Alzheimer's Association, *Activity Programming for Persons with Dementia: A Sourcebook* (Chicago: Alzheimer's Association, 1995).

2. P. Mychack et al., "The Influence of Right Frontotemporal Dysfunction on Social Behavior in Frontotemporal Dementia," *Neurology* 56, no. 11, suppl. 4 (2001): S11–S15.

3. M. Grossman, "A Multidisciplinary Approach to Pick's Disease and Frontotemporal Dementia," *Neurology* 56, no. 11, suppl. 4 (2001): S1–S2.

4. Ibid.;1K. M. Robinson, "Rehabilitation Applications in Caring for Patients with Pick's Disease and Frontotemporal Dementias," *Neurology* 56, no. 11, suppl. 4 (2001): S56–S58.

5. J. W. Rowe and R. L. Kahn, "Successful Aging," in *Healthy Aging: Challenges and Solutions*, ed. K. Dychtwald (Gaithersburg, MD: Aspen, 1999); Zgola, *Doing Things*.

6. C. J. Camp, ed., *Montessori-Based Activities for Persons with Dementia*, vol. 1 (Beachwood, OH: Menorah Park Center for Senior Living, 1999).

7. S. H. Briller et al., "Maximizing Cognitive and Functional Abilities," in *Creating Successful Dementia Care Settings*, ed. M. P. Calkins (Baltimore, MD: Health Professions, 2001).

8. Zgola, *Doing Things*; Alzheimer's Association, *Activity Programming for Persons with Dementia.*

9. American Occupational Therapy Association, *Occupational Therapy Practice Guidelines for Adults with Dementia* (Bethesda, MD: American Occupational Therapy Association, 1999).

10. J. A. Brackley, *Creating Moments of Joy for the Person with Alzheimer's or Dementia* (Polk City, IA: Enhanced Living, 1999); American Occupational Therapy Association, *Occupational Therapy Practice Guidelines for Adults with Dementia.*

11. President's Council on Physical Fitness and Sports Research Digest, *Physical Activity and Aging: Implications for Health and Quality of Life*, series 3, no. 4 (Washington, DC: President's Council on Physical Fitness, 1998).

12. J. Diffendal, "Giving Up the Car Keys: When Are Dementia Patients Unfit to Drive?" *Advance for Occupational Therapy Practitioners* (July 17, 2000).

13. Association for Driver Rehabilitation Specialists, *Fact Sheet on Driving and Alzheimer's/Dementia* (Edgerton, WI: Association for Driver Rehabilitation Specialists, n.d.).

CHAPTER 13

FOSTERING PERSONAL CARE

Hygiene, Dressing, and Eating

Lisa Ann Fagan, MS, OTR/L

For individuals with a progressive neurodegenerative disease such as FTD, the ability to maintain maximal independence in the everyday activities of personal care (such as hygiene and dressing), or the ability of others to provide such care, becomes of paramount importance. Improvements in self-care tasks are not expected. However, the ability to maintain current levels of function is facilitated through strategies to reduce the effort required to achieve tasks or by changing the environment to promote independence. A focus on assisting the individual by doing the personal care tasks *with* the person, instead of doing it *for* the person, is the key to maximizing remaining skills and preventing overdependence on caregivers.

Another critical issue for individuals with FTD and their families is the maintenance of personal safety. In many individuals with dementia, their ability to conduct themselves in a safe manner is lost early in the disease process due to a number of factors, from sensory changes to impulsive behavior. Strategies for maintaining a safe environment for personal care will be discussed.

FACTORS AFFECTING ABILITY TO PARTICIPATE IN PERSONAL CARE

Psychosocial/Emotional Factors

- disinhibition of social norms (doesn't care what others think)
- depression (poor motivation to engage in any activities)

- fear of falling during personal-care activities (limits willingness to move)
- paranoia, embarrassment, or anger

Cognitive Factors

- limited attention span (doesn't remember to complete all steps of an activity)
- decreased awareness of environmental cues (doesn't notice toothbrush in bathroom, forgets to brush teeth before bed)
- difficulty following complex verbal directions
- sequencing difficulty (can't figure out which item to put on first)
- perceptual deficits (puts right arm in left sleeve of a shirt)

Sensory Factors

- doesn't respond to internal cues (need to void, hunger/thirst/fullness, etc.)
- becomes distracted by background noises
- perceives touch as threatening

Physical Factors

- unable to plan body movements (difficulty putting leg in trousers)
- balance or mobility problems (difficulty standing or sitting without support)
- decreased coordination (difficulty fastening buttons)
- decreased endurance or strength from disuse (too tired to assist)

(Adapted from Hellen 1998)

STRATEGIES TO ASSIST INDIVIDUALS WITH PERSONAL-CARE TASKS

1. Timing—know when the individual is best able to assist (showers or baths might be more successful in the evening as opposed in to the morning, or vice versa).

2. Consistency—a familiar caregiver, following a set routine, is often the most successful arrangement.

3. Focus on abilities—involve the individual in assisting as much as possible, and praise attempts (whether successful or not).

4. Cueing—give one-step directions (e.g., "Wash your face" as you hand the individual a washcloth)

5. Distraction—use singing, food, holding an item, etc., if the individual becomes upset during personal-care activities, or to prevent the person from becoming upset.

6. Mirroring—an individual may be able to copy actions demonstrated by the caregiver (such as brushing teeth, combing hair, etc.).

7. Chaining—the caregiver initiates the activity, then the individual completes the task (such as buttoning, washing an arm or leg in the shower, shaving with an electric razor, etc.).

(Adapted from Hellen 1998)

HYGIENE (GROOMING, TOILETING, AND BATHING)

The ability to maintain body cleanliness, as well as complete activities related to elimination of body waste, is important for health and for social acceptance. While cultural norms may dictate higher or lower expectations of cleanliness, basic hygiene is important to prevent odors, infection, and disease. Individuals with dementia may not recognize the need for maintaining good hygiene due to disinhibition of social norms and other psychosocial and emotional factors, decreased sensory awareness, or decreased cognitive skills, as mentioned in the previous section.

Grooming includes the tasks we perform to maintain our appearance and health. These include activities such as toothbrushing and/or denture care; shaving; hair care; nail care; eye care (including applying glasses or contact lenses); ear care (including applying hearing aids); applying deodorant, powders, or lotions; and applying cosmetics.

In the early stages of FTD, environmental strategies such as leaving grooming items in a visible location alongside the sink may cue individuals to use the objects and complete tasks. For some, a daily checklist is helpful, to provide order and organization to the grooming routine.

In later stages, mirroring (demonstrating the tasks) is an effective strategy, as is chaining (initiating the task and letting the individual complete the activity). Limiting the environmental cues can be helpful because too many visible items can cause confusion.

In late stages, assistance from the caregiver is required. Allowing the individual to complete whatever steps of the grooming task he or she can is important to promote feelings of accomplishment and to prevent overdependence on caregivers.

Toileting includes activities related to excretory body functions. Activities include clothing management, managing continence needs (including catheters or colostomies), cleaning the body, and applying protective equipment (such as disposable pads or briefs).

In the early stages of FTD, environmental strategies, such as leaving the bathroom door open, may prompt the individual to use the toilet. Other environmental strategies include painting the wall behind the toilet a contrasting color to increase the visibility of the toilet or installing a floor surface (linoleum, vinyl tile, carpeting) in a contrasting color. Another strategy is to mark a pathway with colored tape on the floor between the bed or chair, etc., and the bathroom, so the individual can follow the trail.

Verbal prompts on a regular basis (before or after meals, for example) can promote continued continence. Clothing that is easier to manage (such as elastic-waist pants instead of zippered trousers) may allow for continued success with toileting.

In the later stages, more environmental modifications may be needed, including grab bars along the toilet to provide stability during transfers, and a raised toilet seat to make transfers easier for the caregiver.

If getting in and out of the bathroom becomes a challenge due to difficulty with transfers or mobility, a commode may be needed. Commodes can be rented or purchased from medical-supply companies. Commodes come in several different styles, and some have armrests that can be removed for sliding transfers.

In the late stages of FTD, the individual may not respond to internal cues to void. Incontinence care may need to be provided, and disposable briefs may be used to avoid accidental soiling of clothing. While the individual is in bed, some caregivers use protective devices to prevent soiling of the bedding. These devices include disposable absorbent pads can be placed on top of the fitted sheet, beneath the individual, and changed as need. Other caregivers prefer to use waterproof mattress pads.

Bathing includes cleansing of body parts (whether in a shower or tub, or by sink, or through use of newer products such as premoistened towelettes) as well as the rinsing and drying of the body. Many individuals with dementia have an aversion to bathing. The reason behind this phenomenon is not fully understood but could be related to several factors:

- fear of water
- modesty
- fear of falling

Whatever the cause of the anxiety, assisting with bathing is one of the most challenging of all personal-care tasks for the caregiver and can be a significant factor in considering the need for professional assistance in the home or facility-based care.

Whatever method of bathing is selected, start by assembling all the necessary items: soap, shampoo or shower cap, washcloth, towels, robe, and any other products needed. Caregivers may want to wear a water-resistant apron or bathing suit to avoid getting their clothes wet. They must make sure they have everything gathered in advance, since some individuals should not be left in the bathtub or shower alone while the caregiver retrieves missing supplies.

Some individuals may be more calm during the bathing routine if soft music is playing or if scented bath products are used. Others dislike being cold and respond best in a warmer ambient temperature. A ceiling-mounted heat lamp may be helpful.

For all methods of bathing, the individual should be encouraged to assist as much as possible, from washing body parts after verbal or visual cues to completing the action once initiated by the caregiver.

For individuals who prefer taking a bath, getting in and out of the tub may be the most difficult and dangerous part of the task. Nonskid strips, decals, or a mat decrease the risk of slips or falls. A hydraulic or mechanical seat that raises and lowers the individual in the tub can be extremely helpful for the caregiver. There are models of bathtubs in which the side wall rolls down to allow the individual to easily enter and exit the tub. These tubs would replace the existing tub, but would fit in the same space.

For assisting individuals who stand while showering, most caregivers report that using a stall shower is an easier option than showering in a bathtub. As with the bathtub, a nonskid floor surface will reduce the risk of slips and falls. Grab bars should be installed in and around the shower stall. They are important wherever the individual would reach for support when entering and exiting the shower stall, and where he would require support while standing during the shower. Grab bars can be installed vertically, horizontally, or on a diagonal, depending on need. An occupational therapist can assist in determining the proper location for grab bars. (See chapter 14 for further details regarding environmental modifications.)

Many individuals are less fearful if they face away from the shower stream, facing toward the opposite wall. A horizontally mounted grab bar on the rear wall can give the individual something to hold onto for an increased feeling of support. A handheld shower is highly recommended by many caregivers, using the following strategies:

- Adjust the water temperature before directing water toward the individual.
- Use a gentle stream or mist of water.
- Start with a less sensitive part of the body, such as the feet.
- Move the water around the individual instead of having the individual move.

(Adapted from Olsen 1993)

For individuals who have difficulty standing, a bath or tub seat may be used. There are several styles from which to choose. A seat with a backrest is almost always preferable to a stool, as it provides more support. Other design factors to consider include armrests, seats that extend over the rim of the tub (to allow an individual to slide over the side of the tub, rather than step in and out of the tub), and padding. The individual's need for support and the available space in the bathroom may influence the decision to choose a style with or without armrests and/or an extended seat.

For individuals who are unable or unwilling to take a shower or bath, thorough cleansing can be accomplished by a sink or sponge bath, or by the use of commercially available premoistened towelettes. Dry shampoo (a powder that is applied to the head and brushed out) can be used if the individual does not like to have her hair washed.

DRESSING

We often dress in a manner that expresses our personal taste and style. For some individuals with dementia, maintaining the same style of dress as before the illness may be important to self-image and self-esteem. A former businessman may prefer to wear a shirt and tie every day; some ladies are accustomed to wearing a dress, jewelry, and makeup at all times. For others, clothing has little personal value.

We often take for granted the complex physical and cognitive skills involved in selecting and donning apparel. Choosing clothing from a full closet or dresser that is appropriate for the weather and that coordinates can be a daunting task for anyone. Limiting choices can be one strategy to simplify dressing. One way to limit choices is by keeping only seasonal items in the closet or hanging complete outfits on one hanger (pants/skirt and shirt/blouse) and letting the individual choose the outfit for the day. Another way to limit choices is by giving the choice between two items when ready to dress (e.g., "Do you want to wear the tan pants or the blue pants today?").

Some individuals prefer to wear the same outfit repeatedly, giving the caregiver little opportunity to clean the clothes. Buying multiples of the same outfit allows the caregiver to wash one set while the other is being worn.

Loose-fitting styles of clothing (such as elastic-waist pants in knit materials) and button-front shirts and sweaters are easier to put on than other styles. Shoes with hook and loop closures may be easier than tying laces. Shoes should have a rubber, non-skid sole and offer stability while walking and transferring.

Some individuals, when faced at one time with all items to be worn (undergarments, clothing, sweater, etc.) have difficulty determining which items to put on first. The proper sequence or order of which item goes on first is not recalled, and pieces of clothing can be skipped or put on top of other items (such as undergarments over pants or shirts). Layering clothing in the order in which it is put on is helpful in preventing such mistakes.

Others need assistance only in starting the process of putting on an item of clothing. After receiving assistance with the initial step (such as putting an arm into a sleeve), they can complete the rest of the task.

Some individuals with FTD may undress themselves at socially inappropriate times. Clothing that is more difficult to remove, such as shirts that have buttons or zippers in the back, offers a greater challenge to the individual with FTD, which might prevent him from removing the clothing at inappropriate times and consequently remain properly clothed for a longer period of time. Avoid putting button-front shirts on backward, as they do not fit correctly and are uncomfortable. Other strategies to prevent inappropriate disrobing include wearing multiple layers of clothing (e.g., undershirt, shirt, and sweater or vest), wearing clothing that is more challenging to remove (such as overalls or jumpsuits), and facing belt buckles toward the back instead of the front of the body.

EATING

We eat for a variety of reasons: to satisfy our hunger, to provide pleasure through our senses of smell and taste, to be polite in certain situations, and several other factors. Individuals with FTD often experience changes in habits and behaviors relating to food. They may overeat or constantly crave certain food items (especially sweets). They may disregard manners and social graces while eating and may try to eat nonfood items.

To curb overeating, some caregivers limit access to the refrigerator or snack drawers through the use of locks on these areas, or they block access to the kitchen. While this may work for a brief period, many caregivers report that their loved ones find ways to obtain food regardless of the method used to prevent access.

To slow the pace at which some individuals consume food, weighted utensils may be used. The added resistance may slow the rate of speed with which they eat. These utensils may be purchased online by doing a search for "weighted utensils."

To reduce the likelihood that individuals may try to help themselves to food from someone else's plate, try using colored tape to mark a zone for each person at the table.

For individuals experiencing difficulty using utensils, a plate guard may be helpful. The device enables the individual to load food onto the utensil by pushing it against the plate guard and onto the fork or spoon. If the plate slides away from the individual, try using a nonskid placemat.

Some individuals with FTD have difficulty holding cups, and a mug may be easier to grasp. Unbreakable cups and mugs should be used when possible.

A bendable straw can also be used if drinking from a cup or mug becomes compromised.

When utensil usage becomes too challenging, an individual may still be capable of feeding him- or herself "finger foods." Fish sticks, chicken fingers, sandwiches, fruit and cereal bars, hard-boiled eggs, and tacos are all fingers foods, but there are many other possibilities as well. Almost any cooked meat can be wrapped in a flour tortilla; a scoop of tuna salad can be put on an ice cream cone. Many foods, while not necessarily neat, can be eaten by hand, including pieces of meatloaf, sausage links, waffles with jelly instead of syrup, and many others. These are but a few examples—use your creativity to think of other options.

SAFETY

Individuals with FTD often have difficulty with self-regulation and safety awareness. They may not realize the potential danger of situations, including cooking, using tools, smoking, and other engaging in other activities.

Some caregivers have a cut-off switch installed on the stove or oven, so that the individual with FTD cannot turn on the range without supervision.

For individuals who use power tools, lawnmowers, and other tools, the basement or garage may need to be locked to prevent unsupervised access to these items.

If the individual smokes cigarettes, cigars, or pipes, he or she may need supervision or assistance with using matches or lighters.

Gentlemen may need supervision while shaving, and a safety razor or an electric shaver should be used.

A lack of attention to sensory cues (such as water temperature in the shower) can lead to accidental scalding. Reducing the temperature setting on the water heater can prevent burns.

ASSISTING WITH TRANSFERS

In the later stages of the disease, individuals may experience limitations in movement. They may require assistance getting up and down from the bed, chair, or toilet, and they may need to use a wheelchair. During transfers, caregivers must be careful to avoid injuring themselves and the individual needing assistance. There are a few basic safety points when assisting with any transfer:

- Make sure each person has nonskid footwear, securely fastened.
- Remember to keep your back as straight as possible—bend from the knees!
- Have the individual "scoot" forward toward the end of the seat.
- Make sure the individual's feet are on the floor, with heels slightly behind the front of the seat if possible.
- Have the individual lean slightly forward and place hands on armrests if available, or on the surface of the seat.
- Prepare the individual to stand (count to three, or give a short direction, such as "Stand up").
- Assist the individual as needed, either from the side (with a hand at or slightly below the waist, or under the arm) or from the front (with hands slightly below the waist). Do not pull the individual up by the arms.
- If you need to lift the individual, a transfer belt may be used.

(Adapted from Zgola 1987)

A physical therapist or occupational therapist can teach you the proper method to assist with transfers so both you and your loved one are safe.

SUMMARY

Assisting individuals to maintain as much independence as possible in self-care tasks is an important part of caregiving. An emphasis on doing *with*, rather than doing *for*, the individual maintains his or her dignity and self-esteem. Simplify activities to allow for continued participation by the individual with FTD, and modify tasks to ensure safety. As each person in the world is unique, so too is each individual with FTD. Not every strategy presented here will be helpful for each person; these suggestions are but a guide.

BIBLIOGRAPHY

American Occupational Therapy Association. *Occupational Therapy Practice Guidelines for Adults with Dementia*. Bethesda, MD: American Occupational Therapy Association, 1999.

Briller, S. H., et al. "Maximizing Cognitive and Functional Abilities." In *Creating Successful Dementia Care Settings*, ed. M. P. Calkins. Baltimore, MD: Health Professions, 2001.

Hellen, C. R. *Alzheimer's Disease: Activity-Focused Care*, 2d ed. Boston, MA: Butterworth-Heinemann, 1998.

Mychack, P., et al. "The Influence of Right Frontotemporal Dysfunction on Social Behavior in Frontotemporal Dementia." *Neurology* 56, no. 11, suppl. 4 (2001): S11–S15.

Olsen, R. V., E. Ehrenkrantz, and B. Hutchings. *Homes That Help: Advice from Caregivers for Creating a Supportive Home*. Newark, NJ: NJIT, 1993.

Perrin, T., and H. May. *Well-Being in Dementia: An Occupational Approach for Therapists and Carers*. Edinburgh, Scotland: Churchill Livingstone, 2000.

Robinson, K. M. "Rehabilitation Applications in Caring for Patients with Pick's Disease and Frontotemporal Dementias." *Neurology* 56, no. 11, suppl. 4 (2001): S56–S58.

Zgola, J. M. *Doing Things: A Guide to Programming Activities for Persons with Alzheimer's Disease and Related Disorders*. Baltimore, MD: Johns Hopkins University Press, 1987.

CHAPTER 14

WITHIN THESE WALLS

Creating a Safe and Supportive Environment

Lisa Ann Fagan, MS, OTR/L

According to interior designer Betsy Brawley, who specializes in designing environments for individuals with dementia, the environment is a "silent partner in caregiving."[1] A well-planned environment can be supportive and promote continued abilities and participation in activities, while a nonsupportive environment can lead to falls, agitation, and a decline in functional skills by limiting opportunities to participate in activities. This chapter will provide an overview of the role of the environment in supporting care and strategies to improve the fit between the individual with frontotemporal degeneration (FTD) and his environment.

Just as no two persons are alike, no two environments are alike. The physical space, the objects in the space, and the interactions of the people in the space make each environment unique. The strategies presented in this chapter are ones that have worked for many individuals but may not be applicable or helpful in all situations. If there is a specific environmental challenge in your home, an occupational-therapy home evaluation may be useful to determine an individualized environmental-modification plan.

The need for environmental modification will change over the course of the illness, as well as in response to the aging process or other medical conditions the individual with FTD experiences. In the early stages of the disease, only minor modifications may be needed to simplify the environment and promote safety. As the disease progresses, more substantial adaptations may be needed, including installing grab bars, or making the home wheelchair accessible. Planning ahead is crucial. If you anticipate needing to make major changes (such as adding a first-floor bedroom or bathroom), it is best to start renovations when the individual is in the earlier stages of dementia. This gives her more time to adjust to the environment before she experiences further declines and is less able to adapt to changes.

CREATING A CALM AND REASSURING ENVIRONMENT

For many caregivers, creating a calming environment to reduce anxious or agitated behavior is the first goal of environmental modifications.[2] Various objects in the environment can frighten or upset the individual with dementia. Sensory overstimulation can also lead to anxiety. When the individual with dementia becomes stressed, he is unable to change the environment to reduce the source of the stress. He may try to escape the environment (wander away or attempt to leave the house), become combative or resistive during care, or become extremely violent. Eliminating the sources of environmental stress can reduce anxiety and promote a calmer atmosphere.

The following can be sources of environmental stress for some individuals. Suggested strategies to reduce the stress follow in italics.

Mirrors
: The individual may not recognize her own reflection and be frightened that a stranger is in the house.
  —*Remove the mirror or cover it with a pull-down shade.*

Photographs
: Some individuals do not recognize current pictures of friends and family members and are confused by them.
  —*Label the photographs or remove the pictures and replace them with photographs the individual recognizes (pictures taken during the years before the onset of the disease).*

Television
: The individual may think there are other people in the room or may not be able to differentiate between reality and the television program.
  —*Do not watch violent or scary programs.*
  —*Try watching nature programs, reruns of favorite shows, or old movies.*

Excess noise
: Too many sources of overlapping noise, such as the television, a barking dog, a ringing telephone, and a radio being played in a nearby room can cause auditory overstimulation.

	—Reduce noise levels throughout the house. Use sound-absorbent materials (carpeting, drapes) to reduce noise levels.
Excess glare	Unfiltered sunlight shining through windows or reflecting off of shiny surfaces, such as floors or mirrors, can cause visual stress.
	—Use light-filtering window coverings (sheers, blinds, or shades).
	—Consider nonglare floor surfaces (carpet, tile).
	—Move mirrors that reflect sunlight.
Too little light/ uneven light levels	Shadows or dark areas within a room may cause fear.
	—Provide increased lighting that covers a room with even levels of light.
Clutter	Too many objects in the environment can overstimulate.
	—Reduce the number of items in the room.
Room temperature	Increased agitation has been reported in environments that were perceived as too cold or too hot by the individual.
	—Regulate room temperature or add/remove a sweater as needed.
Seeing an area they cannot access	Seeing the front yard or back deck but not being able to get there because the doors are locked can cause stress.
	—Provide access to safe areas (fenced backyard) if possible.
	—Cover windows to reduce distractions.
Locked doors	Some individuals are frustrated because they want to be able to open the door and cannot do so.
	—Camouflage the door (paint or wallpaper the door the same as the rest of the wall).
Unable to find the bathroom	Some individuals are unable to remember where the bathroom is located.
	—Keep the bathroom door open.
	—Paint the bathroom door a different color than the other doors in the house.
	—Label the door with a sign that states "Bathroom" or "Toilet" or has a picture of a toilet.

For some individuals, creating an environment that includes pleasurable sensory experiences can be calming. The following strategies may reduce anxiety:

Colors	Pastel or light colors may be more soothing than dark or bright colors.
Sounds	Pleasant sounds, such as soft music or nature sounds, may be calming.
Textures	Pillow, blankets, or other objects in soft textures (velvet, chenille, corduroy, etc.) may be held or stroked to relieve stress.
Aromas	Some scents (vanilla, orange, lavender, and others) have calming properties.

The use of scented bath products or room sprays is safer than burning scented candles or bowls of potpourri, which may appear edible.

CREATING A SAFE ENVIRONMENT

Safety is an essential requirement of all living environments. The prevention of injury is a goal of great importance to caregivers. For individuals with dementia, safety risks can be due to cognitive changes in memory and judgment as well as physical changes in balance and mobility.

Ensuring safety involves a multifaceted approach that reviews potential hazards in each room. Categories of hazards will be reviewed, and a room-by-room guide follows.

Breakable objects	*—Remove glass, ceramic figurines, and other items that could have sharp pieces when broken or place them out of reach.*
Knives	*—Remove knives from accessible locations (countertop knife blocks).*
	—Consider a locked drawer for storage.
Matches/lighters	*—Keep matches and lighters in a locked area.*
	—Supervise the individual while smoking.
Guns	*—It is not sufficient to just unload the gun or use a trigger lock.*

	—*Keep guns and ammunition in two separate, locked areas.*
Medications/vitamins	—*In the early stages of illness, monitor medication usage for accuracy.*
	—*Try a medication organizer.*
	—*In the later stages, keep medication in a locked area to prevent accidental overdose.*
Household poisons	—*Keep cleaning products and other toxic substances (such as pesticides) in a secure location to prevent accidental consumption.*
Liquor	—*For those who consume alcoholic beverages, monitor the rate and amount of consumption to prevent intoxication, which can lead to falls and injury.*
Poisonous plants	—*Some plants and flowers are toxic if ingested. Remove these plants from the environment. Consult your local poison-control center for a list of poisonous plants in your area.*
Appliances	—*Unplug irons, hair dryers, and other appliances when not in use.*
	—*In the later stages, supervise use of appliances to prevent injury.*
Power tools	—*In the early stages, make sure protective equipment (safety goggles, gloves) are used and monitor tools use.*
	—*In later stages, access to tools may need to be restricted.*
Telephones	—*Some individuals with dementia become victims of telemarketing scams. Some caregivers turn down the ringer volume on the telephone before leaving the house, so the individual with dementia does not hear incoming calls.*
Summoning help	—*Some individuals are unable to dial 911 for assistance.*
	—*Consider a pendant-style alarm system, if the individual is capable of learning how to activate such an alarm, and a MedicAlert® + Alzheimer's Association Safe Return® identification bracelet.*

Bathroom doors   *—Some individuals accidentally lock themselves in the bathroom and can't unlock the door. Consider removing the bathroom door lock or changing to a lock that can be opened from the outside with a key.*
—If the bathroom door swings into the bathroom, and the individual falls, she could block access into the bathroom for a caregiver coming to assist her. Consider changing the swing of the door out to the hallway or room instead of into the bathroom.

FALLING HAZARDS

Older adults are at higher risks for falls than the general population due to many changes associated with the aging process. Diminished vision, slowed balance reactions, muscular weakness, and low blood pressure can be contributing factors to falls. For individuals with FTD, decreased judgment and safety awareness, impulsivity, and poor motor planning are also fall risk factors.

The following environmental (extrinsic) factors may lead to falls:

- lighting that is too dark, too dim, has a glare, or promotes shadows
- walking surfaces that are uneven, wet/slippery, have busy patterns, have worn carpets or area rugs that are not secured in place, or are waxed
- stairs with edges that are not defined, have uneven riser height, lack handrails, or have wobbly handrails
- furniture that is too low, too soft, unstable (easily tips or moves), or in the walking path
- clothing that is too long or too loose
- footwear that is too loose, has slippery soles, or is unfastened/untied
- objects on the floor, such as magazine racks, trash cans, small ottomans, or low coffee tables

The solutions to most of the above environmental hazards are simple, and many are no- or low-cost interventions. Please see the room-by-room section of this chapter for further safety ideas.

The following physical (intrinsic) factors can increase the risk of falls:

- medications: sedatives, sleeping aids, some blood-pressure reducers
- being tired/having insomnia: individuals are more likely to fall when fatigued
- vision disorders: limited vision can lead to falls
- ataxia/balance disorders/unsteady gait
- depression
- poor initiation
- foot problems
- fear of falling
- use of alcohol
- sedentary lifestyle/Inactivity

Your medical-care team (neurologist, physiatrist, ophthalmologist, physical therapist, occupational therapist, etc.) can assist with strategies to minimize the impact of these fall risk factors.

CREATING ENVIRONMENTS THAT MAXIMIZE FUNCTIONAL SKILLS

Environments can support independence when they are designed to provide cues to compensate for declining cognitive skills. This is an ongoing process that changes with the course of the disease. Cues that work in the early stages may be confusing in the later stages. There are several strategies to accomplish this goal; several are listed below.

In the early stages of the disease, labeling drawers with a picture or description of the contents can assist an individual in finding objects used in everyday activities. For example, labeling the utensil drawer in the kitchen with a picture of a fork, or the word "forks" in large letters may enable the individual to find the forks when preparing to set the table.

Leaving commonly used items within sight may help in the early stages of the disease. In the bathroom, leaving the toothpaste and toothbrush on the counter may cue the individual to brush his teeth; leaving a hairbrush may prompt the individual to brush his hair. In the middle stages, having too many items in view may be distracting, and the individual may not be able to determine which items are used for a certain task. He may try to brush his hair with the toothbrush if all the above items are still in view. At that stage, only one item should be left in sight at a time.

The use of grab bars in the bathroom can promote continued ability to transfer to the toilet or bathtub. For maximum effectiveness, grab bars should always be of a contrasting color to the wall on which they are placed.

Use color to highlight or minimize attention to areas of the house. Use a solid, contrasting color on the wall behind the toilet to direct attention in the bathroom. Paint in the same color as the rest of the wall a door that you do not want opened, so it appears to blend into the wall.

TECHNOLOGY AND HOME ENVIRONMENTS

Advances in technology can provide assistance in promoting safety and functional skills. Motion detectors can automatically turn on lights as one approaches the bathroom or staircase, or sound an alarm when an individual attempts to leave the house.

These devices are widely available in electronics stores, and the price of these devices is surprisingly affordable.

HOUSEHOLD CHECKLIST

Using the following checklist is a good way to start a home assessment. Some modifications to the home and the related equipment are reimbursable by health-insurance plans, including Medicare. The following list has been noted by a double asterisk (**) where the modification or equipment is reimbursable by some health-insurance plans. A single asterisk (*) notes items that are nonreimbursable by most health-insurance plans. There are other options for funding home modifications besides health insurance. Some other funding programs have age and income qualifications (Community Development Authority (CDA) Block Grants administered by local area agencies on aging, Christmas in April, Volunteers in Medical Engineering, benevolent organizations, etc.), others are available only in certain areas (university projects, demonstration grants, etc.). Another option for those who own their own homes is a home-equity loan or reverse mortgage.

Bathroom

Are throw rugs secured with double-sided tape?
Is there a nonskid mat, strips, or finish on the tub/shower floor?*
Is there a shower chair?*
Is there a handheld shower?*
Are there grab bars to provide support during transfers and while bathing?*
Are the grab bars in the proper location for the individual?*
Are the grab bars in a contrasting color to the wall?*
Are there grab bars near the toilet?*
Is a raised toilet seat needed?**
Is there sufficient lighting in the bathroom?
Is there a ground fault interrupted (GFI) outlet to avoid electrical shocks
    while using an electric shaver, hair dryer, or other appliances in the
    bathroom?*
Is there a phone to summon help if needed?

Bedroom

Is the bed the proper height for the individual?
Is a hospital-style bed needed?**
Is the room cluttered with furniture and accessories?
Is there a place to sit while dressing, other than the bed?
Is there too much clothing in the drawers and closet?
Is there a commode for safer toileting, especially during nighttime?**
Are there night lights?*

Kitchen

Are there childproof locks on all areas containing hazards?*
Is a range cut-off switch needed to prevent use of the stove or oven?*
Is a refrigerator lock needed?

Stairs

Are there handrails on each side of the steps?*
Are the steps even?

If there is carpeting on the steps, is it firmly attached?

Are there nonskid, contrasting edges on the steps?*

Is the lighting sufficient at the top and bottom of the staircase?

Are there unsecured throw rugs at the top or bottom of the staircase?

Living Room

If carpeted, is the carpeting low pile, or are there plastic runners over the carpeting to create level paths?*

Is there a clear path to maneuver around furniture?*

Is there a chair with a firm seat and sturdy arms in which to sit?

Is there a lift chair or cushion for easier sitting to standing?** (This requires a letter of medical necessity.)

Is there glare control at the windows?*

Throughout the Home

Is the home able to accommodate an individual in a wheelchair?

Is one-floor living a possibility? Is there a full bathroom and room for a bedroom on the first floor?

Can stair glides be rented or purchased for safer negotiation of stairs and to continue access to two floors?*

Is a rented or purchased wheelchair needed for more energy-efficient, longer distance mobility?** (Most insurance plans will reimburse the cost of one wheelchair every five years unless there is medical justification to receive one more frequently.)

Would a ceiling-based track-lift system* or portable sling lift (e.g., Hoyer® lift)** facilitate transfers?

Are there one-touch on/off lamps and glow-in-the-dark light switches?*

RESOURCES

Ageless Design—great information on dementia-specific home modifications. www.agelessdesigns.net.

American Association for Retired Persons (AARP)—general information about home modifications. www.aarp.org.

American Occupational Therapy Association—information on home modification and how to contact an occupational therapist. www.aota.org.

healthgrades®—a national directory of occupational therapists. It includes ratings and contact information. www.healthgrades.com.

LifeEase—home-evaluation information. www.lifease.com.

National Directory of Home Modification Resources—information on resources by state. www.usc.edu/dept/gero/nrcshhm/directory.

National Resource Center on Supportive Housing and Home Modifications, University of Southern California, Andrus Gerontology Center (213) 740-1364—home-modification information. http://gero.usc.edu/nrcshhm.

NOTES

1. E. C. Brawley, "Environment—A Silent Partner in Caregiving," in *Behaviors in Dementia: Best Practices for Successful Management*, ed. M. Kaplan and S. B. Hoffman (Baltimore, MD: Health Promotions, 1998).

2. R. V. Olsen, E. Ehrenkrantz, and B. Hutchings, *Homes That Help: Advice from Caregivers for Creating a Supportive Home* (Newark, NJ: NJIT, 1993).

BIBLIOGRAPHY

Brawley, E. C. *Designing for Alzheimer's Disease: Strategies for Creating Better Care Environments*. New York: John Wiley and Sons, 1997.

Calkins, M. P. *Creating Successful Dementia Care Settings*. Baltimore, MD: Health Professions, 2001.

Changing Needs, Changing Homes: A Guide to Resources. Bethesda, MD: American Occupational Therapy Foundation and American Occupational Therapy Association, 1996.

Pynoos, J., J. Sanford, and T. Rosenfelt. "A Team Approach for Home Modification." *OT Practice* 7, no. 7 (2002): 15–19.

Ruga, W. "Designing for the Senses." In *Healthcare Design*, ed. S. Marberry. New York: John Wiley and Sons, 1997.

Sanford, L. "The Importance of Lighting for the Elderly." *Aging and Vision* 11, no. 1 (1999). (Available online at www.lighthouse.org.)

Warner, M. L. *The Complete Guide to Alzheimer's-Proofing Your Home*. West Lafayette, IN: Purdue University Press, 2000.

Wylde, M., A. Baron-Robbins, and S. Clark. *Building for a Lifetime*. Newton, CT: Tauton, 1994.

CHAPTER 15

ALTERED RELATIONSHIPS

Adapting to Emotions and Behavior

Katherine P. Rankin, PhD

INTRODUCTION

As you have already realized from the previous chapters in this volume, one of the most important differences between frontotemporal degeneration syndromes (FTD) and Alzheimer's disease is that FTD typically affects behavior, often early and severely. It is this factor, perhaps more than any other, that makes caring for an FTD sufferer so much more of a challenge. To make things even more complicated, the experiences among FTD caregivers differ considerably because the areas of the brain that are damaged in frontotemporal syndromes vary substantially from patient to patient. One caregiver may be at the end of his rope because he finds himself battling the patient over her excessively rigid, compulsive eating behavior, while another may find that though her loved one is easygoing and complacent, she dreads taking him into public places due to his tendency to make loud, socially inappropriate comments to strangers and friends. As the disease progresses, particular behavioral changes may appear and then disappear later in a manner that researchers are only beginning to understand, much less be able to predict. However, as this family of diseases becomes more widely recognized by the public and the scientific community alike, new resources are becoming available to alleviate some of the burden and isolation experienced by FTD caregivers in the past.

In this chapter, I will describe some of the social and emotional changes particular to patients whose disease affects the frontal and/or temporal lobes of the brain, and will make some suggestions about how to cope with or manage these changes. These symptoms are commonly found in patients with FTD but will also sometimes occur in other diseases such as progressive supranuclear palsy and some progressive aphasias. There already exists considerable literature directed toward dementia caregiving that can provide very helpful guidance in the major principles of behavior management. However, there are a few issues that are worth briefly repeating here. During the course of his or her loved one's disease, each caregiver will experience a series of changes in the patient's manner and behavior over time. The first important step for the caregiver is to learn to notice each change, no matter how gradually it has appeared. This not only is necessary to give the patient's healthcare providers accurate information to aid in treatment decisions, but also is an important issue for maintaining a healthy caregiving relationship. For each change, caregivers must first ask, "How is this behavior affecting quality of life for me, the patient, and others around us?" Second, they must ask, "Is the best course of action to (1) adjust to this new behavior, (2) try to change it, or (3) both?" The caregiver must recognize that not every challenging new behavior really needs to be changed, nor will it even be possible given the nature of the patient's disease. Conversely, however, caregivers must also be honest about the negative impact a behavior may be having on themselves or others and should not choose to overburden themselves unnecessarily by neglecting opportunities to either modify the patient's challenging behavior or obtain additional assistance coping with it. Above all, caregiving for patients with FTD requires flexibility and an awareness that each new problem may need to be handled using a different approach than the problem before.

For instance, a patient may develop an affinity for a particular shirt and will insist on wearing that shirt and no other. After a few weeks of escalating conflict over her attempts to dress the patient differently, one caregiver may decide that other than the mild embarrassment it causes her in social settings, this behavior is having no negative effects on the patient or others. This caregiver chooses to wash the shirt regularly and ceases her attempts to make the patient wear other shirts, thus resolving the problem by choosing to adjust to the behavior rather than changing it. For a different caregiver, however, the added effort of laundering the favorite shirt three to four times per week would be an unreasonable drain on her limited time and energy, and she may opt for a compromise. She agrees to allow the patient to wear the same color and style of shirt daily, adapting to his wishes despite her embarrassment, but she will buy five identical versions of the shirt for the patient to wear. If the patient is bothered by the fact that these are in fact different shirts, it still may require some effort and creativity on the part of the caregiver to convince him to wear them. However, working to slightly modify the patient's behavior will significantly decrease her workload and help protect her quality of life.

The second main caregiving principle that should be reiterated here is that it is crucial for caregivers to monitor themselves and know when to get help. Numerous studies suggest that it is a dementia patient's behavioral disturbance, not their cognitive decline (e.g., poor memory or mental disorganization), that is the most significant predictor of social and emotional distress for caregivers.[1] Clearly, this issue is particularly salient in the case of frontotemporal degeneration caregivers, as the social and behavioral manifestations of the disease are often the primary symptoms and challenge the caregiver on a daily basis. The suggestions entailed in this chapter are only an initial resource for handling the strain of caring for an FTD patient. Chapters 19 through 24 of this volume are dedicated to elucidating the resources available to provide support for caregivers when the patient's emotional and social behaviors become too much to handle alone.

INSIGHT AND AWARENESS

Loss of self-awareness is one of the hallmarks of frontotemporal dementia, and it is often one of the most difficult aspects of the disease for caregivers. Patients can have problems recognizing that they are ill or may appear to be unable to correctly monitor their own behavior or their impact on others. In fact, when FTD patients are asked to describe their current personality and behaviors, many will state that there is "nothing wrong with them" and will describe themselves as they once were, even misreporting factual information about themselves. Though the family members report, for instance, that this once-genial and extraverted woman has become persistently harsh, critical, and uninterested in social engagements, the patient's self-description will match the family's report of her extraverted and pleasant personality before the onset of the disease. She may even say that she likes to go to parties regularly when she has not been willing to attend such an event for years. It is important to realize that this is not a case of psychological denial, as if the patient refuses to admit changes that could be perceived as shortcomings. This is, in fact, a brain-based disorder that prevents patients from accurately perceiving and interpreting new information about their behavior that would challenge their longstanding self-image.

This problem can result from damage to various complex circuits throughout the brain that process and update information about one's physical and emotional state, personal history, and interpersonal relationships. It has long been demonstrated that patients who have strokes damaging the right parietal lobe can lose awareness of their own disease or dysfunction, even to the point where a paralyzed patient will insist that she has never been immobilized, or a blind patient will state that he can see and will create elaborate, inaccurate descriptions of his surroundings. This lack of awareness of one's disease, or *anosognosia*, is often seen in Alzheimer's patients, probably because the parietal lobe typically becomes damaged as a part of this disease. However, patients with damage to the frontal or temporal lobes of the brain also can evidence anosognosia, even without parietal damage. Recent studies suggest that structures in the middle of the frontal lobe, including the anterior cingulate and orbitofrontal cortex, are involved not only in paying attention to oneself but also even in caring enough to bother maintaining an accurate self-image.[2] Both of these structures can be severely damaged in the frontal variant of FTD and can sustain some damage in the temporal variant.[3] However, they are both relatively spared in the nonfluent primary progressive aphasia (left frontal) subtype of FTD,[4] the only subtype in which patients typically retain full awareness of their disease and maintain normal social behavior until late in the disease process.[5]

Caregivers learning to cope with an FTD patient's lack of insight may find that their frustration is partly alleviated when they accept that it will be difficult, if not impossible, for the patient to recognize the truth about himself and his behavior. This is merely a part of the disease, just as failure to lay down new memories is a part of Alzheimer's disease. Maintaining patience and compassion is key. A caregiver's attempts to hold up a mirror to the patient will often result in escalating a fruitless power struggle. And yet caregivers should also recognize that the patient's lack of self-awareness may actually be a blessing in disguise. This lack of insight actually presents much more of a burden for the caregiver than for the patient, who is oblivious to what would probably be devastating information about her progressive loss of abilities and the dramatic change from her previously held standards of behavior.

The practical issue arising from lack of insight that perhaps carries the greatest potential for harm occurs when the patient refuses to participate in evaluation and treatment due to his failure to recognize his illness. At our dementia specialty clinic, I have witnessed instances where the family members were eventually forced to deceive the patient about the true purpose of the visit in order to convince him to cooperate with necessary medical treatment. The ethical issues involved in the treatment of dementia patients are often thorny; however, when it comes to the point where deception and coercion seem necessary, the patient's lack of insight may be interfering with his capacity to make decisions in his best interest. To resolve this issue, the primary caregiver may choose to seek legal guardianship of the patient in order to be allowed to make their medical decisions for him or her. With an FTD patient who manifests this lack of insight early in the disease, before other functional impairments arise, it may require testimony from a specialist in frontotemporal dementia to convince the legal authorities that the patient should have a conservator. In all such cases, it is important to thoroughly discuss the issue with the treatment team in order to determine a course of action that maximizes the dignity and independence of the patient while maintaining appropriate standards for her care.

LOSS OF EMPATHY

Another change that can come as a shock, particularly to family and friends, is that some frontotemporal dementia patients lose their ability to sense or care about what others are feeling, and they may become extraordinarily self-centered as a part of their disease. One caregiver described an incident in which he had accidentally cut off part of his toe with a lawnmower. He was appalled when his wife casually walked over to the neighbor's house to return the borrowed mower before getting into the car to drive him to the hospital. While in the car, she showed no distress over his injury and even told him he was "making too much noise." In another incident, a caregiver who had been very close to his mother before her disease tried to convey to her some very difficult times he'd been having at work. His mother was so preoccupied with turning the topic back to the mundane events of her day that even when the son began to cry describing an incident he had experienced, his mother merely looked bewildered for a moment, then returned to chatting away about her garden. Both of these patients were early in their disease, and neither had yet been diagnosed with frontotemporal dementia, though they were both later found to have a right-temporal variant of FTD. FTD patients are more likely to be perceived as introverted, unempathic, aloof, and even cold-hearted by their caregivers, and these personality changes have been directly linked to the damage to frontal and temporal structures. [6]

Empathy is a complex socioemotional response that involves perceiving another person's emotional signals, mirroring their emotional experience within oneself, and then choosing the best course of action to help or comfort the other.[7] These abilities are primarily mediated by structures in the right hemisphere of the brain, particularly the temporal lobes. Damage to parts of the right temporal lobe can interfere with the patient's capacity to realize that certain facial expressions, body postures, gestures, and voice inflections carry emotional significance, which renders him unable to recognize others' emotions or correctly interpret social signals. Other parts of the right temporal lobe help us generate emotional responses and allow us to "feel with" the other person. Even if these abilities to perceive and feel remain intact, parts of the frontal lobe are required for us to understand those emotions in context, to feel motivated to express those emotions, and to help us choose the right thing to say or do according to the situation.[8] These structures and circuits sustain different degrees of damage in each FTD patient, so very diverse patterns of emotional blunting and empathy loss are seen across individuals, with no one patient acting exactly like another. Right-temporal damage may disrupt the ability to recognize when a situation or memory is supposed to have personal emotional relevance, causing some patients to lose their sense of attachment to loved ones, or even realize that other people "matter."[9] If this problem is compounded by a lack of insight, the patient will not only fail to correctly identify the emotional state of the other, but she will not even realize that she is missing something. This is also one of the reasons some FTD patients make harsh or judgmental comments to friends or strangers, or insist on conversation topics that do not interest their listener.

Humans are by nature social, relational beings, and we tend to gauge who a person is by how he or she interacts with us. Thus, the emotional blunting and loss of emotional attachment that occurs in many FTD patients can make caregivers feel like they are living with a stranger. Again, coping with this change begins with a clear recognition that this is not willful coldness or spitefulness on the part of the patient but is a loss of emotional functioning directly caused by damage to the brain. However, it is natural to feel that such patients are more prickly and difficult to like, and the emotional one-sidedness of the relationship puts additional strain on FTD caregivers on a day-to-day basis. Like the loss of insight described previously, loss of empathic warmth cannot be changed through behavioral interventions, and caregivers must shoulder the burden of adapting to the patient's change in personality. One of the most important things caregivers can do in this situation is to make an honest assessment of the way this change affects them emotionally, and to give themselves the opportunity to mourn this loss. A readjustment of the caregiver's support system is often necessary, recruiting other family members, friends, community members, and counselors to provide the nurture and emotional attentiveness that the patient can no longer supply. Studies show that when family members can learn to view the caregiving relationship with greater distance, taking on a perspective similar to that which is held by nonrelative caregivers, they become happier, better adjusted, and more effective caregivers.[10] Though many frontotemporal dementia patients show decreased empathy, only a small proportion of them become entirely incapable of emotional expression or receptivity, thus most caregivers will still occasionally experience some modified emotional responsiveness from the patient. When a caregiver ceases to expect direct emotional support from the patient and his emotional needs are adequately met elsewhere, he is more likely to appreciate and even enjoy the patient again, making the caregiving relationship less stressful.

APATHY

Another change that may be seen in patients with dementias affecting the frontal lobes of the brain is loss of interest in the activities and people that they used to enjoy. In FTD patients, this apathy is usually distinct from depression, though the two are easily confused by family members and clinicians. Both apathy and depression may cause a decrease in activity, loss of interest and enjoyment, and a general lack of responsiveness. However, typical depression is characterized by somatic symptoms such as loss of appetite, weight loss, and insomnia, as well as negative cognitive preoccupations with worthlessness, hopelessness, sadness, and helplessness. Rather than becoming more preoccupied with negative emotions and thoughts, however, FTD patients with apathy actually cease to be troubled by the things that used to bother them. They begin to generate fewer thoughts and emotions and initiate fewer words and actions. Families of FTD patients will sometimes report that their first indication that something was wrong was that the patient *stopped* worrying and became uncharacteristically complacent and passive. A patient who has been hardworking and conscientious her whole life may suddenly stop bothering to meet deadlines or may quit her job altogether without cause or explanation. Later in the disease, this apathy may become so pervasive that she only speaks when spoken to and moves only when led around, showing very little interest in the events and conversations going on around her, even when she herself is the topic of discussion.

The brain circuit responsible for apathy is centered around the anterior cingulate, a band of tissue in the middle of the frontal cortex involved in motivation. A number of different brain networks converge on the anterior cingulate, which plays roles related to many aspects of behavior, including paying attention to important cues in the environment such as errors, experiencing self-awareness, and mobilizing us to act on a selected plan of action.[11] Patients with strokes limited to this brain area sometimes develop what is called "akinetic mutism," a severe form of apathy where the patient stops moving and speaking altogether despite possessing intact brain systems for language and movement. Studies have directly linked apathy with anterior-cingulate damage in frontotemporal dementia patients.[12] The fact that this structure is significantly atrophied in FTD suggests that patients' apathy may result from an inability to derive motivation from internal cues, coupled with a sense that things that they once found rewarding enough to pursue are no longer worth the trouble.

Apathy can be both a curse and a blessing for caregivers. On the one hand, the patient ceases to be supportive and helpful in the household, often requiring prompting to perform basic self-care tasks, much less do work around the home. He can become dependent and passive, putting more of a burden on the caregiver to step into the role of provider, organizer, and director in the relationship. This can be a particularly difficult transition when the patient once had the dominant role in the relationship, such as in the case of a breadwinner or parent. At first the caregiver may be very reluctant to perform the coaching and prompting that is often necessary with an apathetic patient, and may find that she needs to develop previously unexplored skills, such as attending to financial concerns or housework. On the other hand, apathy tends to make patients more compliant and cooperative with care and treatment, and they are less likely to engage in power struggles with the caregiver. Depending on the degree of apathy, some patients actually become much more easygoing, pleasant, and even friendly than they were before the onset of their disease. The patient is spared the pain of caring about his condition, and he remains comparatively untroubled despite significant loss of function and freedom.

When asked how they feel, apathetic patients will typically respond genuinely that they feel "just fine" and that their symptoms are not bothering them.

Again, the origin of apathy in frontotemporal dementia patients is entirely neurologic and not psychological, and thus is not subject to rehabilitation; however, there are some behavioral interventions that may make it easier for the caregiver to manage the patient. Even in patients for whom the apathy is pervasive, they typically have some preserved likes and dislikes that can be utilized as concrete motivators or rewards. The typical scenario with a very apathetic patient is that the caregiver wishes for the patient to do something, for example, get dressed or bathe, and the patient would really rather not. In such a case, if the caregiver has noted that the patient likes a particular food or television show, he can promise this as a reward for performing the task. Though the patient's cognitive deficits may keep her from focusing on the reward long enough to complete the task, the caregiver may wish to frequently remind the patient of the imminent reward to prime her deficient motivational system. At other times, however, the caregiver must take a good look at his reasons for wanting the patient to perform a particular task and may need to adjust his expectations. For example, he may decide that since the patient is no longer attending regular social events or going to work daily, more infrequent bathing may be adequate and appropriate.

RIGID, BIZARRE, AND SOCIALLY INAPPROPRIATE BEHAVIOR

Perhaps the most infamous aspect of frontotemporal disorders is their tendency to produce odd behavior in some patients. Some patients will develop compulsive behaviors such as playing computer solitaire for hours every day, insisting on eating only very specific foods, or buying a favorite object every time they find one at the store (e.g., pens, stepladders, cans of soup). This compulsivity is often accompanied by mental rigidity, where the patient has certain ideas about how things must be done and is highly resistant to alternatives. She may also become obsessed with a particular place, event, or theme, and will persistently bring the conversation back around to this topic even when her listener has no interest in it or even reminds the patient that he has heard the story many times before. Some patients will develop odd or repetitive movements, such as fidgeting, pacing, walking oddly for no discernible medical reason, putting inedible objects in their mouths, or grimacing. Other patients will show a disregard for social norms, touching themselves or others inappropriately, making inappropriate or rude comments, stealing, or wearing bizarre clothing combinations.

Neuroanatomically, this heterogeneous group of behaviors emerges from a variety of brain circuits, often linked to changes in the right frontal and temporal lobes but sometimes involving damage to subcortical structures and circuits or a neurochemical or hormonal imbalance in the brain. The kinds of complex, stereotypical motor routines often seen in FTD patients (e.g., taking shoes on and off again repeatedly, drumming on tables) has been linked with damage to a set of subcortical structures called the basal ganglia that are involved in automatic movements.[13] Impulse control is mediated by various circuits in the frontal lobes, including the lateral parts of the orbitofrontal cortex, which provide a sense of negative future consequences that works with the anterior cingulate to act as a "stop signal."[14] Behaviors can sometimes be controlled by using pharmacological treatment to increase serotonin, an important neurotransmitter that is commonly diminished in frontotemporal dementia. In particular, compulsive behavior, irritability, impulsivity, and the tendency to consume excessive amounts of sweets and other carbohydrates often respond to treatment with psychotropic medications.[15]

This category of behavior can be cause more frustration, annoyance, and embarrassment for caregivers than any other. As with many other aspects of the disease, caregivers must simply learn to live with some of these behaviors, making sure to monitor their own level of irritation and finding a friend or family member who is willing to provide respite care when the patient's behavior becomes too much to take. However, there are some behavioral interventions that can either modify or limit the effects of the patient's behavior:

Some caregivers find that it is helpful to carry a set of preprinted, business card–sized notes for use in situations where the patient behaves oddly or inappropriately in public. Such a card could read, "My wife has an Alzheimer's-like disease that affects her behavior. Thank you for your patience," and could be handed unobtrusively to the food server who receives an undeserved rambling lecture from the patient or the stranger whose attire is commented on a little too loudly.

Patients who steal items typically do so impulsively rather than because they actually need the item in question. If the caregiver is familiar with the patient's interests and habits, it will become easier to recognize environments that may contain objects the patient might be tempted to steal (e.g., certain types of stores, friends' homes, passing by street vendors with open display cases). The patient may require extra supervision in such an environment. It may be helpful to recruit the help of a second caregiver to monitor the patient if the primary caregiver will be otherwise occupied. Sometimes, physically placing oneself between the patient and the display rack is enough of a deterrent. Also, discreetly checking the patient for stolen items before or immediately after leaving the problem environment may sometimes be necessary to minimize unwanted consequences.

Though rigid, compulsive behavior is by nature resistant to change, compromises can sometimes be reached by bargaining with the patient. Again, this requires having a clear understanding of the patient's interests and preoccupations. The goal is to convince him to give up one desire (e.g., buying a fifth set of socket wrenches) in order to be rewarded with another (e.g., sitting for a half hour in the food court of the mall while the patient plays solitaire on a handheld computer game). It is always a good idea to plan ahead in order to minimize the need to push or rush the patient. Expect even simple activities to require more time than they once did. For instance, some caregivers choose to schedule in an extra hour in the morning on the day of an appointment so that they can negotiate with any of the patient's unanticipated demands or rituals without being late.

NOTES

1. N. Matsumoto, M. Ikeda, R. Fukuhara, et al., "Caregiver Burden Associated with Behavioral and Psychological Symptoms of Dementia in Elderly People in the Local Community," *Dementia and Geriatric Cognitive Disorders* 23, no. 4 (2007): 219–24; J. C. Mourik, S. M. Rosso, M. F. Niermeijer, et al., "Frontotemporal Dementia: Behavioral Symptoms and Caregiver Distress," *Dementia and Geriatric Cognitive Disorders* 18, nos. 3–4 (2004): 299–306; A. Braekhus, A. R. Oksengard, K. Engedal, and K. Laake, "Social and Depressive Stress Suffered by Spouses of Patients with Mild Dementia," *Scandinavian Journal of Primary Health Care* 16, no. 4 (1998): 242–46; L. D. Clyburn, M. J. Stones, T. Hadjistavropoulous, and H. Tuokko, "Predicting Caregiver Burden in Alzheimer's Disease," *Journal of Gerontology* 55B, no. 1 (2000): S2-S13; C. Donaldson , N. Tarrier, and A. Burns, "Determinants of Carer Stress in Alzheimer's Disease," *International Journal of Geriatric Psychiatry* 13 (1998): 248–56.

2. M. Hornberger, B. Yew, S. Gilardoni, et al., "Ventromedial-Frontopolar Prefrontal Cortex Atrophy Correlates with Insight Loss in Frontotemporal Dementia and Alzheimer's

Disease," *Human Brain Mapping* 35, no. 2 (2014): 616–26; T. Shany-Ur, N. Lin, H. J. Rosen, et al., "Self-Awareness in Neurodegenerative Disease Relies on Neural Structures Mediating Reward-Driven Attention," *Brain* (in press 2014); M. F. Mendez and J. S. Shapira, "Loss of Insight and Functional Neuroimaging in Frontotemporal Dementia," *Journal of Neuropsychiatry and Clinical Neurosciences Research* 17, no. 3 (2005): 413–16.

3. H. J. Rosen, M. Gorno-Tempini, W. P. Goldman, et al., "Patterns of Brain Atrophy in Frontotemporal Dementia and Semantic Dementia," *Neurology* 58, no. 20 (2002): 198–208.

4. M. Gorno-Tempini, N. F. Dronkers, K. P. Rankin, et al., "Cognition and Anatomy in Three Variants of Primary Progressive Aphasia," *Annals of Neurology* 55, no. 3 (2004): 335–46.

5. Shany-Ur, Lin, Rosen, et al., "Self-Awareness."

6. M. Sollberger, J. Neuhaus, R. Ketelle, C. M. Stanley, V. Beckman, M. Growdon, J. Jang, B. L. Miller, and K. P. Rankin, "Interpersonal Traits Change as a Function of Disease Type and Severity in Degenerative Brain Diseases," *Journal of Neurology, Neurosurgery, and Psychiatry* 82, no. 7 (2011): 732–39; K. P. Rankin, J. H. Kramer, P. Mychack, and B. L. Miller, "Double Dissociation of Social Functioning in Frontotemporal Dementia," *Neurology* 60, no. 2 (2003): 266–71.

7. Shany-Ur, Lin, Rosen, et al., "Self-Awareness"; Decety J and Michalska KJ., "Neurodevelopmental Changes in the Circuits Underlying Empathy and Sympathy from Childhood to Adulthood," *Developmental Science* 13, no. 6 (2010): 886–99.

8. I. R. Olson, A. Plotzker, and Y. Ezzyat, "The Enigmatic Temporal Pole: A Review of Findings on Social and Emotional Processing," *Brain* 130, no. 7 (2007): 1718–31; K. P. Rankin, M. Gorno-Tempini, S. C. Allison, et al., "Structural Anatomy of Empathy in Neurodegenerative Disease," *Brain* 129 (2006): 2945–56.

9. Rankin, Gorno-Tempini, Allison, et al., "Structural Anatomy"; Van Lancker D., "Personal Relevance and the Human Right Hemisphere," *Brain and Cognition* 17 (1991): 64–92.

10. K. W. Hepburn, J. Tornatore, B. Center, and S. W. Ostwald, "Dementia Family Caregiver Training: Affecting Beliefs about Caregiving and Caregiver Outcomes," *Journal of the American Geriatrics Society* 49 (2001): 450–57.

11. A. D. Craig, "How Do You Feel—Now? The Anterior Insula and Human Awareness," *Nature Reviews in Neuroscience* 10 (2009): 59–70; W. W. Seeley, J. Zhou, and E. J. Kim, "Frontotemporal dementia: What Can the Behavioral Variant Teach Us about Human Brain Organization?" *Neuroscientist: A Review Journal Bringing Neurobiology, Neurology and Psychiatry* (2011); V. E. Sturm, M. Sollberger, W. W. Seeley, et al., "Role of Right Pregenual Anterior Cingulate Cortex in Self-Conscious Emotional Reactivity," *Social Cognitive and Affective Neuroscience* 8, no. 4 (2013): 468–74.

12. L. Massimo, C. Powers, P. Moore, et al., "Neuroanatomy of Apathy and Disinhibition in Frontotemporal Lobar Degeneration," *Dementia and Geriatric Cognitive Disorders* 27, no. 1 (2009): 96–104; W. Liu, B. L. Miller, J. H. Kramer, et al., "Behavioral Disorders in the Frontal and Temporal Variants of Frontotemporal Dementia," *Neurology* 62 (2004): 742–48.

13. K. A. Josephs, J. L. Whitwell, J. E. Parisi, et al., "Caudate Atrophy on MRI Is a Characteristic Feature of FTLD-FUS," *European Journal of Neurology: The Official Journal of the European Federation of Neurological Societies* 17, no. 7 (2010): 969–75.

14. D. J. Sharp, V. Bonnelle, X. De Boissezon, et al., "Distinct Frontal Systems for Response Inhibition, Attentional Capture, and Error Processing," *Proceedings of the National Academy of Sciences of the United States of America* 107, no. 13 (2010): 6106–11; M. L. Kringelbach and E. T. Rolls, "The Functional Neuroanatomy of the Human Orbito-frontal Cortex: Evidence from Neuroimaging and Neuropsychology," *Progress in Neurobiology* 72, no. 5 (2004): 341–72; J. O'Doherty, M. L. Kringelbach, E. T. Rolls, et al., "Abstract Reward and Punishment Representations in the Human Orbitofrontal Cortex," *Nature Neuroscience* 4, no. 120577671 (2001): 95–102.

15. M. Manoochehri and E. D. Huey, "Diagnosis and Management of Behavioral Issues in Frontotemporal Dementia," *Current Neurology and Neuroscience Reports* 12, no. 5 (2012): 528–36.

CHAPTER 16

BEFORE DRUGS

Nonpharmacologic Approach to Symptom Management

Lauren M. Massimo, PhD, AGNP-BC;
and Geri R. Hall, PhD, ARNP, GCNS-BC, FAAN

INTRODUCTION

Frontotemporal degeneration (FTD) accounts for 10 to 20 percent of all neurodegenerative disease (ND) and is thought to be one of the most common causes of ND affecting adults under age sixty-five (Ratnavalli et al. 2002). FTD occurs equally in men and women and has a life expectancy of seven to twelve years from disease onset (Onyike 2011). FTD results from progressive damage to the frontal and temporal lobes of the brain and can be caused by several different pathologies (Massimo and Grossman 2008). Symptom presentations can vary widely depending on the areas of the brain affected, but all types of FTD share many features as the disease progresses. People with FTD experience a gradual, progressive decline in behavior, a decline in the ability to use language, and, in some individuals, losses in motor functioning (National Institute on Aging 2010, www.theaftd.org 2012).

Nonpharmacological approaches to managing FTD are likely to play an important role in delaying functional decline (Yamaguchi, Maki, and Yamagami 2010). Such interventions include a range of activities and strategies that are delivered by caregivers in an effort to support functions that are impaired as a result of FTD. The following chapter will describe common symptoms of FTD and suggested nonpharmacological strategies. Each type of FTD has a number of presentations, each with its own care challenges. Case examples will be used to demonstrate behaviors. The information below is derived from research literature and extensive clinical experience.

TYPES OF FTD

FTD can be classified into three types, depending on the earliest presentation of symptoms:

Behavioral variant FTD (bvFTD): Progressive behavioral and personality decline marked by changes in behavior, emotions, concentration, attention, ability to reason, ability to inhibit, capacity for empathy, and poor judgment.

Primary progressive aphasias (PPA): Progressive language decline characterized by early changes in the ability to speak, understand spoken and written language, and write.

Motor disorders including corticobasal degeneration (CBD), progressive supranuclear palsy (PSP) and frontotemporal degeneration with motor neuron disease (FTD-MND): Progressive difficulty with visual-spatial function and movement including motor planning (apraxia), weakness, poor coordination, and gait change.

BEHAVIORAL VARIANT FRONTOTEMPORAL DEGENERATION (BvFTD)

bvFTD is characterized by profound changes in personality and behavior. There is a gradual decline in function accompanied by insidious personality changes. Persons with bvFTD are often initially diagnosed with depression or bipolar disorder, but behavioral symptoms tend to worsen over time and fail to respond to medications used for the psychiatric disorders. Initially a family may see the following symptoms:

- Changes in emotion: The person may lose his or her "sparkle," anger easily, or cry spontaneously
- Loss of empathy: The person loses the ability to understand, or care about what others are thinking or feeling. This often produces social isolation as friends and family detect a lack of caring.
- The development of stereotyped behaviors including compulsive thoughts and obsessive behaviors: The person may spend large amounts

of money on the computer or televised shopping networks. There may be gambling or hoarding behavior. The person may become agitated if the activities are stopped and may develop ingenious ways to restart the activity. Obsessions can include a specific television program watched over and over; following rigid schedules for laundry, housework, and television viewing; insisting on eating the same food at a meal; fostering a weapon collection; obsessive shopping for clothing and makeup; and continuous overeating.

- Apathy: The person may sit, staring, watching television without being involved with the program, not caring whether he or she interacts with family and friends, neglecting personal hygiene
- Poor judgment: The person may participate in unsafe activities such as brandishing guns, making threats, continuous roaming or bicycling into unsafe areas, or performing unsafe physical stunts near grandchildren
- Disorganization: Individuals' finances may be in chaos; bills not paid; not discarding old newspapers, mail, or refuse; starting many activities but finishing very few.
- Disinhibition: The person may become outspoken or rude despite the feelings of others; shoplifting; removing food from other dining patrons' tables; making inappropriate sexual gestures or statements; having spontaneous bowel movements when in highly stimulating places, such as the supermarket.
- Loss of insight: The person may lose self-awareness; no matter how many people tell the person he or she has a problem, the person with FTD fails to recognize a problem, despite numerous poor outcomes.

Mild-Stage bvFTD

Behavioral symptoms are often worst in early disease and may result in being fired from work and isolation from family members or friends. In the early stages, the person with bvFTD looks and sounds normal, even to health professionals. A hallmark of bvFTD is a lack of insight. People with the disease are unable to understand that they have a problem despite numerous poor outcomes. It is not uncommon for them to take financial risk, as they compulsively invest, shop, spend, gamble, or mismanage funds while denying that there is a problem.

Care Goals in the Mild Stage

In the mild stage of disease, care is focused on properly diagnosing the condition. Unfortunately, FTD goes unrecognized by general physicians, thus, the family should request an evaluation by a "behavioral neurologist," a specialist in degenerative cognitive disorders. Families can locate specialists in their area by contacting the Association for Frontotemporal Degeneration (www. theaftd.org) or the Alzheimer's Association (www.alz.org).

A second care goal in the mild stage is protection of family resources. Lack of insight and compulsive spending behaviors are common in FTD, and affected individuals may spend or gamble away their life savings. In addition, the person with FTD may be fired for poor job performance or inappropriate social interactions with coworkers. It is imperative that the family consult with an "elder-law" attorney to prepare advanced directives and assist with attaining disability insurance. Employers must be notified in order to have the person with FTD placed on disability insurance to obtain the maximum insurance possible. Families are commonly forced to limit the person's access to money, credit cards, and to the Internet.

A third care goal is disclosing the person's illness to essential people—most notably, immediate family members, children, and employers. Placing the person's behavior in the context of an illness can help with decreasing family anger and conflict (Massimo, Evans, and Benner 2013). If there are school-age children in the household, special attention should be given to notifying the guidance counselor and carefully monitoring grades to detect suppressed emotional changes.

The final goal is to help the person with FTD develop an acceptable routine. The family can help with scheduling safe activities that can be followed automatically, day after day. The routine can tap into the person's previous likes and new interests, perhaps even building compulsive behaviors into activities. Unlike AD, where distraction is encouraged to avoid repetitive behaviors; in FTD, the goal is to build the acceptable compulsive behavior into the routine. This may help to decrease anxiety and acting out.

Case Study: Mild Stage

George was a successful financial planner until at age forty-two he began to have difficulty in his work. He was disorganized, made mistakes completing forms, missed appointments with clients, and was accused of sexual harassment after grabbing and kissing a colleague. George spent every evening at a local disco and was arrested for driving under the influence. He denied drinking, despite an elevated blood-alcohol level and tried to bribe the policeman. His license was revoked and he spent some time in jail. Two years later, he was financially broke, as were several of his clients who followed George's poor investment advice.

George's elderly parents pursued neurological evaluation after they visited him and discovered: his diet consisted solely of potato chips, ice cream, and candy bars; he had subscriptions to twenty-four magazines arranged unread in disorganized piles; there were dozens of boxes from television infomercials and shopping networks; and his personal grooming was ignored. George insisted there was nothing wrong with him. After he was diagnosed with bvFTD, a family meeting with the nurse practitioner and social worker was scheduled to begin to map the following care strategy. An elder-law attorney helped the family with advanced directives and applications for Social Security Disability Insurance (SSDI). George's father took over his finances. His ex-wife and parents joined support groups associated with the Association for Frontotemporal Degeneration. He agreed to wear a MedicAlert® + Alzheimer's Association Safe Return® identification bracelet and had a GPS device placed in his shoe after refusing to give up driving. The treatment team assisted George's family to obtain retroactive disability benefits since his inappropriate behavior was due to a neurological disease. His living situation improved with the monitoring and supervision provided by his parents.

Moderate-Stage bvFTD

Moderate FTD is characterized by increasing apathy (Chow et al. 2012). There is a total loss of reasoning, and the person may be less attentive or resistant to personal care, even developing incontinence because of reduced insight and apathy. The person may disengage from and objectify people, even those who are close, and may display anger if demands aren't met immediately. Many individuals in the moderate stage develop a "stare" that appears hostile, yet is not linked with anger.

Compulsive repetitive behaviors such as eating constantly, roaming, watching a particular television show over and over, doing "find the word" puzzles, sorting or tearing paper, or collecting certain items become more pronounced in the moderate stage. The person with bvFTD may have reduced initiation of productive behavior and may be unable to plan and organize any activity except for those that are compulsive.

Diminished speech production, which may be accompanied by reduced comprehension of spoken and written language is also seen in the moderate stage. There may also be signs of problems with a motor apraxia—programming the parts of the body to complete a task.

Care Goals in the Moderate Stage

The primary goal in the moderate stage is safety. Caregivers should anticipate objects that can lead to injury of the person with FTD or others. For example, weapons, including guns, knives, fireplace pokers, and so on, should be removed from the home as the person with FTD may be too unpredictable and impaired to use them safely. Caregivers may have occasional unpleasant interactions with neighbors and police, as the person with FTD may try to take something that catches their immediate attention (for instance, stealing a pretty necklace at a store).

Individuals with FTD may feel the need to walk continuously throughout the day. This is called "roaming" and is quite different than wandering in AD. Individuals who roam move compulsively, unable to stop on their own. Once stopped, the person with FTD may become agitated and possibly aggressive until they are allowed to resume the movement. While generally safe, the person with FTD will be oblivious to common environmental, traffic, and human hazards. Many caregivers report the person with FTD follows a predictable route over and over, throughout the day. A GPS tracking device can be invaluable in monitoring the individual's location. Other compulsive behavior may be manifested by overeating. Many people with bvFTD go through a stage where they eat constantly, including nonfood items. Caregivers report that changing from full meal preparations to hourly presentation of small plates or snacks is helpful. It is not uncommon for a person with bvFTD to raid the pantry or refrigerator, sometimes eating a half-gallon of ice cream or entire package of cookies in one sitting. Compulsive eating behavior can lead to rapid and significant weight gain. Caregivers may want to consider purchasing locks for cupboards and the refrigerator online at the Alzheimer's Store™ (www.alzstore.com).

Another goal is to maintain hygiene. Reminding the persons with FTD to bathe, brush their teeth, change clothing daily, get dressed, and change clothing when soiled can be a regular struggle and may result in caregiver injury from resistance. It is important for caregivers to choose their battles. In some cases, persons with FTD will clean up if they understand that they cannot go out in public unless clean and groomed. Dressing is a complex activity that requires multiple steps, and this may be too overwhelming for persons with FTD. In some cases, a consult for occupational therapy is warranted. Occupational therapists are specifically trained in task simplification to help ease problems with the complexities of activities of daily living. Other recommendations for simplifying complex tasks include making lists of tasks for the person with FTD and crossing them off as they are completed; providing explicit step-by-step directions of tasks to be completed; and reducing options and choices to minimize decision making, which can put stress on the person with FTD who has limited executive function.

Case Study: Moderate Stage

Over the next twenty-four months, George's disease progressed. He initiated very little productive behavior and moved in with his parents due to his inability to care for himself. Although he was generally resistant to personal care, his mother found he would agree when told they would go out for ice cream. He needed to be led into the shower and would shave only when the electric razor was placed in is hand. He refused mouth care, and arrangements were made with the dentist for quarterly cleanings.

George did not spontaneously help with chores; however, he would clear the table and wash the dishes with constant prompting from his mother. George would sometimes get up at night and raid the refrigerator. One night, he ate two half gallons of ice cream and a package of shortbread cookies. His parents locked the fridge and began to store sweets in the garage.

George was occasionally incontinent of urine and bowel, particularly when in public. George's medical team ruled out urinary-tract infection and constipation as the cause of his incontinence. His parents decided to use protective garments for his incontinence. They developed a routine, toileting him on a consistent schedule. Lastly, because overstimulation contributed to George's incontinence, his parents took him on outings only on off hours, when there were fewer people around.

Severe-Stage bvFTD

The clinical symptoms that occur in the severe stage vary widely from person to person. In the severe stage, most individuals require assistance in activities of daily living including grooming, bathing, dressing, and eating. Many require assistance with mobility. Some sit and stare blankly for hours and few participate in activities. Many persons in the severe stage are unable to effectively communicate. Individuals can have difficulties swallowing and begin to hold food in their mouth, producing a choking hazard. Most shuffle or require assistance with walking. Individuals who roamed continue to walk, albeit more slowly.

Disinhibited behavior and poor impulse control continues. Persons in the advanced stage continue with compulsive and simple repetitive behavior including picking nails, grabbing food from others, stacking blocks, and shredding paper (Miller 2012). The "stare" is common among individuals in the severe stage of FTD. It is a blank yet penetrating stare that appears to be angry or hostile to staff members who are often frightened by it. It is, however, not linked to aggression.

Care Goals in the Severe Stage

The primary goal of care in advanced disease is comfort and preparation for end-of- life care. Attention must be paid to maintaining cleanliness, preventing infection and skin breakdown, and maintaining nutrition. One facility incorporates nutrition in all activities, providing small amounts of food at each activity throughout the day. Their residents do not lose weight, and the facility reports fewer episodes of choking.

A second goal is providing for safety. In long-term care facilities, falls and resident-to-resident altercations are not uncommon. While neither can be entirely eliminated, use of adaptive devices and enhanced supervision help to minimize the risk. Physical therapy and alternative activities can help with developing safer ambulation and adaptive equipment.

A third goal is to provide meaningful activities that stimulate the senses.

This is accomplished using food, music, aroma therapy, and simple activities. Sitting one-on-one with the person with FTD may provide a degree of emotional comfort. Families tend to plan simple activities such as playing with blocks, shredding paper, looking at picture books, listening to preferred music, and playing simple videos to engage their loved one.

Case Study: Severe Stage

George was placed in a residential-care facility specializing in memory care. The staff needed extra training to help them understand the differences between George's needs and those of someone with AD. George slowly adjusted to his new routine and allowed staff to help him bathe and dress. His family met with the recreational therapist, and together they developed a daily routine that included a few of George's previous interests that were tailored to his current capabilities.

He no longer spoke but would occasionally shake or nod his head. During this time, George started picking his nails until they bled and grabbing food from the plates of other residents. He began to have spontaneous vocalizations, yelling "NO!" repeatedly throughout the day and night. Staff explored activities that would engage George and try to distract him from picking his nails. They found that he would stop when given blocks to stack and sort. He was more likely to participate when activities were individualized and a staff member sat beside him to get him started.

PRIMARY PROGRESSIVE APHASIA (PPA)

PPA describes a set of conditions that result in a gradual progressive impairment of language production, object naming, and syntax. Persons with PPA lose the ability to comprehend and use spoken language. PPA can be further subcategorized into a nonfluent/agrammatic variant (previously known as progressive nonfluent aphasia), a semantic variant (previously known as semantic dementia), and a logopenic variant (previously known as logopenic progressive aphasia) (Gorno-Tempini et al. 2011). While the dominant feature of PPA is aphasia, persons with PPA may also exhibit symptoms similar to those found in bvFTD (described in the previous section of this chapter) (Modirrousta, Price, and Dickerson 2013).

General Characteristics of PPA:

- trouble speaking and producing words
- slowed, halting speech
- difficulty with word comprehension
- impaired object knowledge
- difficulty finding words
- unable to repeat words or phrases
- generally very aware of difficulties and frustrated

Mild-Stage PPA

In the mild stage of PPA, caregivers may notice their loved one is struggling with finding the word he wants to use or perhaps he has difficulty understanding what others are saying. Some individuals with PPA may have slowed, effortful speech. Other areas of cognition such as memory, visuospatial skills, and executive abilities typically remain preserved in the mild stage.

Care Goals in the Mild Stage

As described in the section above regarding care goals in mild bvFTD, it is imperative to obtain an accurate diagnosis, assemble a treatment team that you trust, and establish legal and financial protections. Additional care goals in mild-stage PPA are aimed at optimizing communicative efficacy. Some individuals with PPA may benefit from the use of a homemade picture dictionary—take pictures of frequently used items and keep them in a book so that pictures can be pointed to when individuals are struggling to find words. Some persons with PPA may find it helpful to communicate through alternative forms of communication, such as written communication or text-to-speech programs on computer-assistive devices, such as a laptop or electronic tablet. Additionally, there is evidence to suggest that speech and language therapy may useful in PPA, especially in those with naming difficulties (Henry et al. 2013; Farrajota et al. 2012; Savage, Piguet, and Hodges 2014).

Case Study: Mild-Stage

Judith was a forty-three-year-old district attorney for a major metropolitan area when she began to have difficulty with speaking. Married to Dave and having two children, ages fifteen and sixteen, Judith was a consummate litigator and a well-liked public official. Initially, Dave noted that Judith appeared to stutter. She knew what she wanted to say and understood what was said to her but struggled to pronounce words—especially if she had to concentrate. This problem did not appear to trouble her, although she became more irritable. She attributed this to her high-stress job. She spoke with her primary-care doctor, who diagnosed the problem as an anxiety disorder and prescribed medication and exercise. Initially this helped, but Judith stopped the medication because it made her feel groggy.

She continued to be angry with Dave when he encouraged her to seek help for her problems. Over the next nine months, the problem worsened to where she needed co-counsel to argue for her. Her written briefs, however, did not deteriorate. Judith remained independent in all activities.

Judith was eventually referred to a behavioral neurologist, who diagnosed her with primary progressive aphasia, non-fluent/agrammatic type. After much encouragement, she stepped down to go on disability. Judith was evaluated by a speech pathologist that specialized in neurodegenerative disorders. The speech-language pathologist (SLP) evaluated Judith's language production, comprehension, ability to read and write, and her swallowing function. The SLP recommended adaptive equipment, and Judith obtained a computer tablet outfitted with a program to produce language to assist in communication.

Judith selected her husband, Dave, as her durable power of attorney, with her parents as backup. Dave helped with filing for disability insurance and SSDI. Judith was turned down for benefits on the initial application, however, after consulting with an attorney who specialized in elder law, the appeal was approved.

Moderate-Stage PPA

Characteristics of moderate-stage PPA include severe problems producing speech and significantly impaired comprehension. Some individuals may be aware of their deficits and consequently may try to compensate by talking around the words they intended to use. The ability to perform instrumental activities and basic activities of daily living diminish in the moderate stage. This may also be accompanied by apathy, where the person will sit inactive until someone actually helps him begin an activity. At this stage, individuals with PPA may develop compulsive behavior including overeating, and other hyperoral behaviors, such as excessive smoking.

Care Goals in the Moderate Stage

In moderate-stage PPA, individuals have more difficulty understanding relationships between words in a sentence (Charles et al. 2014), thus, care goals are aimed at supporting comprehension. Strategies to enhance comprehension include altering the delivery of the communication. This includes speaking at a slowed rate to give the person with PPA time to process the communication. Remember to speak in shorter sentences, using simple language and omitting unnecessary words. Sometimes, you may find that you have to be redundant, changing words until you are finally understood. Speak in context so that if you are having a conversation about lunch, have the conversation in the kitchen. Lastly, the use of hand movements or gestures can clarify meaning and improve understanding.

A secondary goal is to evaluate and assist the individual in activities to maintain function. At this stage, the individual with PPA will not initiate household activities or personal-care activities. Suggesting bath time, supervising grooming, and establishing a consistent daily routine can help to maintain function because it does not require thought and planning.

Case Study: Moderate Stage

Four years into the disease, Judith was experiencing major problems with language. She was unable to repeat words—even her name. Her sentences were shortened to three to four words, yet she still could not pronounce all of the words. She often did not understand what was said to her, but she was able to answer "yes-no" questions appropriately. She was no longer able to use her talking tablet. The speech pathologist ordered a pictured language board to help the family communicate.

Judith was now dependent on others for some activities of daily living and became lax in her personal care. Her husband, Dave, could get her to shower only when he showered with her. She developed an obsession, insisting that she only wear one outfit: a red pair of shorts with a flowered top. Dave would wash them each night so that she could wear them every day. Judith began to make sexually suggestive comments to males, including her children. The couple stopped dining out at peak hours because Judith would approach other tables, taking food from others diners' plates.

Dave enrolled Judith in an adult day health program five days a week. He met with the activities director and staff to provide a better understanding of Judith's behaviors and language difficulty. Judith's attendance at the day program allowed Dave to continue working, and Judith seemed to enjoy the activities. It also provided their children quiet time after school. Dave joined a PPA support group, where he found many care recommendations, support, and understanding from other caregivers.

By the sixth year, Judith was not able to say more than one or two words with great difficulty. She was able to answer "yes" or "no," but she frequently corrected herself. She understood little of what was said to her. Dave and the children now used one or two words and hand gestures to express ideas to her. Lastly, they found that limiting noise and visual distractions in the environment enhanced communication.

Severe-Stage PPA

Advanced PPA renders people mute, unable even to indicate "yes" or "no." Individuals with PPA may grunt or yell spontaneously but have little to no comprehension of language. They may have difficulty with swallowing in the severe stage. The person may stuff her mouth, unable to coordinate a swallow, and needs careful observation to prevent choking.

Activities of daily living are impaired, including bathing, grooming, selecting clothing, dressing, and toileting. The person may have difficulty with balance and may suffer repeated falls. It is not uncommon for people with advanced PPA to become resistant to help with personal care and become combative during care. Using the person's returned primitive grip (the automatic reflex grip we see in childhood development that is suppressed in adulthood may return when cerebral damage or regression occurs) by having them hold an object such as a small stress ball, may help to keep caregivers safe. It is important to remember that the person with advanced PPA may not understand directions given by caregivers and lacks the ability to communicate his fears and needs.

In the severe stage, individuals with PPA may simply sit and stare. There may be a reversal of day/night orientation, mandating the need for twenty-four-hour care. Activities should be undertaken, but very simply and with a minimum of group interaction. Very simple objects, such as colorful blocks, using crayons, or paper towels to shred may occupy their attention for long periods of time. Mild sensory stimulation, such as gentle music or aroma-therapy, may also be helpful. The person should always be supervised to prevent eating the activity materials.

Care Goals in Severe Stage

Dysphagia, or difficulty swallowing, may be present in severe-stage PPA. Initial strategies for those with dysphagia include changing the consistency of food. Textures such as soft foods with thicker liquids should be modified to reduce the risk of aspiration, one of the primary causes of mortality among those with PPA. Provide foods that are high in calorie and rich in protein and fat content to maintain nutrition. Speech-therapy interventions may be useful for recommending swallowing maneuvers and a variety of strategies to maintain safe oral feeding. Lastly, caregivers may need to crush medications. Consult your healthcare provider or pharmacist to determine if crushing is appropriate. Also ask your provider or pharmacist if the medication is available in a liquid form.

An additional goal in severe PPA is to promote emotional and physical comfort. This is accomplished with a consistent routine and, whenever possible, caregiver support. Attention should be paid to potential injuries, such as the onset of decubitus ulcers, perineal infections, skin tears, or pathological fractures. If the person has even mild pain, it should be treated with analgesics on a scheduled basis. Attend to function with the least amount of physical and emotional discomfort to the person. For example, bed or towel baths can be soothing and eliminate the need for showers (Hall, Gallagher, and Hoffman, 2013). All clothing should look alike and be easily applied. At this stage, most individuals are using pull-up briefs. Toileting schedules should be utilized, especially after meals.

Lastly, dental care may also be an issue at this time. The goal is to maintain current dentition with the least amount of restorative care, as dental prosthetics often require a great deal of flossing and care, and to prevent pain. Seek a dentist who has hospital privileges and is willing to provide professional cleanings at least quarterly under procedural sedation. If the person is in long-term care, inquire if there is a dentist who visits the facility.

Case Study: Severe Stage

Judith eventually became entirely mute. She spent most of her time at home sitting at the kitchen table, arranging and rearranging colorful children's blocks. Dave plays soft folk music and easy-listening selections. Four days each week, she attends an adult day health program, but the staff informed Dave that her care was too heavy for them to manage. Judith continued to eat just about anything she could fit into her mouth, which meant that she required constant supervision.

Dave decided to bring more help into the home. He hired a home health aide to help Judith with her activities of daily living such as bathing and meal-time. Together, Dave and the home health aide developed a daily routine for Judith that included a set schedule for mealtimes and bedtime, as well as other consistent simple activities that Judith could anticipate, which reduced her anxiety.

MOVEMENT DISORDERS— CORTICOBASAL DEGENERATION (CBD), PROGRESSIVE SUPRANUCLEAR PALSY (PSP), AND FRONTOTEMPORAL DEGENERATION/ MOTOR NEURON DISEASE (FTD-MND)

FTD presents with a number of distinct types that are highly dependent on affected brain regions and underlying pathology (Grossman et al. 2007). For example, motor features such as slowed and rigid movement make it diffi-cult to perform purposeful actions for persons with corticobasal degenera-tion (CBD) and progressive supranuclear palsy (PSP) (Armstrong et al. 2013). Abilities requiring visuospatial functioning are also sometimes compromised in these two phenotypes. Simply put, visuospatial function refers to the ability of the brain to interpret the world around us, as it relates to the perception of objects in space. Motor neuron disease (MND) such as amyotrophic lateral sclerosis (ALS) is associated with a variety of motor features such as muscle weakness and muscle spasms. FTD-MND describes the dual diagnosis of FTD with MND. This syndrome is characterized by behavioral and language features common in FTD, as well as motor symptoms common in MND such as dysphagia (difficulty swallowing), muscle loss, weakness, and, in some cases, spasticity (Lillo and Hodges 2009).

Mild-Stage Movement Disorder

Visuospatial impairment is often seen in mild CBD and PSP (Borroni et al. 2008). This may include symptoms such as difficulty perceiving visual objects and difficulty with spatial orientation. Many patients will also complain of limb apraxia, or loss of ability to perform purposeful movements. In the mild stage, persons with FTD-MND may experience behavior and language difficulty as well as muscle weakness and atrophy (muscle shrinkage). There may also be some difficulty with fine motor movements (Hsiung et al. 2012).

Care Goals in the Mild Stage

The goals in the mild stage are aimed at maintaining function. A variety of strategies can be used to optimize visuospatial function. These include orienting the person to place and location frequently, especially in new or unfamiliar settings. Use bright-colored tape as a guide for stairs or other hazard areas where falls may occur. Use banisters on the stairs for support (enhanced with bright-colored tape) and backpacks for carrying objects. Remove throw rugs and toys from the floor, which also pose a fall hazard. Create wide walking paths for common walking areas and use only safe walking shoes, such as athletic shoes. For difficulty with fine motor movement, it may be helpful to adapt clothing, such as using Velcro® instead of buttons. Physical therapy and occupational therapy can be good resources for recommendations about adaptive devices and other environmental modifications.

Case Study: Mild Stage

Anthony was a fifty-eight-year-old carpenter who noticed he was particularly clumsy with his right arm. He began having difficulty holding his hammer in his hand and seeing the nails he wanted to strike. A few months later, he noticed his right arm began to jerk unintentionally. He was eventually diagnosed with CBD. Anthony and his wife, Lori, met with the interdisciplinary team, which included his medical doctor, nurse practitioner, social worker, physical thera-pist, occupational therapist, and speech-language pathologist. The team met with Anthony and Lori to discuss strategies for managing his visuospatial and motor difficulties. The physical therapist and occupational therapist visited Anthony's home and made recommendations about how to structure the home to maximize his functioning. While it became unsafe for Anthony to con-tinue working, he began attending an adult health activity program and would perform supervised tasks as a volunteer at his local church. He also enjoyed taking a modified tai chi class at his local community center.

Moderate-Stage Movement Disorder

In the moderate stage of disease, the person with FTD develops more difficulty with activities. You may see a need for more supervision or assistance with personal-care tasks such as dressing and bathing. Mobility may also become more difficult as the disease progresses into the moderate stage.

Care Goals in the Moderate Stage

Special consideration should be given to safety-enhancing interventions in the moderate stage (Talerico and Evans 2001). Patients with movement disor-ders may have difficulty walking independently. Strategies to promote safety include the provision of an injury-safe environment as described in the pre-vious section regarding fall-risk reduction. Assistive devices such as a walker or a cane may provide support for the person with FTD if she is unsteady on her feet. An individualized, home-based exercise program that includes balance training and strengthening exercises, supervised by a physical thera-pist, can maximize balance and mobility in persons with movement disorders (Suttanon et al. 2013, Hauer et al. 2012). Medications including antidepres-sants and antipsychotics (American Geriatrics Society Beers Criteria Update Expert 2012) have been associated with an increased fall risk and, when pos-sible, these medications should be minimized (Epstein et al. 2014). Lastly, gentle range-of-motion exercises can promote blood flow and joint mobility.

Fatigue, a frequent complaint among those with movement disorders, negatively impacts physical and psychological well-being. The identifica-tion of potential causes of fatigue is an important first step in managing this symptom. Common causes of fatigue include dehydration, malnutrition, pain, depression, disturbed sleep, and side effects of medications (Payne, Wiffen, and Martin 2012). Nonpharmacological interventions shown to be effective in reducing fatigue include exercise, adequate sleep, incorporating rest breaks throughout the day, and avoiding conditions that worsen fatigue (i.e., heat) (Krupp and Pollina 1996).

Case Study: Moderate Stage

Four years into the disease, Anthony was having more difficulty with dressing and bathing independently. His walking became unstable, and he fell frequently. His wife, Lori, hired a retired nurse to help her with her caregiving activities, and this also allowed Lori to get some respite. Anthony's physical therapist visited the home to perform a home safety assessment. Anthony's family was advised to keep the walking areas free of clutter. His family also rearranged the furniture to give him wider walking paths. Lastly, they ordered a commode to place on the first floor so that Anthony did not have to navigate the steps to get to the bathroom.

Severe-Stage Movement Disorder

In the severe stage of disease, as the person with FTD loses basic functions; as such, the focus is on quality of life and well-being. At this stage, there are several complications, such as pneumonia, infection, or injury from a fall, that may occur as a result of loss of function (theaftd.org). It is important for caregivers to be aware of these complications and work closely with the healthcare team to manage these issues.

Care Goals in the Severe Stage

The care goals in the severe stage tend to focus on promoting comfort and optimizing quality of life. Oftentimes, in the severe stage, individuals affected with CDB, PSP, and FTD-MND, are often chair-bound. Individuals in the severe stage, thus, may experience musculoskeletal pain because of immobility. Assisted range-of-motion exercises may be effective in reducing pain, and premedication with acetaminophen may be necessary to improve adherence to exercises (Miyasaki 2013). Constipation is another symptom that some may experience due to reduced mobility. Diet modification, such as increased vegetable and fruit intake in combination with good hydration, is the first step that should be taken to address constipation. Constipation may also be treated with standard laxatives and stool softeners, but you should consult your healthcare team about which medication is most appropriate.

Case Study: Severe Stage

Anthony's limited mobility eventually limited him to a wheelchair, and he needed total assistance with activities of daily living. His wife, Lori, decided Anthony needed more care than what she was able to give him in their restrictive home environment. Anthony was transitioned into a nursing facility that was better equipped to manage his physical impairments. Anthony continued to receive physical therapy for range-of-motion and stretching exercises, which reduced his stiffness in his arms and legs. The staff ordered a special bed with a support mattress that helped reduce pressure and friction, factors that contribute to bedsores. The speech-language pathologist made suggestions for altering the consistency of Anthony's food to help him swallow. The staff also provided small, frequent meals for Anthony, and they found that this helped to reduce his fatigue so that he was able to continue to participate in group activities.

END-OF-LIFE CARE IN FTD AND RELATED DISORDERS

Unlike diseases such as cancer, persons with neurodegenerative conditions experience a slow deterioration over time. This uncertain trajectory makes it challenging to predict how much time a person has until death. Medicare's hospice-eligibility criteria for dementia pose additional challenges to timely services for people with FTD because the criteria were built on the progression of AD. Although persons with FTD present differently from each other in the earlier stages depending on the variant, all forms of FTD tend to appear similar at the end of life.

At the end-of-life stage, the person with FTD is bed- or chair-bound and requires assistance for all purposeful movement. The body may be immobile, or joints may be stiff. Individuals may experience significant weight loss and muscle wasting. Body movements are limited. The person may develop complications from immobility, such as deep-vein thrombosis or pulmonary embolism. The person is completely dependent on others for all activities of daily living and is incontinent of bowel and bladder. There is no spontaneous participation in activities. The individual is likely mute or speaks only a few words, however, he may have spontaneous repetitive vocalizations. There may be pooling, choking, or coughing on food/liquid/saliva. Recurrent infections, including pneumonia and urinary-tract infections, are common at the end of life.

Care Goals in the End of Life

Anecdotal evidence suggests that people with FTD and their families are commonly deprived of hospice services until the final weeks before death, thus missing the benefits associated with hospice's interdisciplinary expertise in holistic comfort care and support. The primary goal of end-of-life care is for a peaceful and comfortable death. This includes use of opioids and other medications to control secretions. Good positioning, skin care, and massage can prevent joint pain and skin breakdown. Care with food consistency must be taken in feeding to prevent choking and aspiration.

Case Study: End of Life

A local hospice nurse visited George and his parents. Upon reviewing his medical records, the nurse determined that George fulfilled Medicare's criteria for hospice eligibility due to his significant decline and advanced condition (National Hospice Organization 1996). The nurse explored the goals of care with George's parents. Although they never had a discussion with George about specific details regarding healthcare decisions, his parents used their best substituted judgment to identify that George would not choose aggressive interventions to prolong his life when there was little to any benefit to improve his condition. Each item on the healthcare directives (HCD) was discussed with the support of the hospice staff so that George's parents could make informed decisions to honor their son's wishes. The completed document clearly communicated that George did not choose resuscitation, hospitalization, antibiotics, or a feeding tube. Instead, the goals focused on aggressive comfort care so that George could live out his days safe and comfortable in the company of those who knew him best.

George's medication regime was simplified to include only essential medications to maximize comfort. Routine acetaminophen was prescribed for stiffness and chronic-pain issues, and the staff used a nonverbal pain assessment tool to ensure that every measure was taken to evaluate comfort and respond accordingly. The interdisciplinary hospice team focused on optimizing George's quality of life by providing daily sensory pleasures based on those he enjoyed throughout his lifetime. Favorite music, prayers, and poetry kept him engaged for periods of time throughout the day. His parents were encouraged to visit and talk to or read to George. His diet was liberalized to the items he enjoyed most and tolerated safely, and he was offered them frequently in small amounts. Despite his apparent lack of awareness, George's parents were encouraged to bring in familiar items from the past, such as photos and other touchstones to reminisce about meaningful moments of his life. Staff reported that George's screaming episodes, although not completely eradicated, diminished significantly within days after the aforementioned pharmacological and nonpharmacological comfort measures were initiated.

George eventually developed aspiration pneumonia. He was not admitted to the hospital or administered antibiotics. Instead, his comfort was maximized using medications to address fever, pain, and restlessness, while favorite hymns softly played in the background to create a serene and supportive environment for everyone in the room. Shortly thereafter, George died a peaceful death surrounded by his parents, some favorite long-term facility staff, and his hospice nurse. The hospice team actively supported George's parents and long-term-care staff through the entire process and referred them to the bereavement specialist for thirteen months of follow-up care.

THE FTD CAREGIVING EXPERIENCE

Most of the dementia caregiving literature focuses on caring for persons with AD, but caregivers of persons living with FTD face a set of unique challenges. Some experts believe that extending AD caregiving techniques would be useful for persons with FTD, yet these techniques are only partially successful, as FTD affects different brain structures, and therefore different brain functions. Another barrier to implementing AD interventions for individuals affected by FTD is that services and programs available to older adults, such as adult day programs, in-home support, and some long-term-care programs do not serve younger and middle-aged persons. Public understanding of dementia is largely based on knowledge about AD, and this can be very frustrating for caregivers of persons with FTD (Rosness, Haugen, and Engedal 2008). Studies have consistently demonstrated higher levels of caregiver distress, burden, and depression in FTD caregivers when compared to AD caregivers (Riedijk et al. 2006, Wong et al. 2011, Mioshi et al. 2012, Mioshi et al. 2009). This is likely related to several factors, including behavior, language, and motor changes that are severe early on in the disease. Here, we suggest several interventions that we hope will help you manage some of the difficult aspects of FTD.

Caring for persons with FTD is complex and poorly understood. Until recently, FTD was considered a rare disorder, so there was concern that there would be too few people to study for research. A second concern was that due to lack of self-insight, individuals with FTD would refuse to participate in research. Both of these arguments have proven false, and now there is considerable research in the field of FTD, however, most studies focus on the biologic basis for behaviors. Descriptive studies of behavior often are limited to very few subjects (Hall, Shapira, Gallagher, and Denny 2013; Lavenu and Pasquier 2005; Massimo, Evans, and Benner 2013). As a result, there is little research on the efficacy of nonpharmacological interventions for FTD. The interventions described in this chapter were the result of clinical experience and tips from real caregivers who have faced these challenges with grace and ingenuity.

BIBLIOGRAPHY

Alzheimer's Association. 2012. MedicAlert® + Alzheimer's Association Safe Return®. http://www.alz.org/care/dementia-medic-alert-safe-return.asp.

American Geriatrics Society Beers Criteria Update Expert Panel. "American Geriatrics Society Updated Beers Criteria for Potentially Inappropriate Medication Use in Older Adults." *Journal of the American Geriatric Society* 60, no. 4 (2012): 616–31.

Armstrong, M. J., I. Litvan, A. E. Lang, et al. "Criteria for the Diagnosis of Corticobasal Degeneration." *Neurology* 80, no. 5 (2013): 496–503.

Arvanitakis, Z. "Update on Frontotemporal Dementia." *Neurologist* 16, no. 1 (2010): 16–22.

The Association for Frontotemporal Degeneration. 2014. www.theaftd.org.

Borroni, B., M. Turla, V. Bertasi, et al. "Cognitive and Behavioral Assessment in the Early Stages of Neurodegenerative Extrapyramidal Syndromes." *Archives of Gerontology and Geriatrics* 7, no. 1 (2008): 53–61.

Boxer, A., et al. "A 26-Week, Randomized, Multicenter, Placebo-Controlled Trial of Memantine for Behavioral Variant Frontotemporal Dementia and Semantic Variant Primary Progressive Aphasia." Paper presented at the 8th International Conference on Frontotemporal Dementias, Manchester, England. September 5, 2012.

Charles, D., C. Olm, J. Powers, et al. "Grammatical Comprehension Deficits in Non-fluent/Agrammatic Primary Progressive Aphasia." *Journal of Neurology, Neurosurgery & Psychiatry* 85, no. 3 (2014): 249–56.

Chow, T. W., J. D. Fridhandler, M. A. Binns, A. Lee, J. Merrilees, H. J. Rosen, R. Ketelle, and B. L. Miller. "Trajectories of Behavioral Disturbance in Dementia." *Journal of Alzheimer's Disease* 31, no. 1 (2012): 143–49.

Epstein, N. U., R. Guo, M. R. Farlow, J. P. Singh, and M. Fisher. "Medication for Alzheimer's Disease and Associated Fall Hazard: A Retrospective Cohort Study from the Alzheimer's Disease Neuroimaging Initiative." *Drugs Aging* 31, no. 2 (2014): 125–29.

Farrajota, L., C. Maruta, J. Maroco, et al. "Speech Therapy in Primary Progressive Aphasia: A Pilot Study." *Dementia and Geriatric Cognitive Disorders Extra* 2, no. 1 (2012): 321–31.

Folstein, M. F., S. E. Folstein, and P. R. McHugh. "'Mini-Mental State': A Practical Method for Grading the Cognitive State of Patients for the Clinician." *Journal of Psychiatric Research* 12 (1975): 189–98.

Gallagher, M., A. McLean, and R. Wilson. 2011. "Discussion of Hospice and End-of-Life Symptoms in FTD" [PowerPoint® slides]. Retrieved from the AFTD website at http://www.theaftd.org/support-resources/managing-health-care/hospice-end-of-life/hospice-and-end-of-life-symptoms.

Garcin, B, P. Lillo, M. Hornberger, et al. "Determinants of Survival in Behavioral Variant Frontotemporal Dementia." *Neurology* 73 (2009): 656–1661.

Gorno-Tempini, M. L., et al. 2011. "Classification of Primary Progressive Aphasia and Its Variants." *Neurology* 76, no. 11:1006–14.

Grossman, M., et al. "Distinct Antemortem Profiles in Patients with Pathologically Defined Frontotemporal Dementia." *Archives of Neurology* 64, no. 11 (2007): 1601–1609.

Grossman, M. 2002. "Frontotemporal Dementia: An Update." *Journal of International Neuropsychological Society* 8: 566–83.

Hall, G. R., J. Shapira, M. Gallagher, and S. Denny. "Clinical Concepts: Managing Differences: Care of the Person with Frontotemporal Degeneration (FTD)." *Journal of Gerontological Nursing* 39, no. 3 (2013): 10–14.

Hauer, K., M. Schwenk, T. Zieschang, et al. "Physical Training Improves Motor Performance in People with Dementia: A Randomized Controlled Trial." *Journal of the American Geriatrics Society* 60, no. 1 (2012): 8–15.

Henry, M. L., M. V. Meese, S. Truong, et al. "Treatment for Apraxia of Speech in Nonfluent Variant Primary Progressive Aphasia." *Behavioural Neurology* 26, nos. 1–2 (2013): 77–88.

Hsiung, G. Y., et al. "Clinical and Pathological Features of Familial Frontotemporal Dementia Caused by *C9orf72* Mutation on Chromosome 9p." *Brain* 135, pt. 3 (2012): 709–22.

Krupp, L. B., and D. A. Pollina. "Mechanisms and Management of Fatigue in Progressive Neurological Disorders." *Current Opinion in Neurology* 9, no. 6 (1996): 456–60.

Lillo, P., and J. R. Hodges. "Frontotemporal Dementia and Motor Neurone Disease: Overlapping Clinic-Pathological Disorders." *Journal of Clinical Neuroscience* 16, no. 9 (2009): 1131–35.

Massimo, L., L. K. Evans, and P. Benner. "Caring for Loved Ones with Frontotemporal Degeneration: The Lived Experiences of Spouses." *Geriatric Nursing* 34, no. 4 (2013): 302–306.

Massimo, L., and M. Grossman. "Patient Care and Management of Frontotemporal Lobar Degeneration." *American Journal of Alzheimer's Disease & Other Dementias* 23, no. 2 (2008): 125–31.

Mendez, M. F., and J. S. Shapira. "Loss of Emotional Insight in Behavioral Variant Frontotemporal Dementia or 'Frontal Anosodiaphoria.'" *Conscious Cognition* 20, no. 4 (2011): 1690–96. Epub September 29, 2011.

Mendez MF, J. S. Shapira, A. McMurtray, E. Licht. "Preliminary Findings: Behavioral Worsening on Donepezil in Patients with Frontotemporal Dementia." *The American Journal of Geriatric Psychiatry* 15, no. 1 (2007): 84–87.

Merrilees, J., and R. Ketelle. "Advanced Practice Nursing: Meeting the Caregiving Challenges for Families of Persons with Frontotemporal Dementia." *Clinical Nurse Specialist* 24, no. 5 (2010): 245–51.

Miller, B. 2012. "Progression of FTD." UCSF Memory and Aging Center. http://memory.ucsf.edu/ftd/overview/ftd/progression/multiple.

Mioshi, E., M. Bristow, R. Cook, and J. R. Hodges. "Factors Underlying Caregiver Stress in Frontotemporal Dementia and Alzheimer's Disease." *Dementia and Geriatric Cognitive Disorders* 27, no. 1 (2009): 76–81.

Mioshi, E., D. Foxe, F. Leslie, et al. "The Impact of Dementia Severity on Caregiver Burden in Frontotemporal Dementia and Alzheimer Disease." *Alzheimer's Disease & Associated Disorders* 27, no. 1 (2013): 68–73.

Miyasaki, J. M. "Palliative Care in Parkinson's Disease." *Current Neurology and Neuroscience Reports* 13, no. 8 (2013): 67.

Modirrousta, M., B. H. Price, and B. C. Dickerson. "Neuropsychiatric Symptoms in Primary Progressive Aphasia: Phenomenology, Pathophysiology, and Approach to Assessment and Treatment." *Neurodegenerative Disease Management* 3, no. 2 (2013): 133–46.

Nasreddine, Z. S., et al. "The Montreal Cognitive Assessment, MoCA: A Brief Screening Tool for Mild Cognitive Impairment." *Journal of the American Geriatrics Society* 53, no. 4 (2005): 695–99.

National Hospice Organization. *Medical Guidelines for Determining Prognosis in Selected Non-Cancer Diseases.* 2nd ed. Arlington, VA: National Hospice Organization, 1996.

National Institute on Aging. *Frontotemporal Disorders: Information for Patients, Families, and Caregivers.* Washington DC: National Institutes of Health and Human Services, 2010. http://www.nia.nih.gov/sites/default/files/frontotemporal_disorders_information_for_patients_families_and_caregivers_0.pdf. Accessed November 15, 2012.

Onyike, C. U. "What Is the Life Expectancy in Frontotemporal Lobar Degeneration?" *Neuroepidemiology* 37, nos. 3–4 (2011): 166–67.

Papatrianafyllou, J., I. Viscontact, S. Papagegeorgiou, et al. "Difficulties in Detecting

Behavioral Symptoms or Frontotemporal Lobar Degeneration across Cultures." *Alzheimer's Disease & Associated Disorders* 23, no. 1 (2009): 77–81.

Payne, C., P. J. Wiffen, and S. Martin. "Interventions for Fatigue and Weight Loss in Adults with Advanced Progressive Illness." *Cochrane Database of Systematic Reviews* 1 (2012): CD008427.

Rascovsky, K., J. R. Hodges, D. Knopman, et al. "Sensitivity of Revised Diagnostic Criteria for the Behavioural Variant of Frontotemporal Dementia." *Brain* 134, pt. 9 (2011): 2456–77.

Ratnavalli, E., C. Brayne, K. Dawson, and J. R. Hodges. "The Prevalence of Frontotemporal Dementia." *Neurology* 58 (2002): 1615–21.

Riedijk, S. R., M. E. de Vugt, H. J. Duivenvoorden, et al. "Caregiver Burden, Health-Related Quality of Life and Coping in Dementia Caregivers: A Comparison of Frontotemporal Dementia and Alzheimer's Disease." *Dementia and Geriatric Cognitive Disorders* 22, nos. 5–6 (2006): 405–12.

Rosness, T. A., P. K. Haugen, and K. Engedal. "Support to Family Carers of Patients with Frontotemporal Dementia." *Aging & Mental Health* 12, no. 4 (2008): 462–66.

Savage, S. A., O. Piguet, and J. R. Hodges. 2014. "Giving Words New Life: Generalization of Word Retraining Outcomes in Semantic Dementia." *Journal of Alzheimer's Disease* 49, no 7 (2013): 1823–32.

Suttanon, P., K. D. Hill, C. M. Said, et al. "Feasibility, Safety and Preliminary Evidence of the Effectiveness of a Home-Based Exercise Programme for Older People with Alzheimer's Disease: A Pilot Randomized Controlled Trial." *Clinical Rehabilitation* 27, no. 5 (2013): 427–38.

Talerico, K. A., and L. K. Evans. "Responding to Safety Issues in Frontotemporal Dementias." *Neurology* 56, no. 11, suppl. 4 (2001): S52–5.

Wong, C., J. Merrilees, R. Ketelle, et al. "The Experience of Caregiving: Differences between Behavioral Variant of Frontotemporal Dementia and Alzheimer Disease." *American Journal of Geriatric Psychiatry: Official Journal of the American Association for Geriatric Psychiatry* 20, no. 8 (2012): 724–28.

Yamaguchi, H., Y. Maki, and T. Yamagami. "Overview of Non-pharmacological Intervention for Dementia and Principles of Brain-Activating Rehabilitation." *Psychogeriatrics* 10, no. 4 (2010): 206–13.

CHAPTER 17

A BALANCE OF HEALTH

Maintaining General Medical-Care Practices

Bruce L. Miller, MD;
and Rosalie Gearhart, RN, MS, CS

What will he be like after surgery?
Is cancer screening important at this point? If the test is positive, what will
   happen next?
What are the alternatives?

The goal of this chapter is to outline some guiding principles to support you
through the ongoing decision-making process regarding health issues as a caregiver for a person with frontotemporal degeneration (FTD). Because FTD is
still a relatively understudied disorder, there are few research studies or tested
theories that are available to guide you. We all learn as we go along this difficult
journey, and much of what is shared in this chapter comes from the experiences,
stories, and writings of patients and families who have waged a fight against
this devastating illness. They have championed this cause to help others avoid
the traumatic experiences that they have gone through with FTD. Due to their
courage, we are fast approaching the day when we will no longer receive calls
from caregivers reporting that "they don't know much about FTD around here."

   This chapter is based on the overarching goal of helping caregivers make
effective decisions for their loved ones. Rarely in the caregiving world do
we take the time to reflect on how we got here and how we worked through
so many difficult decisions. How do we know what is the right thing to do?
Simply stated, there is no single right answer. Rather, we always need to take
a step backward to think about how to tailor care based on the individual's
values and preferences, ethnicity, cultural background, and spiritual practices.
The lifetime of conversations and joint experiences, and the shared family
values will give you special insights that no physician, nurse, social worker, or
psychologist will have. Your own instincts will serve you well!

Of course, caregiving for FTD is a job that no one ever expected, so usually there has been no training for this role, and no prior planning. Initially, the addition of caregiver duties to existing family responsibilities can be overwhelming. It is hard enough to make up our own minds about our personal health choices, but what do we do when someone else's mind is changing so that we need to make decisions for him or her as well? And what do we do when that person is no longer able to discuss his or her preferences and participate effectively in healthcare decisions?

The guidelines and principles outlined in this chapter can help you to structure an organized and focused approach to anticipated and unanticipated healthcare decisions. It is important for patients, families, and clinicians to make decisions together about treatment plans and treatment goals. Caring for an impaired individual requires a team that will divide the work that is required to accomplish the plan. There will be a stage when joint decisions with the patient are no longer possible. Ongoing assessment and input from the clinicians involved will help to determine when this occurs and you need not feel like you must handle any decision alone. You should choose your physician and other advisors carefully so that you are comfortable with their advice. (See chapter 4 for more information.) Finally, it is important to have realistic expectations for the ill person as the disease progresses.

PATIENTS' RIGHTS

All healthcare organizations adopt some version of patients' rights for staff to follow in the delivery of care to patients. Patients' rights were first developed in response to the need to ensure consistent and fair care to all. In response to the special needs of dementia patients and their families, caregivers have developed a "The Best Friends™ Dementia Bill of Rights"[1]:

Every person diagnosed with Alzheimer's disease or other dementia deserves:

- To be informed of one's diagnosis.
- To have appropriate, ongoing medical care.
- To be treated as an adult, listened to, and afforded respect for one's feelings and point of view.
- To be with individuals who know one's life story, including cultural and spiritual traditions.

- To experience meaningful engagement throughout the day.
- To live in a safe and stimulating environment.
- To be outdoors on a regular basis.
- To be free from psychotropic medications whenever possible.
- To have welcomed physical contact, including hugging, caressing, and handholding.
- To be an advocate for oneself and others.
- To be part of a local, global, or online community.
- To have care partners well trained in dementia care.

You are a key person in assessing the patients' ability to make decisions for themselves along with the professional healthcare providers. This requires an ongoing assessment that can be guided by the following questions. Among the many losses patients with dementia inevitably experience is loss of competency to make decisions for themselves.

- What is the patient's understanding of the illness?
- What is the patient's current level of participation in his care?
- Can the patient show an appreciation of the risks and the benefits involved?
- Can the patient provide rational reasons for the decision?

Patients' rights are available to you to support your advocacy for your loved ones across all settings: clinics, hospitals, assistive living facilities, and long-term-care facilities. This all means that you are not alone in this process.

ETHICAL PRINCIPLES

The moral principles involved in dementia care have been widely reviewed in the bioethical literature. Many novel terms have been developed specific to the progressive degenerative nature of the diseases. Dementia-specific terms regarding competence and treatments that extend the course but do not cure the disease—such as "the then self" and "negotiated autonomy" are used by ethicists. Ethical principles are utilized to govern care and to lead one's life. Often there are conflicts between one, or more than one, of the bioethical principles of autonomy, confidentiality, truth telling, beneficence, and justice when caring for a demented person. These conflicts come up regularly in day-to-day decisions. For example, it is common to see an FTD patient who wants to continue to drive (autonomy), yet we must also protect his or her personal safety as well as the general public's safety (beneficence). The ethical issues commonly encountered by caregivers in decision making include autonomy, competency, consent, advance directives, truth telling, genetic testing, artificial (tube) feeding, behavior control, research, and end-of-life care.

Most bioethical discussions regarding dementia have focused on professionals. There is little written about the ethical issues from the perspective of family caregivers, yet many of the problems faced by caregivers require the same ethical considerations faced by professionals. Unlike issues for professionals, issues for caregivers arise from a personal context and are often shaped by long-term relationships.

We all use guiding principles and belief systems to live our lives and to relate to others. Our society has established certain rules and norms, many based on our best interests and designed to protect our autonomy. Caring for an adult with dementia often forces us to readdress these principles. As we strive to avoid being overly paternalistic in the delivery of our care, we must also protect the patient from harm or risks that the disease has created secondary to lack of insight, poor judgment, and impaired reasoning.

CAREGIVER ROLES IN HEALTH DECISIONS

Unlike many other adult-onset illnesses, FTD requires that the family play an essential role in the diagnostic process and care on an intimate level. Identifying the roles of all caregivers involved can be helpful in sharing the job. Identify the strengths and, yes, the weaknesses of the caregivers involved. Some family members may have a more sophisticated knowledge of the healthcare delivery systems, and they can be identified as the ones to talk with the multiple healthcare providers involved. Others may have the most patience and empathy, and these skills can be used to spend the time providing direct daily care, listening and talking with the patient. It is important to utilize each individual's expertise and strengths and to constantly reassess whether the family is the best choice as caregiver or if a nonfamily alternative caregiver is indicated. We have found that FTD patients are often made more pliant and trusting by their illness as it progresses, which, in turn, may make them particularly accepting of new caregivers who are not within the family.

There are no published studies of the reactions, experiences, or burdens involved in caregiving for a loved one with FTD. No doubt, as with Alzheimer's disease, FTD caregiving is an emotional roller coaster. Adding to this problem is the fact that our society undervalues the role of caregiving. Caregivers may feel proud of their accomplishments and strengthened by their love and commitment to their loved one, as well as frustrated, exhausted, and depressed. In everyday life it is difficult to separate the needs and preferences of the patient from the needs and best interests of the caregivers. The effect that caregiving has on the relationship with the patient cannot be overlooked. The value of the family's participation in the healthcare of the patient is indisputable, but it is known to place strain on the dynamics of adult relationships. It is important to focus on the strengths of the patients as well as the caregivers. People need acknowledgment of their successes and accomplishments when faced with such challenging situations and stress.

ANTICIPATING HEALTHCARE DECISIONS THROUGH THE COURSE OF THE DISEASE

Early planning for decisions, when possible, is the key to making successful choices and reducing stress. Discussing choices with the patient early in the disease is helpful but can be difficult and sometimes even counterproductive due to the patient's deficits in judgment and insight. Asking help from a professional to guide this discussion can be very constructive and supportive. It is vital to collect information and to ask all the questions you need but to be careful not to let information collection harmfully delay your decisions. It is vital to establish the goals of care based on the current stage of the disease and life expectancy. Each informed decision must weigh the risks and benefits regarding the possible outcomes. The goal is to optimize the level of function and the quality of life for all involved.

Setting the Scene

Whether it is a routine health-related visit or an unexpected visit to the emergency room, some planning and thought will need to be given to ensure the most successful outcomes. Personality and behavioral changes are hallmarks of this disease. As the primary caregiver, you most likely have the best understanding of how your loved one may react during a medical visit. If possible, discuss your needs and concerns ahead of time. Discuss with staff the optimal forms of communication and potential avenues for decision making. Discuss the possible role of medication. Ensure that your loved one feels included in discussions related to her healthcare. Also, talking to other families of FTD patients may give you additional ideas of what works. Having a durable power of attorney for healthcare acknowledges the role of the assigned decision maker in the event that the person with FTD loses the capacity to make informed decisions. (See chapter 22 for more information.)

Being prepared for the visits to health providers optimizes the use of the face-to-face time with the healthcare provider in an environment where third-party payers (insurance) are shortening the time allotted for visits. Maintain a record of the names of all healthcare providers, their contact information, and the dates of service. It can be very helpful to spend the time to write up the history of the illness so that important details and events are not forgotten. Also keep a list of all medications and note the response to the medications or any side effects and the response when off medications. Maintain health-insurance information, policy numbers, and telephone numbers in an organized manner.

Probably one of the most important management tools for caring for a FTD patient is keeping track of any changes in behavior or personality. This behavior log will be extremely helpful to healthcare providers when administering selected treatments and interventions. It is also helpful to caregivers as it assists in identifying patterns or potentially causative factors that may lead to disturbed behaviors. A behavior log can also be very valuable in helping caregivers to realize that it is not their own personal issues at fault. They can quietly sit and review at a calm moment several weeks of notes that clearly confirm their worries and suspicions. FTD is a behaviorally loaded disease, and it can be very challenging to self-reflect and acknowledge your own emotions and reactions to the behaviors of a person with a brain disease that causes drastic changes in expected behaviors and characteristics.

Patients with FTD often have no insight into their condition and, therefore, concerned family members often have a difficult time getting them to seek help. This is where distractions can be of help. Often caregivers will ask the patient to come to the doctor's appointment for another problem that the patient is concerned about. We have had many visits to our memory clinic for knee pain or new glasses. They are important needs to address as well but certainly are not always the primary reason for the visit. Another strategy to get resistant patients into a clinic for help is to refocus their attention on someone else. Ask them to come along for you. Say you need to talk to someone about a problem. Also, since a person with FTD may have a good memory, a promised reward may work as an incentive. For example, a stop at a favorite spot on the trip home may lead to cooperation. Staff at dementia centers can be very helpful. Do not hesitate to call and ask for suggestions or guidance.

Health Maintenance

How do I get him to the dentist?
I'm not sure if she can't understand me or can't hear me.
What about alternative treatments?

A person's values and beliefs, as well as her ability to access care, influence screening for health-related problems. You and your family should develop a close working relationship with your primary-care provider to ensure that thoughtful decisions are made that reflect your values and beliefs. In general, the adoption of sound nutritional practices, exercise, and adequate rest promote health and well-being and may help prevent illness and disability. It is also important to remember that, while behavioral changes are a key feature in FTD, sudden changes may indicate an illness, such as the flu or urinary-tract infection, or adverse effects of medication, and medical evaluation should be sought. It is critical for all of us to maintain our health at an optimal level. Making sure all sensory systems are functioning at their best is very important. Routine eye exams, hearing exams, podiatry exams, and dental care can prevent problems and improve quality of life. There are standard health screenings, such as colonoscopy or mammography, that are recommended. Decisions regarding the benefits for these screenings will be based on the stage of the illness and the potential outcomes. For example, a decision to screen for prostate or breast cancer should include a discussion on what will be done if results are positive. Will surgery or treatment be considered, or would they not be an option because of the stage of dementia?

Interventions and Treatment

What new FTD-management issues can be anticipated and when?

What changes are atypical and deserve evaluation for a superimposed problem?

How long will it take before we know the treatment is working?

At what stage of the disease would you consider it inappropriate to continue use of any of the treatment options?

How long will the patient benefit from this invasive procedure?

There are some general rules to follow when planning treatment and discussing treatment options with healthcare providers. The first is to start with one change at a time. For example, if your loved one is experiencing problems with both mood and cognition and you have decided to use a medication, it is always best to pick the most bothersome problem and to initiate treatment of one problem at a time with one medication at a time. This is the best way to tell whether the medication is having the desired effect. Additional medications may be needed, but when two or more are started at the same time, it is difficult to determine which medication is effective or is causing side effects.

Another rule to follow regarding medication usage is to start low and go slow. In this way, the lowest, yet most therapeutic, dose of medication can be used. Also, in selecting pharmacological treatments it is important to consider the simplest dosing schedule possible. It is easier to take a pill once a day than four times a day. Another helpful guideline is to discuss with the prescribing physician drugs with side effects that may be used to a therapeutic advantage. For example, an antidepressant with sedating properties may be a better choice for someone with both depression and trouble sleeping. Everyone should seek evaluation for symptoms that are causing distress; some examples include shortness of breath and pain. No one should be expected to suffer from symptoms when effective forms for managing those symptoms exist.

Treatment of Secondary and Existing Conditions

Of course, patients with FTD also have other medical conditions common to their age group, such as cardiovascular disease, diabetes, hypertension, arthritis, and cancer. FTD patients may have trouble describing specific symptoms, so the caregiver and physician must be vigilant and consider the possibility that new behavioral symptoms are medical in origin. Recently, we witnessed a woman with a urinary catheter whose rhythmic writhing was due to a urinary-tract infection, not the advance of her FTD. Similarly, tooth pain can lead to agitation and aggression in a patient who is unable to describe his or her discomfort. Conversely, repeated visits to the bathroom often represent a compulsion that may be relieved by a serotonin-boosting antidepressant and is not another medical illness.

Many FTD patients will develop symptoms of Parkinson's disease or amyotrophic lateral sclerosis (ALS)—Lou Gehrig's disease. The addition of Parkinsonian symptoms can make the patient prone to falls, and loss of insight into this deficit is particularly problematic with FTD. Patients whose voices weaken or who begin to develop problems with swallowing may be manifesting early symptoms of ALS. When either deficits of movement or ALS occur, life expectancy is markedly diminished and goals and expectations need to be reconsidered.

Medications, particularly SSRIs (selective serotonin reuptake inhibitors), are often helpful for the FTD patient, as discussed in chapter 5. Because of the vulnerability of FTD patients to Parkinsonian symptoms or ALS, it is important to realize that traditional antipsychotic medications such as chlorpromazine or haloperidol can have devastating effects on the FTD patient. Even the atypical antipsychotic medications such as Zyprexa® and Risperdal® can exacerbate swallowing deficits. This increases the need to use tiny doses of medications to avoid choking. In addition, we have found that Ritalin® can precipitate confusion and agitation. It is often the caregiver who is left with monitoring the different treatments recommended by various specialists.

Participating in Research

There is still so much to learn about FTD. Continued and expanded research is needed regarding causes, prevention, medication management, nonpharmacologic methods for managing behavioral problems, as well as the needs of, and effects on, family members providing care to loved ones with FTD. Ideally, it is best to discuss one's interest in research early in the disease. Each opportunity for participation in research projects must be thoughtfully considered, weighing the risks and benefits for all involved. Participating in a research study should be considered as long as it is not unduly burdensome for the patient and family. Participation in research is often personally rewarding as well as significantly beneficial to future generations. (For more information, see chapters 5, 8, and 9.)

SUMMARY

Caregiving is admirable and rewarding. We hope this chapter has provided some general guidelines to support your efforts throughout the course of this disease as you make multiple, thoughtful decisions with your loved one's health and your own health in mind. The golden rule is to keep the patient's wishes in mind and give yourself permission to reassess the situation. Tough decisions you felt were clearly set may need to be modified when the actual time comes, based on the circumstances faced at that time. Use the support of friends and professionals, and base your decisions on your shared beliefs and an organized and focused system of decision making.

Summary addendum

There are many new technologies in various stages of development aimed at improving dementia care, enhancing patient independence, and supporting caregivers. These utilize mobile technology, home-based technology, and social networking to positively impact care and support for individuals with dementia. Examples include intelligent assistive devices, communication devices, activity sensors, and biomedical monitoring. Also available are web-based resources currently available to help prepare both patients and caregivers as they face care choices and to guide healthcare decisions and planning.

RESOURCES FOR SHARED DECISION-MAKING AIDS

Prepare: www.prepareforyourcare.org.
Informed Medical Decisions: www.informedmedicaldecisions.org/patient-page.

NOTE

1. David Troxel and Virginia Bell, "The Best Friends™ Dementia Bill of Rights," Virginia Bell and David Troxel's Best Friends™ Approach to Alzheimer's Care, 2013, http://bestfriendsapproach.com/about/the-best-friends-bill-of-rights/ (accessed July 16, 2014). (The Best Friends™ Dementia Bill of Rights by Virginia Bell & David Troxel. Copyright © 2013 Health Professions Press, Inc.)

CHAPTER 18

FINAL CHOICES

Successfully Navigating Challenges in Advanced and End-of-Life Care

Maribeth Gallagher, DNP, PMHNP-BC, FAAN;
and Jeannette Castellane

This chapter addresses many of the common concerns associated with caring for those with advanced frontotemporal degeneration (FTD) nearing the end-of-life stage. It focuses on maximizing comfort and optimizing quality of life; identifying and upholding the final wishes of the person with FTD; and equipping care partners with the knowledge and skills necessary to successfully navigate challenges that arise. Highlights include exploring realistic options for where loved ones will be cared for during their last days, clarifying health-care decisions at the end of life and discussing the ethical issues around life-prolonging measures. Specific topics will include the importance of a power of attorney; living wills and advance directives; long-term-care (LTC) place-ment, hospitalizations, palliative care and hospice services; and considerations regarding the use of CPR, tube feedings, and treatment options for infections and secondary illnesses.

Caregivers may be able to verbalize that FTD is terminal, but many are still caught by surprise and left unprepared when their loved one reaches the final stages of the disease. Perhaps some caregivers are so consumed in the arduous daily tasks of creatively responding to the seemingly endless series of unexpected challenges that arise as FTD caregivers that they never get a chance to see what is coming their way. Many have witnessed their loved one survive numerous threats along the way, which may have led to a false belief that their loved one will survive any situation.

It is important to take a moment and realize that when the person with FTD enters the final decline and dies, it does not imply failure as a caregiver.

Decline and death in FTD is an inevitable part of the journey, but until the end we can successfully accompany the person every step of the way, safely surrounding them with comfort and love. The following pages will provide information and hopefully assist you in making informed decisions about how best to care for a loved one with FTD and to prepare for the final days. Caregiving for someone with a prolonged illness can be difficult, but caregiving for a person with frontotemporal dementia presents unique challenges many of us have never encountered before.

IT'S NEVER TOO EARLY TO PLAN AHEAD

To date, there are no established methods to cure or halt the progressive deterioration that accompanies FTD, and thus it remains classified as a terminal illness. Although end-of-life decisions may be uncomfortable and extremely difficult to consider, they are vitally important to address as soon after diagnosis as possible so that before decision-making capacity becomes severely impaired, the person with FTD can actively participate in identifying and communicating how he or she wants the final months to unfold.

It is never too early to gather information and initiate discussions about specific plans as they pertain to the end of life. All details should be clarified by having frank and informed discussions whenever possible, followed by securing the information in legal documents (see chapter 22). Copies of the documented details should be given to all those identified as potential proxy decision makers for the person with FTD so that when unforeseen critical medical events arise, the health directives will be readily available to clearly guide and direct the plan of care. In addition to clearly designating a medical power of attorney (MPOA), in many states a mental health power of attorney (MHPOA) is required in the event that the person with FTD needs admission to a psychiatric facility for the treatment of severe agitation or aggression. Failure to obtain the MHPOA can result in expensive, time-consuming efforts to secure guardianship at the exact time the family is in crisis, so be sure to investigate your state's specific regulations.

OPTIMAL ENVIRONMENTS

Environments have the power to influence our thoughts and emotions in significant ways and can trigger moods, perceptions, and behaviors. People with advanced and end-stage FTD are particularly vulnerable to their surroundings as their severe impairments cause them to struggle even more with deciphering and responding to what is going on around them. In their vulnerable and weakened condition they lack any control to modify their world or escape it. Environments, including the people in them, can determine the formidable differences between someone with advanced FTD who feels safe and comfortable, and one who is driven by primitive urges such as fight, flight, or freeze.

Familiar versus Unfamiliar

To a certain extent, we all fear the unknown. Under normal circumstances, new situations may cause anxiety whereas familiar environments and situations provide more stability, security, and sense of emotional well- being. To people with FTD, being in new environments can be particularly upsetting, frightening, and threatening experiences. Unfamiliar places and routines may produce anxiety, frustration, and confusion and trigger escalating emotional expressions and distressing behaviors. Therefore, care partners must play a pivotal role as fierce advocates for creating a comfortable and familiar environment regardless of where the person with FTD resides at the end-of-life stage. Ideally, persons with FTD would never have to leave the comfort and familiarity of their homes, but realistically, due to disease progression and the subsequent need for intensive around-the-clock care, most people with FTD will ultimately require placement outside the home.

In the advanced stage of FTD, whether the person is at home or in a LTC setting such as a residential facility or group home, it is essential to establish environments where they see familiar faces and have familiar routines. It is most important that they are surrounded by people who know how to approach them in a comfortable manner, anticipate their unmet needs, and modify the environment to maintain a sense of calm and safety. Person-centered care approaches that suit the unique needs of the individual with advanced FTD should be the goal, so that in spite of the severity of disease progression and total dependence on others, we do our best to optimize their quality of life well into their last days.

For care partners exploring LTC placement options, remember that familiarity and continuity of staff are important factors to explore. When interviewing potential facilities for your loved one, ask about consistency in the direct caregiving staff and have them share examples of how they implement the concepts of person-centered care for each resident. Because environmental change is distressing, it is ideal to never have to relocate the person with FTD again, so inquire as to whether the facility will be able to provide care into the final days.

Cost of Care

Any illness is costly. A dementia illness is very costly. With dementia, the family is looking at an illness that may go on for many years. Decisions must be made at this time as to what financial resources are available and what are the financial concerns for the future. Refer to chapter 22 for detailed coverage of financial preparation, but here are a few critical things to think about.

Begin by looking into the patient's assets and financial resources. How much income do Social Security, pensions, stocks and dividends, savings accounts, rental property, and any other sources provide?

1. Calculate what it will cost to keep the patient at home with in-home care and/ or modifications to the home. What are the yearly costs for LTC versus being at home?
2. What are the costs for medical care going to be? Will insurance policies help pay for any of these costs?
3. If you need in-home help or respite care, what is this going to cost?
4. What about meal preparation and assistance with feeding costs?
5. Are there any legal fees?
6. If the patient remains at home, what are the annual taxes?
7. What are additional costs in LTC, such as hair care, medications, laundry, etc.? Will the person be able to reside in the facility until he or she dies?
8. Will there be cars or other types of transportation required?
9. What are clothing expenses and other miscellaneous items?

The Internal Revenue Service can assist by explaining tax breaks available for the elderly or disabled and persons caring for a family member with dementia. Spending money on a good financial or tax consultant and elder-law or estate-planning attorney may be well worth the investment (see chapter 22 for more information).

LTC can be very expensive. The average nursing home can cost $70,000 or more per year for a semiprivate room. Financially, this can bankrupt a middle-income family in a short time. Medicare covers acute care but not long-term care. Some coexisting medical conditions may be covered by Medicare and provide for intensive nursing or rehabilitation. Ask a Medicare representative if any condition your loved one has will be covered. Some insurance policies will cover LTC costs but they may exclude people with a dementia. The Veterans Administration may also extend benefits to veterans.

Once a person has exhausted his or her financial resources, he or she becomes eligible to apply for Medicaid. A social worker and the business manager of the LTC can assist you in applying for Medicaid. The Area Agency on Aging is also a good resource.

At-Home Care

Many families wish they could keep their loved ones with advanced FTD at home until they die, for any number of reasons, some of which follow.

1. The family members may feel strongly that they can give better care than an institution can. They know their loved one's habits and needs better than anyone else. The person with dementia may not be able to communicate, but seeing a familiar face and being in a familiar environment is reassuring and calming to them.
2. Some spouses or partners feel that the marriage vows they took or promises they made to care for each other in sickness and health mean just that. They may have made a promise to their loved one never to put them in a nursing home. Breaking that promise may cause them to have considerable guilt.
3. Some cultures expect the family to care for their loved one at home until death occurs. It is expected that members of the close-knit family will help with the care.
4. Some caregivers feel that caring for someone else is the most meaningful thing they can do. They are not looking for praise. They are doing this out of love and respect for the individual. You could almost say it is a vocation for them.

However valid the aforementioned reasons may be, caregivers are urged to seriously consider how they will realistically meet the intensive and around-the-clock demands of caring for someone with advanced FTD at home. Some things to consider when making this decision are:

1. Make sure you have thoroughly discussed your decision to keep your loved one at home with those you trust and respect—family, healthcare providers, clergy, and other important people in your life.
2. Thoroughly understand the disease process and specific demands that will arise as the disease progresses.
3. Know what resources are available in the community should you need them. Are there reliable family and friends who can fill in when necessary? Do you have financial resources to afford home healthcare agencies to provide a homemaker or personal-care aide who can take on some of the duties?
4. Be aware of how the stress of caregiving may impact you in body, mind, and spirit.
5. In the event that something happens and you are unavailable to provide care, what plans have you made for someone else to oversee your loved one's care in the future?

When It's Time for Caregiving Assistance

It is important to understand that it is rare for any one person to be the sole caregiver for someone with FTD throughout the entire trajectory of the illness. This is particularly true when the person with FTD reaches the advanced stage when he or she is completely dependent on others to get every need met and be kept safe. This monumental task "takes a village." Recognizing that one can no longer do this alone is not a sign of giving up, abandonment, or weakness. Quite the contrary, recognizing that assistance is needed reflects insight and good judgment. Requiring assistance or placing a loved one in LTC does not indicate a lack of love and devotion, nor imply a flaw of character, but simply reflects our human limitations and frailties that mandate that we must care for ourselves if we are to remain healthy and functional.

Placing a loved one where he or she will be safe and have 24/7 care has its benefits. As many books on long-term caregiving remind us, the best way we care for our loved ones is to take good care of ourselves. When we have more time to maintain our own well-being, we can genuinely give more of ourselves when we are present with our loved ones, particularly during this precious time as death draws closer. We are freed from our roles performing countless custodial caregiving tasks and invited to resume the original desired relationship of one who simply cherishes the presence of another.

HOSPITALIZATIONS AND THE PERSON WITH FTD

Persons in the later stages of dementia are usually admitted to a hospital because of another acute condition like a fractured hip, urinary-tract infection, dehydration, or pneumonia. These conditions do not necessarily require hospitalization when the goals of care are palliative and identified as "comfort only." In the event that the person with FTD is transferred to the emergency department or hospital, here are some considerations.

Make sure you bring the documents that appoint you as the person's medical power of attorney (MPOA) (otherwise known as healthcare proxy). Also share a copy of the person's healthcare advanced directives (otherwise known as a living will) that clearly identify the patient's specific wishes for medical care. One state's advanced directives do not always work in another state, so make sure the paperwork is updated to be effective when and where it may be needed. Be aware of a little-known fact that if emergency technicians are called (dialing 911), they are required to do whatever is necessary to stabilize a patient and cannot comply with living wills. Only after the patient is evaluated by a physician in the ER can the health directives be implemented.

Admission to a hospital is anxiety-provoking under normal conditions. A person with FTD may find it to be a particularly distressing experience. She may not understand where she is and what is being said or done, and she will not recognize the people who are probing and examining her. In their confusion and frustration, individuals with FTD may feel anger or the need to protect themselves by trying to bite, kick, or punch the staff. In this state of escalating confusion, the person may try to pull out intravenous lines and catheters or climb out of bed and feel a desperate need to escape. Hospitals may use physical and/or chemical restraints to subdue resistive patients, but utilizing these methods frequently adds to the person's confusion and distress while increasing risks for significant injuries.

Families understandably find it upsetting to visit their loved one and see him more confused than when he was in a familiar environment. Hospitals are not experts in treating patients with FTD but are beginning to educate staff on using more patience, respect, flexibility, and compassion when caring for the confused adult. Hospitalized patients with FTD may need one-on-one staffing to keep them reassured, calm, and safe. Most hospitals don't have the time or staff available to do this. Ideally, loved ones can take turns staying with the patient to provide the familiar presence of one who more easily anticipates needs and understands behaviors in the person with FTD. For those with available financial resources, hiring private-duty care may be a good investment as a short-term solution until discharge.

Once a hospitalized patient is stabilized, the caseworker will talk in further detail to the family and/or the LTC facility about discharge (if the patient has come to the hospital from LTC). From the first day in the hospital, discharge plans should begin. If the family has been caring for the patient at home, this is the time to seriously consider placement in an LTC facility that can provide the necessary 24/7 safe care. Another alternative is to consider hiring services that provide in-home assistance so that family caregivers can get the rest they need. Be sure to utilize the caseworker's skills in helping to access available supportive legal and financial resources along with information about adult day-care centers, caregiver support groups, and professional organizations such as the Association of Frontotemporal Degeneration, the Alzheimer's Association, or your area agency on aging. Chapters 20 and 21 provide information on professional services and places to get support.

Optimally, the family has been looking into LTC facilities during earlier stages of the illness, so family members are prepared to make the best choice when one is needed. Visiting various facilities, asking the right questions, and putting the patient's name on a waiting list will help to expedite placement if and when it is necessary. Lack of planning can lead to hasty placement that may not be in the best interests of an individual with special needs. Chapter 20 covers long-term-care placement in great detail.

Avoiding Preventable Hospitalizations

The professional literature reveals a scarcity of information associated with issues concerning advanced and end-of-life care for people with FTD, but studies exploring the same issues in persons with Alzheimer's disease and related dementias may serve as some general frame of reference in areas that lack specific FTD evidence until more scientifically based FTD information emerges.

Hospitalized dementia patients are more likely to have adverse outcomes including: delirium, inadequate pain control, restraints, incontinence, pressure sores, infection, deconditioning, and decreased quality of life. When considering hospitalizations for the person with dementia, keep in mind that transfers from the home to a hospital run the risks of further decline, falls, and more confusion, and use this information to help determine what the person with FTD would have chosen given the realities of the situation.

Studies of people with AD or related dementias suggest that they experience three times the amount of visits to emergency rooms and hospitalizations as compared to those their age without dementia. One factor that contributes to this is the uncertainty that arises from a lack of completed healthcare decisions to clearly guide treatment choices when issues arise. Additionally, many clinicians and dementia caregivers lack awareness that x-rays, laboratory evaluations, and treatment for infections or other illnesses may sometimes be provided in settings other than the hospital, such as at LTC, out-patient clinics and in the home.

As you can see, there is much to consider when it comes to understanding how best to uphold the final healthcare decisions for your loved one with FTD. Therefore, gather as much information as you can and make time to frankly discuss the risks and benefits of all treatment options with knowledgeable healthcare providers to determine if they honor the person's goals of care.

COMFORT CARE

Studies of people with advanced AD and related dementias reveal that a large numbers of them receive aggressive medical interventions at the end of life that demonstrate little to no clinical benefit, cause increased patient discomfort and distress, and result in significantly higher medical expenditures. Consider this fact juxtaposed with the reality that most proxy decision makers say their loved ones with advanced dementia would choose "comfort measures only" as the primary goal of care because they have a terminal neurodegenerative disease that holds no hope of restoration to one's previous condition. Given the discrepancies between patients' identified goals of care and what they actually receive, how do we begin to bridge the gap to ensure that loved ones with advanced dementia avoid aggressive and burdensome medical interventions that have little to no proven clinical benefit? Evidence suggests one way is to raise awareness in professional and family caregivers that there are alternative approaches offered by palliative and hospice services.

Palliative Care

Palliative care is a term that is becoming more widely recognized by healthcare consumers. It means "comfort care" and is offered by a growing number of healthcare organizations with palliative specialists who serve people with serious illnesses. Palliative care can be provided for those who are still pursuing aggressive medical interventions. It does not require a limited life expectancy. Regardless of whether or not one has recently been diagnosed with FTD or has had it for years, palliative care may offer benefits to maximize comfort and quality of life. If interested, check with your insurance provider to determine whether palliative services are covered for your loved one.

Hospice Care

> *"You matter because you are you, and you matter to the end of your life. We will do all we can not only to help you die peacefully, but also to live until you die."*
> —Dame Dr. Cicely Saunders, nurse, physician,
> writer, and founder of the hospice movement (1918–2005)

Hospice is not a new concept in modern society. It had its roots back in medieval times when it was a shelter for the sick or weary who were traveling great distances. The basis for hospice, as we know it today, originated in London. In 1967, Dame Dr. Cicely Saunders founded St. Christopher's Hospice to care for dying patients. This concept spread to the United States and now can be found in many different settings here and throughout the rest of the world.

Although many people associate hospice with cancer care, hospice care is offered to people of all ages who are in the final six months of life due to any kind of terminal illness or injury. Hospice is a philosophy of care that emphasizes compassionate care and comfort management for pain and other symptoms. Hospice focuses on quality of life rather than quantity of days; on caring rather than curing. Hospice delivers its services wherever the person resides. It does not provide twenty-four-hour care or a permanent residence where hospice patients live until they die, but when needed, patients can visit an inpatient hospice unit for the treatment of difficult-to-manage symptoms or to provide brief respite for caregivers.

Hospice services can provide significant benefits for both patients and their families, and link the gap in care delivery between what people want at the end of life and the care that they actually receive. They can assist caregivers in proactively identifying how to confidently respond to future medical decisions. Hospice embraces not only the patient but the caregivers as well. A specialized interdisciplinary team of professionals educated in the hospice philosophy work collaboratively to meet the holistic needs of patients and their loved ones. This includes customizing approaches to honor and uphold the individual's unique psychological, emotional, physical, cultural, and spiritual needs. The team consists of nurses, doctors, aides, chaplains, social workers, trained volunteers, and bereavement counselors. Other support personnel, such as a physical therapist or an occupational therapist, may be called in if needed.

Studies suggest that hospice services are beneficial for persons with advanced dementia by improving symptom management, decreasing preventable hospitalizations, reducing the amount of interventions that offer little to no clinical benefit, and helping people die in their place of choice. Hospice services benefit family members by providing an interdisciplinary support team, periodic respite care, and bereavement counseling for thirteen months following the patient's death. Families report high satisfaction with hospice's quality of care and its treatment of the dying process. Overall, know that throughout the end-of-life process, hospice services offer skilled professionals who will walk every step of the journey with you and your loved one.

Hospice services are covered by Medicare Part A, Medicaid, most insurance plans, HMOs and managed care organizations. To receive Medicare hospice services, the patient must meet three conditions:

1. The physician and the hospice medical director certify that the patient is terminally ill and is expected to live six months or less should the disease run its natural course.
2. The patient or surrogate chooses to use hospice instead of the standard Medicare benefits.
3. The hospice care must be given by a hospice certified by Medicare.

Medicare divides its costs into benefit periods. At the end of each period, patients are reevaluated to determine if they still meet criteria for services. For more detailed information about hospice, contact your healthcare providers, local hospitals, Medicare-certified hospices in your area, insurance plans, and/or the local health department, or call the National Hospice and Palliative Care Organization help line (800-658-8898) or visit the organization on the web at www.nhpco.org.

MEDICARE'S DEMENTIA CRITERIA FOR ELIGIBILITY TO HOSPICE

To be eligible for hospice services, Medicare regulations require the patient to meet certain clinical criteria that suggest the last six months of life have approached. The criteria vary depending on the terminal diagnosis. For dementia, the criteria include the following elements:

- life expectancy is six months or less if disease runs its natural course
- the person is unable to ambulate, bathe, or dress independently
- urinary or fecal incontinence, intermittent or constant
- no consistently meaningful verbal communication—stereotypical phrases only or speech limited to six or fewer words
- one or more of the following has occurred in the past year:
  ° aspiration pneumonia
  ° kidney/upper urinary-tract infection
  ° septicemia
  ° recurring fever after antibiotics
  ° decubitus ulcers (pressure sores), multiple stage 3–4
  ° unexplained weight loss of 10 percent or more in the past six months
  ° blood levels of albumin concentration measure less than 2.5 mg/dl, which is commonly associated with malnourishment or malabsorption.

FTD's Unique Challenges in Meeting Hospice Criteria

Experts suspect that people with FTD and their families do not receive hospice services until the final weeks before death, thus missing the months of benefits associated with comfort care and support. Medicare's current hospice-eligibility criteria for dementia pose challenges to timely services for people with FTD because the criteria were built on the progression of Alzheimer's disease (AD). People with FTD present differently than those with AD because FTD initially impacts different areas of the brain and strikes people who are generally younger with fewer coexisting chronic illnesses. Memory impairment may not be as severe as with AD, and the ability to function and ambulate typically lasts longer, although the risk for falls and significant injury are high. These differences from AD may mistakenly lead clinicians unfamiliar with the clinical progression of FTD to believe patients with FTD are not near the end-of-life stage because they "still look pretty good."

There is a critical need to raise awareness as to common signs and symptoms that may indicate the end of life in persons with FTD. Professional and family caregivers are urged to assume leadership roles for educating society on how these signs and symptoms differ from those of AD in order to establish easier access to palliative and hospice supportive services. Families may need to assertively communicate with healthcare providers to advocate for the initiation of hospice services. Sharing information from this book and the Association for Frontotemporal Degeneration (AFTD) website are means of raising awareness in those who are unfamiliar with FTD. Ultimately the goal is to ensure that people with FTD and their families receive the same timely, expert end-of-life care afforded those with more commonly recognized terminal illnesses.

Predictors of the Final Stage

Although it is common for caregivers to desperately desire some semblance of a predictable timeline for when the end of life may occur, it is very difficult for clinicians to prognosticate the final six months of life in a person with any form of advanced dementia. The advanced stage can be fraught with shifts between plateaus and sharp, unexpected declines that may suggest the beginning of the end. FTD experts propose that life expectancy varies for people with FTD but that disease severity is the greatest predictor of the final stage of life. Generally, the disease lasts approximately six to eight years. The course of FTD with motor neuron disease progresses more rapidly. Although various forms of FTD present differently from one another in the earlier stages, persons in the end stage tend to demonstrate more similarities than differences.

Death usually results from complications related to chewing, swallowing, moving, and incontinence of bowel and bladder. People with end-stage FTD require around-the-clock care because they are completely dependent on others for assistance with all activities of daily living (ADL). They may be bed- or chair-bound, or they may possibly have some limited ability to rise and walk, but their gait will be very unsteady and will require constant assistance to minimize falls. The person is generally incontinent of bowel and bladder, is nonverbal or speaks very few words, and demonstrates stiffness in joints and body movements.

At this stage, persons with FTD are at high risk for aspiration pneumonia and significant weight loss due to frequent difficulties with coordination of effective chewing and swallowing. The person may have widespread fasciculations (involuntary muscle twitching that can be observed under the skin). Infections may occur more frequently even following treatment with antibiotics, signifying the weakening of the body's immune system. There may be complications due to immobility, such as deep-vein thrombosis or pulmonary embolism. The most immediate cause for death is typically infection, usually in the lungs, urinary tract, or skin.

Common Changes Observed in the Dying Person

Although each person's dying experience is unique and influenced by many factors, here are common changes that occur as humans near death. Patients typically begin to show less desire for food and fluids, and they may sleep for longer durations. It is important to note that refusal of oral intake does not create feelings of "starvation" in the patient and that avoiding IV fluid replacement will actually help prevent further discomfort caused by fluid retention. As kidney functions slow down, the body no longer desires food and fluids, and the person naturally declines oral intake. Bowel and bladder output is scant. The vital signs (blood pressure, heart rate, respirations, and temperature) may fluctuate, and increased restlessness may be observed, along with signs of delirium (acute confusion).

In the Days and Hours Prior to Death

When the person enters the active phase of dying, there are signs of decreased circulation, such as cool skin and the appearance of mottling (red or purple patches under the skin) that typically begin in the extremities. Blood-pressure readings lower, and pulse and respirations may have an irregular rate. Sometimes congested breathing sounds are caused by thicker secretions in the back of the throat, but the sound is typically more distressing to the caregiver than the secretions are to the patient. Medications may be effective to help decrease secretions. Suctioning is generally avoided because it may cause distress to the patient. Signs of discomfort related to mouth breathing (dry mouth and lips) can be remedied using lubricants for the lips and gentle oral care.

Patients may continue to hear and feel even when they do not appear to be awake or conscious, so loved ones can continue to talk softly, play the person's favorite music, or recite prayers, and touch the patient to create an atmosphere of calmness. Again, remember that this is a natural progression where we can best serve the person by remaining a steady, loving, and gentle supportive presence, rather than interfering with the process. Patients sometimes hallucinate that people or loved ones come to visit them. Caregivers who become upset by this may consider how such hallucinations may actually bring comfort to the dying person. Should the person experience distressing hallucinations, medications will be available to reduce or eradicate them. Medications are administered to target any possible discomfort, and, over time, death occurs when the person stops breathing.

Palliative care and hospice professionals are skilled in providing interventions for symptom relief. Medications targeting specific issues will be skillfully used to manage any discomfort from fever, pain, restlessness, and/or delirium. The changes witnessed in the person at the end of life sometimes cause inexperienced caregivers to feel anxious and afraid. Remember that it is all part of a natural process signaling the body's shutting down. The hospice team will educate caregivers about the end-of-life process so that everyone can do his or her best to accompany the patient through the final stage in ways that facilitates a comfortable, compassionate, and peaceful passing.

ETHICS

What Is Ethics?

Webster's New World Dictionary of the American Language defines *ethics* as, "the study of standards of conduct and moral judgment; moral philosophy." As one delves deeper into the meaning of ethics, many different ideas come into play. In dealing with issues at the end of life, caregivers are asked to make decisions on what should be done based on information provided to them by the patient, the healthcare provider, their religion and culture, and other codes of ethics shared by the community.

When an ethical question arises, it is called a dilemma. The caregiver, in the absence of a competent patient, is called upon to resolve an issue and choose a course of action. This is not an easy task. Family members may not be in total agreement, medical staff may have different opinions, and the institution itself may be opposed to a caregiver's decision. When such dilemmas occur, an ethics committee may be asked to assist in resolving the dilemma.

Ethics committees are purely advisory. They are made up of staff from within the facility as well as people from the community. It is their responsibility to provide other options, explain policies of the facility, review the dilemma with other similar cases, and provide recommendations that may help to resolve the dilemma. Ethics committees cannot make decisions; they can only advise. What an ethics committee studies about the dilemma, and what the committee recommends to the caregiver, is always confidential.

How does a caregiver reach a decision at the end of life? In Hank Dunn's book, *Hard Choices for Loving People*, he asks four questions to help make this decision. These are:

1. "What does the patient want?"[1] This answer can be found in the advance directive, talking with family and friends, and remembering what the patient may have said in a conversation regarding a feeding tube, CPR, etc.
2. "What is in the best interest of the patient?" It is a question of values to keep the patient alive at all costs versus allowing her to die.
3. "What are the prognosis and probable consequences if a certain treatment plan is followed?" The healthcare provider needs to discuss all the pros and cons of the treatment. Maybe death with dignity is a better option than treating a condition that may allow the patient to live longer, but will not keep him comfortable or help him to respond to his environment.
4. "Can I let go?" This is a difficult question for the caregiver. We may want to keep our loved ones around, even though we know their condition is going to get worse. Keep in mind at all times what the patient would have wanted under these circumstances. It is normal to feel

guilt, and it is difficult to make some tough decisions at the end of life. However, once the decision is made, remember that you made an informed decision based on gathering all the facts about realistic outcomes for the situation and used your best judgment to choose what the person with FTD would have chosen for himself. You have made the right decision for the dilemma as it was presented to you.

Allowing Natural Death versus Prolonging Life

There comes a point in a person's life when the question arises whether a treatment should be started or ended, or if the person should be allowed to die. This question is made easier if the person has a durable power of attorney for healthcare. Many people do not have these documents. Having a living will and/or a medical durable power of attorney for healthcare decision making is crucial. (See chapter 22 for more information.)

A durable power of attorney for healthcare makes it so much easier for a family to reach a consensus when a loved one is unable to speak for herself. Knowing her wishes and recollecting conversations when she was able to discuss what she wanted eases the decisions at hand. It can be difficult for families to remember that the decision being made is what the patient wants and not what the family may want. It is very hard for loved ones to let go, but they must remember at all times what the patient would want if she were able to make a choice. When a patient does not have a durable power of attorney for healthcare, it is possible for the court to appoint a legal guardian.

Whether a guardian is making treatment choices or a durable power of attorney for medical care is in place, the person making the decision must always weigh the benefits and burdens of a particular treatment. What does the advance directive say, what were conversations that the patient had with the decision maker over the years, and what kind of choices had the patient made throughout his life?

From the time of the diagnosis through the progression of the illness, loved ones consciously or unconsciously have been saying their good-byes as the patient gradually becomes someone they have difficulty recognizing. Remember, the decision being made is what the patient would have wanted, not what the decision maker would want.

Honoring What the Person Would Want

You will find that during the gradual decline of someone with FTD, you will be called upon over and over again to make difficult decisions. Each change of condition must be made keeping in mind what the patient would have wanted. How do you go about this?

1. Discuss all questions with the patient's healthcare providers.
2. Ask them if interventions will return the patient to a previous level of care or delay further progression of the illness.
3. Ask if the realistic outcomes for any of the interventions pose significant risks for increased discomfort or distress and determine if they are worth the risk given the progressive, terminal nature of FTD.
4. Will the patient understand enough to allow the treatment to be initiated and continued?
5. Are there alternative treatments?
6. Discuss all options with the family before making a decision, and clearly communicate that the highest priority is to honor whatever it is that the patient would have chosen rather than what the family would want.

There comes a critical time when medical interventions can no longer achieve the positive results we desire and our biological nature takes over the process of decline toward death. The focus can shift from futile aggressive medical interventions to those that maximize comfort and optimize any remaining quality of life. If the person with FTD has chosen the goal of care to focus on "comfort measures only," then it is morally and ethically the right course of action to ensure that they are followed. These decisions may be very difficult to uphold, but they must be honored as one of our last caregiving duties.

FINAL CHOICES

Studies show that families may generally understand the patient's final goals of care but still lack specific information on how to best respect and carry out choices that arise at the end of life. For example, some healthcare directives (HCD) may specify whether or not to perform CPR but do not specifically identify future decisions regarding hospitalization, feeding tubes, and/or use of antibiotics. Families that know their loved one would choose "comfort care only" sometimes feel they are being neglectful when they opt to forego antibiotic treatments or feeding tubes, but in fact these interventions may cause additional suffering to patients.

Hospitalization and Medical Interventions

Typically, the decision to seek care at an emergency room or hospital is an urgent response to medical crises that arises for our loved ones. The earlier section on avoiding preventable hospitalizations in persons with FTD presents new considerations as to whether choosing alternatives to hospitalization may prove to be a better choice for your loved one. Hospitalized patients receive aggressive medical treatments because hospitals generally aim to cure or improve an illness. Hospitals are required to provide certain life-sustaining procedures, but in the case of a person with FTD, we should pause and ask the critical question, "At this point are we choosing to hospitalize him simply to prolong his life? Is there an alternative approach to uphold his medical directives, preserve his dignity, maximize his comfort, and enhance what little quality of life he may have left?"

If the person with FTD could see herself as she is now, would she choose to be hospitalized for surgery, such as reparation of a broken hip, or might she opt to switch the focus to aggressive comfort management and stay in her familiar environment with those who know her best? Caregivers are urged to discuss this with healthcare providers so that everyone involved understands the risks and realistic benefits associated with treatment options and determines whether they align with the person's medical directives. If the person with advanced FTD develops additional medical issues that require more intensive and ongoing treatments that cannot be managed at home or in LTC, then discuss palliative and hospice options with the family and healthcare providers, as this may be the critical indicator that it is time to refocus care to that of palliative approaches.

Again, the caregiver must weigh all options of benefits versus burdens with every change in the patient's condition and every care decision. By avoiding interventions that involve tubes and needle sticks, and simplifying all unnecessary medications and treatments, patients will be spared additional discomfort and caregivers may better spend their time to provide a caring presence and opportunities for meaningful connection with patients. As the person enters the advanced stage, all medications should be reconsidered in light of their risks and benefits. This includes agents that provide long-term benefits to control issues such as blood pressure, cardiac conditions, glucose levels, lipid levels, and anticoagulant therapy. At the end of life, the benefits from such medications are often outweighed by the risk of adverse effects.

Studies of people with AD or related dementias suggest that when the person's healthcare directives specify that they are to receive antibiotic treatments for infections, oral agents may be best as there is no evidence of significant difference in outcomes related to route of administration (i.e., intramuscular injection or intravenous administration). Survival time is similar whether treatment for infection is provided in long-term care or in a hospital. Oral agents are less costly and burdensome to administer and can be given wherever the person resides, thus preventing an unnecessary transition to an unfamiliar environment. Some patients clearly specify on their advanced directives that they do not want antibiotics when infections arise. This may cause caregivers to fear that the patient may suffer more if antibiotics are not given, but rest assured that hospice teams will skillfully administer medications to allay any possible causes of discomfort such as fever and pain.

Pain is commonly under-recognized and undertreated in people with advanced dementia due to cognitive and verbal deficits that prevent communication of discomfort. Pain can be caused by immobility and comorbid conditions and is commonly exacerbated with movement, so consider pain as a trigger for resistive behaviors that arise when caregivers provide assistance with personal care or with any movement of the body (e.g., transferring, dressing, repositioning, brief changing). Consider using a nonverbal pain observation tool to monitor for discomfort, and report signs and symptoms to the healthcare provider so that effective interventions are established. When pain appears to be persistent, discuss the use of scheduled administration of medications around the clock in order to ensure that patients are kept comfortable.

In spite of the impending descent toward death, it is possible for patients and their families to experience moments of shared meaningful connection as the final days unfold. Sensory experiences may continue to bring pleasure and a sense of meaningful connection for the person with FTD, so explore the use of their favorite tastes, smells, sounds, and tactile and visual objects to determine if they bring enjoyment or comfort. For example, try playing the person's preferred music, as it may serve as a source of entertainment and relaxation while creating a sense of familiarity amidst an increasingly confusing world.

Treatment Withdrawal and Refusal

Many caregivers, as well as healthcare providers, feel that to withdraw a treatment is to cause the death of the patient. What must be remembered is that the patient has an underlying disease that is causing his body to slowly die. Whether the treatment has begun or is being withdrawn, this underlying disease is going to prove fatal.

Treatments will not work the same way for everyone. Other medical conditions may make it inadvisable to consider a treatment. If a treatment is useless, there is no moral obligation to begin it. One must weigh the benefits and burdens of all treatments. Each case must be decided on its own merits. Whatever decision is made regarding withdrawal or refusal of treatment, the emphasis should be placed on making the patient comfortable and allowing her to have a peaceful death.

CPR or Cardiopulmonary Resuscitation

The issue of CPR can be controversial. Most cognitively intact people will say no to CPR: "When my time is up, just let me go." Loved ones may get upset hearing this, since they don't want to let go. Some will try to persuade their loved one to change his mind, while others will accept the patient's decision. For a person with FTD, the advanced directives can supply the answer.

What happens when there is no advance directive and the patient has never discussed CPR? Begin by asking what CPR is and how it is administered. CPR involves very aggressive chest compressions that may cause fractured ribs, a punctured lung, and perhaps other physical damage. Also consider AD research that suggests CPR is three times less successful in people who have advanced dementia and that the majority of those successfully resuscitated will die within twenty-four hours in an ICU. Ask whether the patient will derive any meaningful benefit from having CPR initiated. If CPR is initiated and is successful, will the quality of life be improved for the patient? Are we doing CPR for the caregiver's benefit or because we think the patient, even with an advanced dementia, would have wanted it? CPR may prolong survival by keeping the patient alive on a respirator. Is this the peaceful death the patient may have wanted?

When a person is admitted to a hospital or LTC, the question is always asked: Do you want CPR? If CPR is not wanted, make sure the medical providers write "No CPR" or "DNR" (do not resuscitate) in the patient's chart, otherwise CPR will be initiated.

Artificial Hydration and Nutrition

This is probably one of most controversial ethical dilemmas. Food and water are the mainstays of our existence. When a person is dying, many believe everything must be done to maintain nourishment and hydration. Caregivers must be educated that as the body shuts down its systems, it is also providing a relatively comfortable dying process. Sometimes what we decide to do to prolong a life only creates more distress for the dying patient.

Ethically, using feeding tubes to keep someone alive over a long period of time becomes very controversial. Studies reveal that feeding tubes in people with AD and related dementias result in more discomfort and do not improve quality of life or prevent aspiration pneumonia, malnutrition, weight loss, or muscle wasting. They are associated with complications such as nausea, leakage, infections, and skin irritation. Carefully hand-fed patients with advanced dementia have similar survival rates as those with feeding tubes.

If a feeding tube is inserted, be aware of your state's legal position on specifically who may or may not authorize decisions as to whether the tube may be withdrawn. Ask the medical providers about the benefits and burdens of feeding tubes for someone with FTD. Ultimately the choice depends on the wishes of the individual. Again, go back to what the patient would have wanted. Would she prefer to be kept alive at all costs, even if it meant discomfort and increased risk for infection that may lead to other medical problems? Or would the patient prefer to die naturally with all interventions focusing solely on comfort and safety?

In deciding what to do for a person with late-stage dementia, remember that she doesn't understand what is happening to her. Tube feedings can be invasive and frightening. They may increase her agitation, causing her to pull out the tube. To counteract this, restraints may be used. This is not the way most people would choose to end their life, suffering from indignity and emotional distress.

Studies also suggest carefully hand-fed patients with advanced dementia had increased satisfaction, social interactions, and pleasure. Food may be one of the last pleasures available to a person with advanced dementia. Psychologically, tube feedings take away the soothing sensory experiences of taste and decrease opportunities for personal interactions that provide human touch. Even in the advanced stage of dementia, the person responds to touch and love.

Perhaps Hank Dunn sums up the question of a feeding tube best. He states, "Unless the patient has given specific instructions preferring a feeding tube, I believe artificial feeding of those with Alzheimer's disease or other dementias is a totally inappropriate treatment. It does not cure the underlying disease, it does not prevent death, it does not even offer a longer life than for those who do not receive a tube, and the numerous burdens of a feeding tube for these patients are not counterbalanced by any benefit."[2]

Letting Go

All of our life we have been practicing forms of letting go.

It is natural for us to cling to that which brings us comfort and pleasure. It is natural to resist letting go of someone we love. However, there comes a time when a decision must be made to let go of a loved one who is suffering from a terminal illness. How we handle this decision will depend on how we have faced difficult times before. Perhaps it depends on how we face our own mortality or how we are influenced by spiritual beliefs. Are we able to say to our loved one, "I love you but now I must let you go"? We cannot stop death, but we can learn to acknowledge it no matter how painful it may be.

Families of people with a dementia describe a slow letting go and grieving that starts at the time of diagnosis. It is a painful experience to see our loved ones progressively change before our eyes. Without realizing it, caregivers have been going through a sort of dying process themselves as they practice letting go over and over again throughout the progression of the disease.

Caregivers may find themselves with very complicated, mixed emotions that are actually quite a natural response to the situation. They want their loved one to be with them forever, but at the same time, they want to see an end to the loved one's suffering. Caregivers will admit that they don't know how much longer they can continue caregiving and wonder when this will all be over. They question whether they can make it to the finish line. On the one hand, they want control of their lives back and for this painful process to end, while simultaneously, on the other hand, they dread the signs that will indicate that the final days are near. The dichotomous emotions can evoke guilt and make the caregiver feel like the worst person on the planet for having such thoughts. If you identify with this statement, please know that you are not alone.

Are you ready to let go? If we are honest with ourselves, the answer will probably be a mixed "yes and no." However, there comes a time to let go. You will never have to let go of the good memories and love you have shared.

When your loved one dies, you may find yourself with some sense of relief that the arduous caregiving experience is over, and yet it may mingle with missing the person intensely and yearning for one more day with him or her. You have done the best you knew how to do in the face of probably the most challenging experience in your life. Understand that it is essential for you to pause to breathe and now focus some of those keenly developed caregiving skills inwardly to replenish yourself with the healing gifts of gentleness and compassion for all you have endured.

You now have rich experiences that may benefit others. Take your lessons and pass them forward if you feel compelled to do so. Until we can celebrate the arrival of scientific breakthroughs that offer hope for prevention, treatments, and cures for FTD, the journey from diagnosis to death will continue to be a strenuous and deeply challenging experience on many levels. FTD caregivers whose loved ones have died report that their caregiving journey was transformative, that they are different than they were before the entire experience. Their bigger perspective has led them to realize that they would do it again because they discovered a life of deep meaning and extreme expressions of living love as a verb. As we support each other through the caregiving process, may we continue to acquire and generously share wisdom and experiences so that we continue to enrich our abilities to serve those with FTD and their loved ones. And may we remember to ceaselessly advocate for bringing the very best of both the art and science of caring to make a significant, positive impact.

NOTES

1. H. Dunn, *Hard Choices for Loving People: CPR, Artificial Feeding, Comfort Measures Only, and the Elderly Patient* (Landsdowne, VA: A and A Publishers, 2009), p. 47.
2. Ibid., pp. 52–53.

BIBLIOGRAPHY

Association for Frontotemporal Degeneration. http://www.theaftd.org/?s=hospice. Accessed December 26, 2013.

Brodaty, H., K. Seeher, and L. Gibson. "Dementia Time to Death: A Systematic Literature Review on Survival Time and Years of Life Lost in People with Dementia." *International Psychogeriatrics* 24 (2012): 1034–45.

Casey, D., C. Northcutt, K. Stowell, L. Shihabuddin, and M. Rodriguez-Suarez. "Dementia and Palliative Care." *Clinical Geriatrics* 2, no. 1 (2012): 36–41.

Dunn, H. *Hard Choices for Loving People: CPR, Artificial Feeding, Comfort Measures Only, and the Elderly Patient.* Landsdowne, VA: A and A Publishers, 2009.

Fulton, A. T., J. Rhodes-Kropf, A. M. Corcoran, D. Char, E. Kerdovits, and E. H. Castillo. "Palliative Care for Patients with Dementia in Long-Term Care." *Clinical Geriatrics Medicine* 27 (2011): 153–70.

Gallagher, M., McLean, A., and Wilson, R. "Hospice Care: Maximizing Comfort and Enhancing Quality of Life in Persons with FTD and Their Families." PowerPoint® slides. 2011. http://www.theaftd.org/wp-content/uploads/2011/10/Hospice-and-FTD_Hospice-of-the-Valley-2011-ppt-online-version.pdf. Accessed January 10, 2014.

Givens, J. , R. Jones, M. L. Shaffer, D. Kiely, and S. Mitchell. "Survival and Comfort after Treatment of Pneumonia in Advanced Dementia." *Archives of Internal Medicine* 170, no. 13 (2010): 1102–1107.

Hanson, L. C. "Tube Feeding versus Assisted Oral Feeding for Persons with Dementia: Using Evidence to Support Decision-Making." *Annals of Long-Term Care: Clinical Care and Aging* 21, no. 1 (2013): 36–39.

Idziak, J. *Dilemmas in Long-Term Care.* Study edition. Dubuque, IA: Simon and Kolz Publishing, 2000.

Karnes, Barbara. *Gone from My Sight: The Dying Experience.* Depoe Bay, OR: Barbara Karnes Publishing, 1987.

Miller, Bruce. Frontotemporal Dementia: Disease Progression. 2012. http://memory.ucsf.edu/ftd/overview/ftd/progression/multiple. Accessed January 5, 2014.

Mitchell, S. D., et al. "The Clinical Course of Advanced Dementia." *New England Journal of Medicine* 361, no. 16 (2009): 1529–38.

Mitchell, S. D., S. Kiely, S. Miller, C. Connor, and J. Teno. "Hospice Care for Patients with Dementia." *Journal of Pain and Symptom Management* 34, no. 1 (2007): 7–16.

National Hospice Organization. *Medical Guidelines for Determining Prognosis in Selected Non-cancer Diseases.* 2nd ed. Arlington, VA: National Hospice Organization, 1996.

National Institute on Aging. Frontotemporal Disorders: Information for Patients, Families and Caregivers. 2010. http://www.nia.nih.gov/sites/default/files/frontotemporal_disorders_information_for_patients_families_and_caregivers_0.pdf. Accessed January 5, 2014.

Onyike, C. U. "What Is the Life Expectancy in Frontotemporal Lobar Degeneration?" *Neuroepidemiology* 37, no. 166 (2011): 166–67.

Phelan, E., S. Borson, L. Grothaus, S. Balch, and E. Larson. "Association of Incident Dementia with Hospitalizations." *Journal of the American Medical Association* 307, no. 2 (2012): 165–72.

Post, A. *The Moral Challenges of Alzheimer's Disease.* 2nd ed. Baltimore, MD: Johns Hopkins University Press, 2000.

Shega, J., and C Tozer. "Improving the Care of People with Dementia at the End of Life: The Role of Hospice and the U.S. Experience." *Dementia* 8, no. 3 (2009): 377–89.

Shega, J., G Hougham, C Stocking , D. Cox-Hayley, and G. Sachs. "Patients Dying with Dementia: Experience at the End of Life and Impact of Hospice Care." *Journal of Pain and Symptom Management* 35, no. 5 (2008): 499–507.

Takeda, M., T. Tanaka, M. Okochi, and H. Kazui. "Non-Pharmacological Intervention for Dementia Patients." *Psychiatry and Clinical Neuroscience* 66 (2012): 1–7.

Teno, J. M., et al. "Does Hospice Improve Quality of Care for Persons Dying from Dementia?" *Journal of the American Geriatrics Society* 59, no. 8 (2011): 1532–36.

Torke, A., et al. "Palliative Care for Patients with Dementia: A National Survey." *Journal of the American Geriatrics Society* 58, no. 7 (2010): 2114–21.

US Department of Health and Human Services, Centers for Medicaid and Medicare Services. Medicare Hospice Services. 2013. http://www.alz.org/national/documents/endoflifelitreview.pdf. Accessed January 3, 2014.

Volicer, L. "End-of-Life Care for People with Dementia in Long-Term Care Settings." *Alzheimer's Care Today* 9, no. 2 (2008): 84–102.

Volicer, L. End-of-Life Care for People with Dementia in Residential Care Settings. 2005. http://www.alz.org/national/documents/endoflifelitreview.pdf. Accessed January 3, 2014.

Warren, Jason D., Jonathan D. Rohrer, and Martin Rossor. "Clinical Review: Frontotemporal Dementia." 2013. http://www.bmj.com/content/347/bmj.f4827. Accessed January 3, 2013.

Webster's New World Dictionary of the American Language. 3rd college ed. New York: Simon and Schuster, 1988.

PART 3

CAREGIVER RESOURCES

CHAPTER 19

CAREGIVING

Obtaining the Help You Need
from Health and Community Services

Darby Morhardt, PhD, LCSW;
and Mary O'Hara, AM, LCSW

INTRODUCTION

Families caring for persons with frontotemporal degeneration (FTD) cannot do it alone. Patients and families can benefit from health and community support services; however, there are challenges to accessing appropriate care as the disease continues to progress. The service system is complicated and there is much confusion about what is available both nationally and locally. This chapter will explain the services available to persons with FTD and their families from the perspective of both the aging and disability networks and eligibility for Medicare and other forms of insurance. How to obtain in-home care services and adult day services will be described, in addition to the importance of finding a knowledgeable interdisciplinary healthcare team. Case examples of persons with behavior variant FTD (bvFTD) and the language variant primary progressive aphasia (PPA) illustrate how patients and families use these services, including the barriers and challenges they face.

SIGNIFICANCE AND BACKGROUND

A handful of studies have examined the psychosocial impact on and needs of families of persons diagnosed with FTD. So far, these few studies have consistently demonstrated that caregivers caring for persons with FTD experience more stress and burden than persons caring for those with other forms of dementia (Wong et al. 2012, Svanberg et al. 2011, Boutoleau-Bretonniere et al. 2008, de Vugt et al. 2006). Reasons include the distress caused by FTD's primary symptoms of personality changes, behavioral and emotional disturbance, and significant language decline.

Obtaining a diagnosis for FTD symptoms is particularly challenging. Initial symptoms are commonly misdiagnosed as psychiatric disorders, resulting in a delay of several years between the onset of presenting symptoms and a correct diagnosis. This can cause much stress for the patient and family. The onset of speech difficulties, loss of memory, or the changes in personality and behavior in persons are often thought to be a result of anxiety, depression, or "midlife stress." Particularly in someone younger, most physicians do not expect the person to be suffering from a neurodegenerative disease, and many individuals experience several evaluations and numerous expensive tests before an accurate diagnosis is reached. Oftentimes, the person with behavior and personality changes lacks awareness of his or her condition, making it challenging for families to pursue the most appropriate care and support.

Due to the younger onset of frontotemporal disorders; that is, typically in the forties, fifties, and early sixties, the psychological, social, family, and financial issues occur at a developmental stage of life where young children may still be living at home and/or leaving for college. Perhaps more than at any time across the life course, the diagnosis of dementia in younger people is likely to have a complex range of effects on all family members. Dependent children or young adults living in the home are often thrust into caregiving for their parent and also being of support to the well parent.

Persons with FTD have to stop working at a time when they are probably in the prime of their working career, saving for retirement and supporting their younger family. People with associated personality and behavior problems may engage in poor financial management and make inappropriate financial decisions. Individuals are at risk of receiving poor performance evaluations and may be terminated from their positions before the illness is understood.

As a result, financial concerns are abundant. Because of the loss of employment, the well spouse may need to seek additional work to meet the family's financial needs. Formal education costs for children need to be considered, as well as the general expenses of supporting a family. Some teenagers and young adults are naturally trying to "leave home," and the decisions around this will likely be affected by their parent's illness. There are also situations where an older parent who may have his or her own frailties is caring for a middle-aged child with FTD. The loss of income impacts the affordability of future long-term care. After a diagnosis is made, it is too late to obtain long-term-care insurance.

ESTABLISHING A CARE TEAM

As discussed, many individuals with FTD are misdiagnosed for years prior to receiving a proper diagnosis. Once the diagnosis is established and due to additional challenges inherent within the healthcare system, it is vital for families to establish a knowledgeable medical-care team. Together this care team works with family caregivers to provide ongoing guidance, care, and support as they navigate the progression of the disease and the resources available to them. Families are sometimes faced with having to educate providers about the condition. The Association for Frontotemporal Degeneration's (AFTD) Partners in FTD Care program aims to raise awareness of the disease among providers in the field.

Below is a list of possible care team members. The care team is different for each individual based on his or her needs and local available social services. Note that all of the professionals listed below may not be available in your area, covered by your health insurance, or familiar with FTD.

The FTD Medical and Psychosocial Care Team

SPECIALTY	DESCRIPTION OF CARE
Primary-Care Team	This team may consist of a medical doctor (such as an internist, geriatrician, or family medicine physician), nurse practitioner, or physician's assistant who will provide ongoing care and treatment for a variety of common medical conditions. This team will still be in charge of your overall care, even if you see a specialist for a particular condition.

Neurologist	This clinician specializes in illnesses related to the nervous system. A behavioral neurologist is specially trained in neurological disorders that affect cognition and behavior. They are most often found in university healthcare settings. The neurologist is typically the first to diagnose FTD or PPA and is central to monitoring and evaluating the progression of the disorder.
Neuro-psychologist	This clinician evaluates a person's cognitive abilities using specialized paper-and-pencil tests that pinpoint the exact areas of cognition that are affected and to what degree. These tests help the neurologist make a diagnosis or understand more specifically what may be causing the symptoms.
Geriatric Psychiatrist or Neuro-psychiatrist	This clinician specializes in evaluating behaviors and moods of individuals and may prescribe medications to modify challenging behaviors and moods.
Social Worker	This clinician provides information about a diagnosis, linkage to local resources, patient and family counseling, advocacy, and support. Social workers help patients and family members understand the diagnosis, find resources in the community, and cope with changes.
Speech Language Pathologist (SLP) or Speech Therapist	This clinician sees individuals with language and other cognitive changes and their families. They evaluate different aspects of cognition and language in detail and can make recommendations and offer compensatory strategies. SLPs help the patient and family members maintain essential communication for as long as possible. Ideally, the SLP should have an understanding of PPA or be willing to learn more about the condition to design the most effective treatment plan.
Occupational Therapist (OT)	This clinician works with individual patients and family members to improve or maintain the patient's daily functioning by developing ways to modify or adapt activities of everyday life. This can be particularly helpful for patients with visuospatial, movement, or motor changes.

Physical Therapist (PT)	A physical therapist works with individuals to maximize functioning through building strength, improving balance, preventing falls, conducting home-safety assessments, and implementing physical-exercise techniques tailored to each individual. Maintaining the highest level of functioning possible positively impacts the quality of life for both the patient and the family.

The care team differs for each person's needs and by each geographic area, and it expands as a person needs additional services or assistance. For example, speech and occupational therapists can become integral members of the care team as they provide out-patient or in-home services; a care manager begins to work with the clinicians and family to coordinate care as needs increase; additionally, a hired companion or caregiver can also become a member of the care team as this level of care is introduced.

One purpose of the care team is to provide guidance so that families do not have to guess what services are most appropriate, struggle alone with transitions in care, wonder what more they could be doing, or experience distress about planning for future care. Together, a care team addresses these concerns for both the person and the family.

FINDING SUPPORT AND CARE SERVICES

There is a general lack of understanding of frontotemporal disorders among healthcare providers and social-service agencies that are far more familiar with Alzheimer's disease and the older demographic. As a result, it is difficult to find appropriate home- and community-based services willing and able to care for persons with FTD.

Long-term-care services can include in-home care companions, adult day services, and respite programs for those who are trying to maintain living in their own homes. More intense supports such as assisted living and nursing home care may be used as the disease progresses. As the disease reaches the more advanced stages, it is important to help families understand the benefits of palliative care and hospice. The funding sources for these different types of services and supports may vary, which is another reason why proper and prompt diagnosis is important to allow people with FTD and their families plan accordingly.

Long-term-care services can be accessed and financed through private payment or private long-term-care insurance, as well as through various publicly funded aging and disability programs. The types of services, eligibility requirements, and what funding is available for them can vary widely from program to program and location to location. For example, some people with FTD might be able to access Medicaid waiver programs, depending on in which state they live. It's important to recognize that when the Older Americans Act was reauthorized in 2006, the National Family Caregiver Support Program was expanded to allow for service to caregivers of people with dementia of any age. However, types and available amounts of Older Americans Act services may vary. There are other state and local sources that may be available, too. Contacting your local area agency on aging (AAA) or aging and disability resource center (ADRC) is recommended to find out what's available, and the Eldercare locator link, www.eldercare.gov, will give you that local contact information for anywhere in the country.

While a care team can provide essential guidance, it is important for families to understand available resources. For those who can afford to hire a private companion, a barrier is finding professional caregivers with training or experience in the care of persons with FTD. The Association for Frontotemporal Degeneration, in 2011, established Partners in FTD Care, an education initiative that brings together healthcare professionals, experts in FTD disorders, and caregiving families to promote an understanding of the various forms of FTD and to develop best practices in community care. AFTD provides educational materials, quarterly e-newsletters featuring case studies in FTD, and a professionals-only on-line forum for discussion and interaction to help guide professionals in the effective treatment and care of persons with FTD and their families.

Below is a chart that describes different types of care, where to find the care, and various forms of financial coverage for care. If the services in your community lack awareness of FTD, please direct them to AFTD and the Partners in FTD Care initiative.

AVAILABLE COMMUNITY SERVICES

SERVICE	DESCRIPTION	COVERAGE
Disability Resources Services www.eldercare.gov (search by zip code)	Individuals under age sixty who qualify for disability may be eligible for benefits through the local disability offices. These services differ by geographic location.	Based on disability Based on financial eligibility
Private-Duty Home Care www.homecareaoa.org www.eldercare.gov	Private-duty home care staff members are paid professionals who provide a range of services from companion services to skilled nursing care. Licensed agencies should meet criteria for the highest ethical standards and staff training.	Long-term-care insurance* Private pay Some veteran's benefits*
Out-Patient or In-Home Health Services www.medicare.gov/ homehealthcompare	Includes physical, speech, and occupational therapies, skilled and behavioral-health nursing, and social work. Services are temporary, short-term, and provided in the home, outpatient setting, or a facility. One must be "homebound" to be eligible for in-home healthcare.	Medicare Medicaid Private insurance
Care Management www.caremanager.org	Professional care managers provide assistance managing, organizing, and overseeing care. They facilitate transitions in care and are especially helpful for long-distance caregivers and families in conflict.	Long-term-care insurance* Private pay

Individual Therapy
www.helpstartshere.org
www.alz.org
  (contact your local
  chapter)
Creative Arts Therapies
www.arttherapy.org
www.musictherapy.org
www.adta.org
  (or request local
  referrals from your care
  team)
	This clinician can work with either the patient or a family member to develop coping skills and work through the emotional changes brought on by FTD. Counseling helps the patient and family adapt to and cope with the significant changes that occur as a result of the diagnosis and accompanying symptoms. Music and art therapies can be helpful when working with individuals whose ability to communicate verbally is limited. Ideally the therapist should have an understanding of FTD. However, if this is not an option, the AFTD is an excellent educational resource.	(Differs by
		  therapist)
		Private pay
		Medicare
		Private
		  insurance

Adult Day Services
www.nadsa.org
www.alz.org
  (contact your local
  chapter)
www.eldercare.gov
	A structured day program that provides meals, supervision, stimulating and structured activity, and social engagement. Some offer assistance with personal and medical care and transportation.	Long-term-care
		  insurance*
		Private pay
		Some veteran's
		  benefits
		(ask about
		  sliding-scale
		  fees/financial
		  assistance)

Assisted Living
www.seniorhousingfinder
  .org
www.alz.org
  (contact your local
  chapter)
	Assisted living facilities provide assistance with basic activities of daily living such as bathing, grooming, and dressing. Most offer structured social activity, and some provide medication assistance. Assisted-living facilities do not offer complex medical services.	Long-term-care
		  insurance*
		Private pay
		Some veteran's
		  benefits

Nursing Home Care
www.medicare.gov/
  nhcompare
www.communityresource
  finder.org
www.alz.org
  (contact your local
  chapter)
	A nursing home is normally the highest level of care outside of a hospital. Nursing homes provide what is called custodial care, including getting in and out of bed, and assistance with feeding, bathing, and dressing. Nursing homes also provide skilled nursing and a high level of medical care. Some provide security to prevent wandering.	Long-term-care
		  insurance*
		Some veteran's
		  benefits
		Private pay
		Medicare
		  (limited
		  benefits)
		Medicaid

Hospice and Palliative
  Care
www.nhpco.org
www.eldercare.gov
	Care that promotes dignity and comfort at the end of life. Provides therapies and support for diagnosed individuals and families and focuses on pro-viding patients with relief from the symptoms, pain, and stress of a serious illness, whatever the diagnosis.	Medicare
		Medicaid
		Private
		  insurance

*Each plan is different. Refer to your long-term care insurance policy or contact your local Veteran's Administration for specific benefit details.

SOCIAL SECURITY DISABILITY INSURANCE

Historically, persons with FTD have had a very grueling and lengthy Social Security Disability Insurance (SSDI) application process, usually with multiple denials and appeals. However, in 2009, faced with an unprecedented backlog of 2.8 million claims and longer wait times for applicants, the Social Security Administration (SSA) rolled out its Compassionate Allowances (CAL) program in an effort to provide benefits quickly to applicants whose medical conditions are so serious that their conditions obviously meet disability standards. Due to successful advocacy efforts by the Association for Frontotemporal Degeneration in March 2009, FTD was one of the first fifty conditions named in SSA's Compassionate Allowances list. The language variant of FTD, primary progressive aphasia (PPA), was one of the thirty-eight conditions subsequently added in 2010. The motor variants of FTD, progressive supranuclear palsy (PSP) and corticobasal degeneration (CBD), were added in 2011. This was a major advancement toward helping persons with young-onset dementia quickly get on track for Medicare, rather than languishing in the application process.

However, after approval of Social Security Disability Insurance (SSDI), patients must wait two years before they are eligible for Medicare benefits. This two-year waiting period was created in 1972 in order to keep costs down and preserve Medicare for long-term, severe disabilities. Unfortunately, during this waiting period, some individuals can go bankrupt, and nearly a quarter of those caught in the two-year waiting period between SSDI and Medicare have gone the entire two years without insurance. Others have put together a patchwork of coverage to cope financially.

Many disabled people dealing with this two-year wait welcomed the news of the passage of healthcare reform. The Affordable Care Act (ACA) has not explicitly addressed the Medicare two-year waiting period, but it has made some changes to address the problems associated with this gap. Starting in 2014, individuals who find themselves in this waiting period have access to expanded insurance options through state-based insurance exchanges and expanded Medicaid eligibility.

IMPLEMENTING CHANGES IN CARE

Whether in the early, middle, or late stages of the disease, changes in care should occur when:

1. There are concerns about the person's safety.
2. There are concerns about the person's health and well-being.
3. There are concerns about the health, well-being, and safety of the family member(s) providing care.

While not always possible, it is important to introduce additional care gradually. Knowing options for the next level of care and being aware of safety concerns will allow family members to plan as best they can for the transitions ahead. With guidance from the FTD care team, families can make the sometimes difficult adjustments as smooth as possible.

RESPITE CARE

Respite provides short-term breaks that can relieve stress, restore energy, and promote life balance. The following signs of stress may indicate that it is time for a caregiver to take a break.

- feel you have no time to yourself
- unable to see friends/family
- change in appetite
- feel lonely
- lack of interest in things once enjoyed
- experience changes in mood
- poor or disrupted sleep
- putting off own medical visits
- low energy
- trouble focusing or concentrating
- physical pain

Arranging for respite care often requires a change in care arrangements for both the person and the family. While sometimes difficult to implement, additional care and support will result in better support for the person with FTD and relief to families. Your care team can assist you in arranging for, accessing, and implementing essential respite.

Following are two case examples that describe the challenges families face living with FTD and their experience accessing appropriate and affordable care.

CASE EXAMPLE: PPA—FRED AND CAROL

Fred is a fifty-five-year-old male who lives with his wife, Carol, in Chicago. After experiencing two years of word-finding problems, he was diagnosed with PPA by a local neurologist. At the time of diagnosis, he also established care with a social worker and psychiatrist and enrolled into a PPA research program. Soon after the diagnosis, he was forced to modify his role at work at an advertising firm. While he was able to continue in a management role with staff, he began to limit his interaction with clients due to his word-finding difficulties. He and his wife began to explore what his short-term and long-term disability plans offered as well as the process for applying for Social Security Disability Insurance. They also met with an attorney to begin the process of establishing his advanced directives. His neurologist arranged for Fred to begin working with an out-patient speech therapist who identified ways of compensating for the deficits and suggestions for augmenting communication, such as smart-phone applications that could assist him. Because his memory remained intact, Fred was able to learn to use a tablet to navigate these new communication applications.

As language became more impaired and his employer began to question Fred's decision-making abilities, he began to transition out of his work. Because his awareness of the progression of the disease and sadness about the loss of his job placed him at an increased risk of depression, his psychiatrist monitored his mood closely during this time. Fred and his wife continued to work with the social worker, who encouraged him to apply for Social Security benefits once he stopped working and invited him to join a PPA support group to connect with other families living with a diagnosis. They also explored ideas about how he might spend his free time and began discussions around future transitions, such as driving, wearing an ID bracelet, and safety issues in the home.

Fred began to spend more time on his hobby of photography. While his wife worked, she hired his nephew to spend time with him and also arranged for friends and neighbors to visit or check in regularly. Fred's wife established a structured and predictable routine throughout the week. While Fred did not feel he needed the supervision of his family and friends, he enjoyed their company, and they spent time doing physical activities together that were not dependent on language. When it was determined that Fred should no longer drive, his nephew and friends were available to provide him with transportation.

Fred's wife looked into a local adult day program. Unfortunately, Fred's language impairment limited how much he could participate in the activities, which were designed for people with memory problems. Additionally, Fred was reluctant to attend out of discomfort that he was the youngest person there.

Fred began to experience more severe language impairments as behavioral, motor, and cognitive symptoms also emerged. He got turned around during a walk in a familiar area, his gait became more unsteady, he became fixated with certain personal-care rituals, and he was unable follow instructions. An occupational therapist worked with him and his wife, Carol, in the home to identify what Fred was able to do independently with some modifications as well as what was no longer safe for him to do alone. Eventually, it was determined that Fred could not be left home alone due to safety concerns.

Fred's wife explored the services available through the local Department of Rehabilitation for persons under sixty with a disability. However, because Fred needed more supervision than assistance in the home, it was determined that these services were not appropriate. Since these community services were unavailable to them, Fred's wife hired a professional companion to spend more time with him during the week and on weekends. Since this person was unfamiliar with PPA, Carol had to educate the companion about the diagnosis and symptoms as the disease progressed.

Fred began to experience agitation and anxiety as he lost the ability to comprehend what others were saying. Ongoing visits and communication with his neurologist, social worker, and psychiatrist identified ways of keeping him calm, ways his wife could respond to these behaviors, and a plan for his wife to access additional respite care. Additionally, speech therapy, occupational therapy, and behavioral home health were ordered to work with Fred and his wife together in their home. At this time, Carol elected to take a leave of absence from her job for three months through the Family Medical Leave Act (FMLA). She continued to attend a local support group and began seeing an individual therapist to process her grief over the losses in their life, her anxiety about their future, and the changes in their relationship.

When Fred became incontinent and began to have more difficulty with walking and swallowing, the social worker on their team arranged for a palliative- and hospice-care team to begin working with the family to focus on Fred's comfort and preservation of dignity as he entered the final stages of the disease. Carol received additional support from this team while she prepared for Fred's passing. Fred passed away at home with his family by his side after seven years of living with PPA.

CASE EXAMPLE: BvFTD—JOAN

Joan was a fifty-eight-year-old single woman who lived alone when her family and coworkers began to notice changes in her behavior and personality. Once a conservative and reserved person, Joan became impulsive in her decisions and purchases and seemed to have no regard for the consequences of her actions. She began giving money away to a sweepstakes scam and became fixated on connecting with people from her past. She would only eat certain foods and insisted on stopping to speak with any child she passed. Her sister was directed to have Joan see a psychiatrist, who misdiagnosed her with bipolar disorder. Soon after, Joan was fired from her job for making inappropriate comments to clients and coworkers. At this time, her sister discovered that she had been giving away large sums of money to the scam, including most of her retirement savings.

As the symptoms continued to worsen, Joan's sister insisted that she see a neurologist, who diagnosed her with behavioral variant FTD. Joan's sister met with the clinic social worker alone to discuss the diagnosis, the next steps in connecting Joan with disability benefits, keeping Joan safe, and obtaining available support from the family. Joan's sister was advised to seek guardianship to protect her sister financially. The clinic psychiatrist monitored her obsessive and anxious behaviors. Due to her impaired judgment, the team recommended that Joan stop driving and receive twenty-four-hour supervision. They provided support to the sister in implementing these changes. Unfortunately, due to her lack of insight, Joan was unable to participate in certain discussions around her care needs and was unable to appreciate how these limitations were designed to keep her safe. She insisted that she could return to work, manage her finances, drive safely, and live alone.

Joan soon moved in with her sister. Because her sister worked during the day, she contacted the local disability office to see what services they could provide Joan in her sister's home. Due to her ability to carry out her own personal care, cleaning, and meal preparation, it was determined that Joan was not eligible for these in-home services. Family and friends arranged a schedule to provide her with activity, companionship, and supervision each day.

Ongoing meetings with the social worker as the disease progressed focused on responding to behaviors, planning for the next level of care, as well as making a plan for her long-term-care needs. When it became harder for family and friends to provide this ongoing supervision, Joan's sister arranged for Joan to attend a local adult day program five days a week. Due to her limited financial resources, Joan qualified for financial assistance to attend the program, which provided activity, stimulation, structure, and supervision.

Joan attended the day program until the staff was unable to meet her physical-care needs. At this time, she was now dependent in self-care, dressing, and bathing. Her speech was limited to a few words, she became incontinent, and she began to experience falls. Her sister took a family medical leave from her work through the FMLA and cared for Joan at home with the assistance of Department on Aging services, since Joan was now sixty years old and newly eligible. While limited in the hours it could offer, this support service allowed Joan to remain in her sister's home until a fall resulted in a hospitalization and later discharge to a nursing home facility (paid for by Medicaid) for twenty-four-hour care. Hospice care was introduced in the nursing home when Joan began to have difficulty swallowing and walking. Joan passed away with the support of hospice care.

CONCLUSION

Families living with FTD are in a state of constant transition throughout the course of the illness. Because the health and social-service system currently lack the type of safety net for these families that is available for the older-adult population, FTD families are excluded from many dementia services and left to advocate and educate on behalf of their loved one to ensure the most appropriate care. When possible, establishing a care team knowledgeable regarding FTD can provide ongoing guidance and support as care needs increase and additional care and services are sought.

There is a great need for more information, support, and resources for families with FTD. As research works to better understand the mechanisms of the disease, dementia-care providers must work alongside families to better understand their needs and how these can be met to ensure the best care and support as they live with FTD.

BIBLIOGRAPHY

Boutoleau-Bretonniere C., M. Vercelletto, C. Volteau, P. Renou, and E. Lamy. "Zarit Burden Inventory and Activities of Daily Living in the Behavioral Variant of Frontotemporal Dementia." *Dementia and Geriatric Cognitive Disorders* 25 (2008): 272–77.

de Vugt M. E., S. R. Riedijk, P. Aalten, A. Tibben, J. C. van Swieten, and F. R. Verhey. "Impact of Behavioural Problems on Spousal Caregivers: A Comparison between Alzheimer's Disease and Frontotemporal Dementia." *Dementia and Geriatric Cognitive Disorders* 22 (2006): 35–41.

Svanberg, E., A. Spector, and J. Stott: "The Impact of Young Onset Dementia on the Family: A Literature Review." *International Psychogeriatrics* 23, no. 3 (2011): 356–71.

Wong, C., J. Merrilees, R. Ketelle, C. Barton, M. Wallhagen, and B. Miller: "The Experiences of Caregiving: Differences between Behavioral Variant of Fronto-temporal Dementia and Alzheimer's Disease." *The American Journal of Geriatric Psychiatry* 20, no. 8 (2012): 724–28.

CHAPTER 20

NURSING HOME CARE AND ASSISTED LIVING OPTIONS

Warnings and Wise Choices

Morris J. Kaplan, Esq., NHA

IS A NURSING HOME REALLY NECESSARY?

Deciding whether to place a loved one in a nursing home can be one of the most difficult decisions a caregiver can face. The mere thought can arouse overwhelming feelings of guilt, failure, helplessness, and fear. This chapter will provide a framework for a caregiver to examine objectively whether nursing home placement is in the best interest of a loved one with dementia. This is followed by a discussion of how to find a good nursing home, specifically, (1) how to use publicly available information on state and federal government websites, (2) exactly what to look for on-site and sources to contact, and (3) a description of successful programs and practices found at best-care facilities. The discussion will also include important information about the epidemic of overmedication of nursing home residents with dementia and of best-care practices and behavioral management programs that allow for minimal use of antipsychotic medications in these residents.

Excellent care can most often be provided at home. However, certain conditions and situations can arise over the course of a neurodegenerative illness that suggest additional interventions are needed to ensure a person's highest level of functioning and comfort. Key areas of concern are weight loss, skin ulcers, overmedication, incontinence, and personal safety. When problems arise in these areas, the caregiver needs to determine whether corrective interventions can be more effectively implemented at home or in a nursing facility that has adopted best-care practices.

KEY DETERMINING FACTORS

Significant weight loss (5 percent in the last thirty days or 10 percent in the last 180 days) is something that needs to be addressed and corrected. Significant weight loss is not a normal part of a dementia illness until the very end stage of life when swallowing difficulties can impede nutritional intake. Interventions such as special high-calorie and high-protein foods and supplements, together with specialized feeding-assistance programs and techniques, can and should be instituted to reverse the weight loss and maintain adequate nutrition and hydration. Weight loss should be seen by the caregiver as an avoidable condition. The caregiver needs to determine whether proper nutrition and assistance with eating at each meal can be provided or implemented at home. Weight loss and malnutrition can lead to the development of pressure ulcers, weakness, overall decline, and death.

Pressure ulcers (bedsores) are not a normal part of aging. Good toileting care, incontinence care, skin care, nutrition and hydration, and proper positioning and pressure relief should prevent most pressure ulcers except in the end stages of life. Persistent reddened areas on the skin indicate an immediate high risk for sores. Preventive skin care, nutritional interventions, and pressure-relieving interventions (discussed later in the chapter) should be an integral part of the ongoing care program. When a pressure ulcer develops, the interventions must be intensified and skillfully implemented to heal the wound. The presence of pressure ulcers is often a significant indicator of *avoidable* decline in health. It should be acknowledged by the caregiver as a signal that action must be taken either at home or in an appropriately capable nursing facility with a proven record of consistently low incidence of pressure ulcers.

Overmedicating with antipsychotics is another avoidable and common condition among persons with dementia. As discussed below, antipsychotic medications promote falls, lethargy, and a major decline in activities of daily living. Often psychotropic drugs are used or misused to control or diminish undesired behaviors in the person with dementia. At home, caregivers may find little alternative to dispensing a "calming" medication to allow for some respite or sleep for the caregiver and/or patient. Signs of unsteady gait, lethargy, and/or an acute decrease in verbal, cognitive, and functional abilities may be caused by prolonged use of antipsychotics. Alternatively, a good facility will have staff experienced in identifying and correcting instances of overmedication and using person-centered best-care practices and extensive activity programming as alternatives to antipsychotic medication.

Incontinence will likely occur in the middle or later stages of dementia. The onset of incontinence can often be delayed. A few of the critical interventions in delaying the onset of incontinence are these: not using any kind of physical restraint; correcting and avoiding overmedication; providing appropriate prompting, cueing, and cueing aids (e.g., reminder and location signs); and providing regular, scheduled physical assistance to, and on and off of, the toilet, according to the resident's regular pattern and verbal and nonverbal cues. The preservation of bowel and bladder continence should be an ongoing, closely monitored goal of the caregiver. The primary caregiver should assess whether these interventions are being provided at home. If they are not, consideration should be given to identifying an appropriately capable nursing facility.

Personal safety is an important consideration. If a person wanders or easily gets lost when leaving the home, special automatic door-locking devices (that disengage in case of fire) may be needed. Becoming lost outside the home may not only traumatize the person with dementia and the caregiver but also may lead to serious injury. If this does happen, the caregiver should either equip the home with an effective egress restricting system (e.g., Wanderguard® System) or consider placement in a facility that is properly equipped.

A caregiver must also consider safety inside the home. Access to dangerous items such as poisonous liquids, sharp knives and instruments, matches, and the like, should be restricted. If there has been any incidence of unsafe use of appliances, especially in the kitchen, the caregiver must take steps to prevent catastrophes like fire. These can include keeping appliances unplugged, disabled, or locked. The caregiver should consider a secure facility if the home cannot be made secure for the person with dementia.

Sometimes, a caregiver's response to wandering, abusive behavior, or frequent falling is to physically restrain the patient. Physical restraint use is dangerous and can lead to serious injury or death. In addition, there is nothing more effective in promoting incontinence, overall physical decline, mood and psychosocial decline, despair, fear, and agitation than tying a person down. There are safe and effective alternatives to physically restraining a person (a discussion of which is beyond the scope of this chapter). If the caregiver has resorted to tying down the person with dementia (with a seatbelt, a tied vest, a lap tray, lap cushion, roller bar, two side rails in bed, etc.), that caregiver should consider placement in a facility that is restraint-free.

Certainly, treatment such as wound care, tube feeding, IV medications, and rehabilitation therapy all indicate that skilled nursing or rehabilitation care must be provided. This can be done either by bringing in professional nurses or therapists from home care agencies or by finding, even temporarily, placement in a nursing facility.

If, after considering the issues of weight loss, skin ulcers, overmedication, incontinence, and personal safety, a caregiver has concluded that interventions are needed that cannot be provided in the home, the caregiver's next task is to identify a facility where best-care practices have been successfully implemented. Finding a nursing facility where these methods have been adopted requires careful research. The next section will identify essential sources of information and how to use them.

HOW DO YOU FIND A GOOD NURSING FACILITY?

Unlike Korean culture, which reveres its elders and treats them with the utmost kindness and respect throughout aging and dying, American culture reveres youth and healthy bodies and, typically and unfortunately, shuns things old and worn. The realities of aging and of physical and cognitive decline are often kept shuttered by ignorance and fear or behind the doors of professional care facilities. Sadly, the care in most American nursing homes is quite disappointing and inadequate. So, faced with the need for nursing home placement, how do you find a good nursing home? How can you tell that it *is* a good home, particularly for an elder with dementia?

FIVE-STAR RATING SYSTEM

The first place to look is the federal government's "Five Star" rating system for nursing homes. This information can be found on the "Nursing Home Compare" web page of the Medicare.gov website of the US Department of Health and Human Services, Centers for Medicare & Medicaid Services (CMS), www.medicare.gov/nursinghomecompare. After entering a location, you will see a list of nursing homes in that area. Each nursing home is given an "Overall Rating" ranging from one star ("much below average") to five stars ("much above average"). Slightly more than 10 percent of the nation's approximately sixteen thousand nursing homes earn the highest rating of five stars. Separate sub-ratings (with one to five stars each) are given for the categories "Health Inspections," "Quality Measures," and "Staffing." The Overall Rating is based on a formula that gives different weights and values to certain quality measures, health-inspection results, and staffing. It is not a perfect formula and the ratings are not necessarily reliable. However, certain information provided on Nursing Home Compare, can be very revealing about a facility's quality of care or lack of it. *A better nursing home will have an "Overall Rating" of four or five stars, though this rating alone does not ensure that it is a good facility.* By analyzing the particular data on Nursing Home Compare as discussed below, consumers can determine whether the facility deserves the government's star rating, whether the facility has demonstrated good care outcomes, or whether there are indications of deficient care delivery.[1]

HEALTH INSPECTIONS

The first subcategory rating is "Health Inspections." Each nursing home in the country is inspected annually by the state's Department of Health. The state-inspection report or "survey report" must be posted in each facility. It is also summarized on the Nursing Home Compare website in the "Health Inspections" section. It is based on a surveyor's interpretation of the facility's compliance with state and federal regulations. Unfortunately, there often can be significant variation in the interpretation of these regulations by surveyors and regulatory offices. This results in frequent inconsistency in the quality and reliability of survey reports and in enforcement action against nursing homes.

The "Health Inspections" information can be helpful, or it can be misleading. Surveyors can be either too lenient or too harsh. It is often impossible for a consumer to tell the difference just from the health-inspections information. However, if the Nursing Home Compare website notes that a sanction has been imposed as a result of the survey (such as a monetary fine, a ban on admissions, a ban on Medicaid or Medicare payments, or a termination of the facility's nursing-assistant training program), that should be seen as a dangerous sign that very serious care problems were found. It should be noted that the absence of such sanctions does not at all suggest that there are not serious care problems.

If the facility has below four stars in this category, you will want to investigate further why the facility has had problems with state Department of Health inspection(s). In all cases, it is important to read the summary on Nursing Home Compare or to ask the nursing home for a full copy of the most recent report. If the survey report indicates widespread care-delivery problems (as opposed to isolated, infrequent, and minor issues) or problems that directly caused harm to residents, you will want to investigate the details further. You should ask to see evidence that deficient practices have been appropriately corrected and that new practices have been effectively and adequately implemented. (Or you may conclude that your search for a good home has not yet ended and keep on looking.)

QUALITY MEASURES

The next section on Nursing Home Compare, "Quality Measures," is the most valuable section and can often tell you whether the "Health Inspections" information accurately reflects the care. *The "Quality Measures" information can often tell you what the care is like at a nursing home without you even having to set foot in it.* It highlights specific objective measures of quality by noting the prevalence or absence of certain conditions among the nursing home's residents. Most significant, it shows how that nursing home compares to the state and national averages. These characteristics or "quality measures" have been selected by CMS as key areas that can indicate either quality or lack of quality in a nursing home's delivery of care. The "Quality Measures" information on Nursing Home Compare is updated quarterly. However, each nursing home's quality measures are updated weekly and appear on the "CASPER Report—MDS 3.0 Facility Level Quality Measure Report." This more current report is not online but can be obtained directly from the nursing home.

It should be noted that the star rating given to the "Quality Measures" subcategory is not helpful by itself. Unfortunately, the methodology for calculating the star rating for this subcategory is flawed in certain aspects and needs to be corrected by CMS. It is most helpful, instead, to look directly at certain of the individual quality measures listed under the "Quality Measures" section. The information shows the percent of residents with a particular health condition in the facility, the state average, and the national average. *You want to find a facility where the key quality measures are significantly lower than the state and national averages.*

It should also be noted that under "Quality Measures," there are separate listings for "short-stay" and "long-stay" residents. Residents with dementia are almost always long-stay residents (as opposed to short-stay rehab patients who return home following therapy), so your focus should be on that category.

The six most significant of the "Quality Measures" for long-stay residents that are the most revealing about the level of quality at a nursing home are the following: the percent of residents who lose too much weight, the percent of residents with pressure ulcers, the percent of residents who lose control of bowel or bladder, the percent of residents who received an antipsychotic medication, the percent of residents physically restrained, and the percent of residents with urinary-tract infection.

Over time, people with dementia decline and need assistance with activities of daily living (e.g., eating, dressing, toileting, transferring, ambulation). They need reminding, cueing, directing, and prompting. Eventually, they will need someone's assistance to do part or all of these activities. If given the needed assistance, however, a person with dementia (and no other advanced-stage disease or wasting illness) should not, until the very end stages of life, experience unintended significant weight loss, malnutrition, dehydration, pressure sores, or drug-induced lethargy. These conditions are generally preventable. Unfortunately, they are also the conditions that far too many people with dementia decline rapidly from—and often die from—in nursing and assisted living facilities. A nursing home that provides a sufficient number of staff and proper staff training, and that uses recognized best-care practices will have significantly less prevalence of malnutrition, bed sores, and other possible signs of inadequate care. The public posting of these particular quality measures has exposed the extent of previously impossible-to-know conditions in nursing homes, conditions that very often are highly preventable.

Significant Weight Loss

The percent of long-stay residents who lose too much weight is an especially revealing piece of data that reflects in a crude but reliable way the kind of care provided to people with dementia. If a facility provides enough staff, and sufficient time, to slowly and patiently help people eat, along with providing good and nutritious food, the only residents who will lose weight are those who are dying or who are in the later stages of serious illness. If staffing levels are inadequate and meals are served in a hurried manner and with little assistance given (cueing or spoon-feeding as needed), there will be much more weight loss in that facility. Alternatively, a facility with appropriate staffing and dining-assistance programs will have significantly less weight loss.

The national average for weight loss in nursing homes is 7.6 percent.[2] A better nursing home will have an incidence of weight loss that is significantly less than the state and national averages. These numbers are all listed under the "Quality Measures" tab on Nursing Home Compare.

If a facility representative claims that the residents there are sicker and that is why they have a higher incidence of weight loss, ask if you can visit at lunch or dinner. Watch in the dining rooms and in resident rooms. Look for residents who appear very disabled and handicapped and others who are not eating by themselves and are just sitting there. Look to see if staff members are actually sitting with them and giving them cueing, prompting, and assistance with feeding. Most residents with advanced dementia need this help. Without it, their uneaten meals will be returned to the kitchen and weight loss and malnutrition, likely followed by the development of pressure sores, will result.

Pressure Ulcers

Like the weight-loss quality measure, the pressure-ulcer quality measure can reflect good care practices and adequate staffing or it can reveal the lack of it. While certain skin ulcers like venous ulcers and stasis ulcers are unavoidable and can result from poor circulation, vascular disease, and diabetes, bed sores or pressure ulcers can often be the result of neglectful or deficient care. Adequate staffing (i.e., enough certified nursing assistants, nurses, and supplemental staff trained as feeders) is absolutely critical to ensuring proper nutrition and hydration, assistance with toileting and incontinence care, and mobility (ambulation, range-of-motion exercises, etc.) and positioning. Adequate staffing and the provision of these care services is what prevent pressure ulcers.

If there are not enough staff members to help feed people who are too confused to feed themselves, or to keep incontinent people clean and dry, or to reposition or provide exercise to people who would otherwise be immobile, then there will be a high rate of pressure ulcers in the facility. The national average for residents with pressure ulcers is 6.3 percent.[3] A best-practices nursing home will have an incidence of pressure ulcers for long-stay residents that is significantly less than the state and national averages as shown on Nursing Home Compare.

It should be noted that if a resident is at the end stage of his or her illness and life, or where a resident is admitted to a facility in a highly compromised condition with severe weight loss and malnutrition, immobility, and very little body mass or muscle, it can be very difficult or impossible to prevent the development of, or fully heal, a pressure ulcer. As will be described in the "Best Practices" section below, however, steps can be taken to prevent further breakdown and to minimize discomfort and prevent potentially lethal infection.

Bowel and Bladder Control

The next quality measure on Nursing Home Compare to examine is long-stay residents who lose control of their bowels or bladder. Most people with dementia will eventually lose the ability to use a toilet by themselves. The ability to recognize the need to toilet, the recollection of where the toilet is, and the ability to take oneself to the toilet and to use it properly are lost over time. How quickly that happens, however, can be greatly influenced by the amount of staff assistance a resident is provided. Most nursing homes do not provide sufficient staffing. It is actually far less expensive and much faster for the nursing home to have staff change a resident's diaper at the staff's convenience than it is for staff to regularly prompt the resident to toilet, transfer the resident to the bathroom, assist the resident onto the toilet, watch for safety to prevent falls, provide cleaning care, put clothes back on, and transfer off the toilet and back to a bed or chair. Helping to preserve a resident's continence costs more and takes more time. A best-practices facility with steady staff and permanent assignments will tend to recognize the resident's signs of needing to use the bathroom and respond with assistance.

If a resident can no longer express the need to toilet and if the staff doesn't proactively ask and prompt the resident to use the bathroom, the resident will be left to urinate or defecate while clothed wherever he or she is. When a person who needs prompting and assistance to the toilet is left in a diaper and not taken to the toilet, that person will lose whatever ability he or she had to preserve continence.

If there is adequate staffing and staff knows the resident's regular routine and disposition and regularly offers to assist the resident to the toilet, the incidence of loss of bowel and bladder control in the facility will be far lower. The national average for loss of bowel and bladder control for long-stay residents is a whopping 43 percent. A best-practices nursing home will have an incidence of loss of bowel and bladder control that is significantly less than the state and national averages as shown on Nursing Home Compare.

Chemical Restraints: Overmedication with Antipsychotics

The quality measure "long-stay residents who received an antipsychotic medication" is critically important for families of people with dementia to examine. It is important to note that the use of antipsychotic medication can be the only effective option for some people with dementia and their caregivers where they are living at home and in cases where the person suffers from early- to middle-stage frontotemporal degeneration (FTD). Living at home lacks the benefits of a staffed and secured building with activities and distractions. The caregiver is often a spouse or child (sometimes still in the workforce) whose job never ceases and who needs periodic rest and rejuvenation in order to care for the infirm partner.

It may be more necessary to use antipsychotic medications with people suffering from early- and middle-stage FTD. People with FTD are often affected by the illness at a much younger age than most people with dementia and can, in some cases, exhibit significant disruptive behavioral symptoms. When extreme behavioral symptoms are exhibited by younger people of generally good health and strength, it can present a significant threat of harm to the personal safety of much older, more frail, and immobile residents in close proximity. If the person with FTD is significantly younger, stronger, healthier, and better able to ambulate independently than the other nursing home residents, this could present a significant problem if that person becomes very agitated easily. Such a person may require the use of antipsychotic or other medication if he or she repeatedly suddenly and without warning or avoidable provocation becomes extremely agitated, combative, or physically inappropriate toward others.

It is important that the lowest possible dose of antipsychotic medication be used for the shortest possible duration and that attempts at gradual dose reduction be made as appropriate. This is appropriate where it helps to maintain the resident's highest level of psychosocial and physical well-being (something that should be reevaluated regularly by the family and nursing home staff). Also, in some instances very short-term, limited use of antianxiety medication, instead of antipsychotics, can be necessary and helpful for some residents with FTD having extreme behavioral outbursts.

However, most nursing home residents with dementia, including those with late-stage FTD don't require antipsychotic medications and may likely be more harmed than helped by them. These medications can be highly toxic to people in the later stages of dementia in particular. The black-box warning that comes with antipsychotics states that they can increase the risk of death in elderly patients with dementia by six to seven times. It is doubtful that anyone would ever consider giving a child a drug with such risks just because a doctor suggested it might help with behavior.

Prolonged antipsychotic use in elderly patients with dementia can cause significantly increased risk of death; a life-threatening nervous-system disorder called neuroleptic malignant syndrome (NMS), which can cause a high fever, stiff muscles, sweating, irregular heartbeat, changes in blood pressure, kidney problems, and confusion; and a movement disorder called tardive dyskinesia (TD) that can involve muscle movement that cannot be stopped. Other symptoms of antipsychotic use can include lethargy, stiffness, stooped and unsteady gait, increased falls, decreased appetite and significant weight loss, confusion, zombielike affect, loss of interest, indifference, significant change in personality, and steady decline in the ability to perform activities of daily living such as eating, toileting, ambulating, and transferring safely. *The use of antipsychotics in elderly people with dementia significantly quickens the decline in their overall functioning.*

Both the American Psychiatric Association[4] and the American Medical Directors Association[5] have declared that doctors are overprescribing antipsychotic medicines in people with dementia. They urge that antipsychotics not be the first treatment for elderly people with dementia and stress the importance of assessing for an underlying cause of behavioral symptoms.

Nevertheless, the Office of the Inspector General of the US Department of Health and Human Services found that 88 percent of antipsychotic drug claims were not for people with schizophrenia or bipolar disorder—they were for people with dementia[6] There have been penalties and jury awards in the billions of dollars against drug manufacturers for improper marketing of antipsychotic drugs.[7]

CMS's recent initiatives to improve care for nursing home residents with dementia and to reduce the inappropriate use of antipsychotics include a vast educational and collaborative approach and a revision of surveyor guidance on dementia care and antipsychotic use for health inspections and enforcement. This is an important and laudable initiative to unchain the bodies and free the minds of frail elders. Yet it has been over twenty-six years since the Nursing Home Reform Act of 1987 and the start of the campaign to end physical and chemical restraints in nursing homes.

The inappropriate drugging of elders in nursing facilities with antipsychotic medications, especially elders with dementia, is epidemic. The average use of antipsychotics in nursing homes in this country in July 2012 was about 24 percent, almost one in four nursing home residents. After three decades of nursing home experience, this author knows that one in four nursing home residents does NOT need an antipsychotic.[8]

The problem is that in the late 1980s, when most facilities began to remove the variety of physical restraints that were used to tie people to chairs and to beds, they substituted them with chemical restraints like antipsychotic medications. Perhaps another factor in the widespread use of antipsychotics in nursing homes was revealed in a *Wall Street Journal* story about the efforts of CMS to improve dementia care and to reduce the use of antipsychotics in nursing home residents.[9] The *Wall Street Journal* noted that $7.6 billion was spent by Medicare Part D on antipsychotics alone in 2011.

Hopefully, state survey agencies will follow CMS's new initiative. Enforcement tools should be used as necessary to ensure that chemical restraints are finally eradicated from our nation's nursing facilities.

When level-appropriate activity throughout the day is provided for people with dementia and people in the later stages of FTD, where they can thrive, and when we make them feel happy and good about themselves, the incidence of significant behavioral symptoms can be reduced. When significant behavioral symptoms are reduced, the need for antipsychotic, antianxiety, and hypnotic medications is reduced. When the use of these medications is reduced, the risk of fall, perhaps the number one threat to elders at home or in facilities, is also reduced.

Very often behavioral symptoms are an expression of an unmet need that requires attention or a transitory state of discomfort that can be gently redirected and alleviated. Residents with dementia can exhibit agitation, aggression, and what can look like—but is not—psychosis. The key to minimizing these behaviors is finding out what caused the behaviors. Often the resident is trying to tell us something. The staff, together with the family, must play the role of investigator and identify possible causes of the agitation and effective responses. The behavior can be due to a physical illness or condition, the effect of a medication, an infection, pain, the need to toilet, or constipation.

The resident can strike out, yell, or hit as a means of communicating discomfort. Staff must be trained to identify symptoms and to respond appropriately. Behavioral symptoms can also be due to nonmedical, nonphysical causes. They can be the result of emotional distress or frustration from not being able to express either what he or she wants or what he or she wants to say. A person with FTD may actually be saying things that may sound disruptive but that can be very easily redirected with pleasantness and offering different things based on the known preferences (food, activity, routine, etc.) of that particular resident (person-centered care).

The key to nonpharmacologic approaches to behavioral symptoms is, with the help of the family and by interacting with the resident, *knowing* the *resident*—the resident's personal preferences, routine, lifetime occupations and roles, recent loss or long-ago loss that may be affecting the resident, likes and dislikes, and, especially, things that help to distract, engage, or calm the resident. Knowing the resident is the foundation of person-centered care.

Also critical to minimizing behavioral symptoms and avoiding the use of antipsychotics is providing day-long activity programming that helps to guide residents with dementia through their day by keeping them active, engaged, and monitored in level-appropriate activities (while allowing them to take naps and breaks when desired). Behavioral symptoms can be observed, anticipated, redirected, and minimized, and the use of antipsychotic medications can be reduced or avoided. (This is described more in the "Best Practices" section).

Physical Restraints

The quality measure for "long-stay residents who were physically restrained" should be zero percent except in extremely unusual cases. Vest restraints, lap trays that prevent egress, lap bars, belts, and bedside rails all constitute physical restraints. Physical restraints, like chemical restraints, are recognized as horribly detrimental to residents' medical, physical, and psychosocial health and have been prohibited by law since the Nursing Home Reform Act of 1987 was enacted. The national average of physical restraint among residents is 1.4 percent.[10]

Urinary-Tract Infections

Finally, the quality measure for the percent of long-stay residents with a urinary-tract infection can also give an important suggestion about the overall care in a facility, especially for people in the late stages of dementia. Urinary-tract infections can often, but not always, be due to the lack of sufficient assistance with drinking (resulting in dehydration) or to being left wet and soiled in a diaper for extended periods of time due to inadequate staffing. A best-practices nursing home will have an incidence of urinary-tract infection that is less (and preferably significantly less) than the state and national averages as shown on Nursing Home Compare.

If a nursing home has consistently scored four or five stars on each of the six of the quality measures identified above, that is a very strong indication that it is a good nursing home that uses best-care practices.

The Staffing Quality Measure

The information provided in the "Staffing" subcategory on Nursing Home Compare is only somewhat helpful. The staffing data that this is based on is not audited, nor is it based on verified attendance records or payroll information. In most cases, it is based on the findings of only one random day or week at the time of the inspection.

For various reasons, the staffing information reported on Nursing Home Compare is not always consistent with the staffing data collected by state Departments of Health or reported on DOH websites. For this reason, less emphasis should be given to the information provided on this section of Nursing Home Compare. The best way to determine if there is adequate staffing at a facility is to ask a certified nursing assistant (CNA) working there. Ask the CNA how many residents she has to care for and compare that to the recommended CNA staffing levels in the "Best Practices" section below. Also, ask the CNA if she usually has enough staff or whether she usually works short-staffed. The answer you get will be far more reliable than answers you may get from the admissions office.

Other Sources

Each year, *U.S. News & World Report* publishes its list of America's "Best Nursing Homes." *U.S. News* selects its list of "Best Nursing Homes" based on the US government's Five-Star rating system information with some modification. Generally, in order to earn the *U.S. News* "Best Nursing Home" rating, a facility has to have a rating of five stars for at least the three prior consecutive quarters. The *U.S. News & World Report* ratings and articles also contain much valuable information on nursing home care and placement and can be found at www.usnews.com/best-nursing-homes.

It should be noted that several states have websites that provide information on nursing homes, often including full copies of the health-inspection reports. Other valuable sources of information are the local offices of the area agency on aging and the ombudsman in the county where you are looking. You can find the office of area agency on aging in the phone book under "local government" or online. The agency can provide you with a list of nursing homes in the county. The ombudsman, usually a part of the agency, is the person who is available to represent nursing home residents and their families in addressing problems at nursing homes. The ombudsman can be an invaluable resource in steering you toward or away from certain facilities. If the ombudsman is not forthcoming, ask which facilities he or she is regularly called upon to visit. That is an indication of facilities that may have more complaints.

The local chapter of the Alzheimer's Association[11] or the Association for Frontotemporal Degeneration[12] (AFTD) can be a valuable resource in identifying good nursing facilities. The association office may direct you to individuals who have personal experience with certain facilities or to local caregiver support groups. The people in support groups often have loved ones in facilities and can give you firsthand information about them. *There is no better source of information about a facility than the family of a resident.* Another very valuable resource is the National Consumer Voice for Quality Long Term Care a.k.a. Consumer Voice (formerly the National Citizen's Coalition for Nursing Home Reform [NCCNHR]).[13] Consumer Voice is the premier national consumer organization that advocates for the rights and interests of nursing home residents and their families. Consumer Voice will direct you to individuals or local advocacy groups in your state that can help steer you in the right direction.

VISITING HOMES IN PERSON

After checking the above resources, your next step is visiting the nursing home. You will need to call and schedule an appointment to get a complete tour and information about prices and availability. But you can also make an unannounced visit. This section will identify important things to observe, questions to ask staff and families, and specific care programs to investigate.

When you visit the nursing home, look at the interaction between the staff and residents and between the staff and you. Is it a friendly and warm place? As you walk through the home, do people greet you and make you feel welcome? Are staff members speaking to residents, holding their hands, hugging them, keeping them company, giving assistance in a caring, compassionate way? Focus more on the way the staff interacts with the residents and less on the elegance of the furnishings.

Are the residents dressed neatly and in clean clothes? Are their fingernails trimmed? Are the men shaved? Are staff members responding to residents who may be calling for help? Is the home clean? Does it smell clean, or is there an unpleasant odor? Is the home a lively place with different activities going on? Are residents involved in group programs? Are people walking or ambulating with wheelchairs freely throughout the building, or are they physically restrained in some way (a seat belt, a tray or cushion across their wheelchair, or a vest restraint)? Are residents confined in bed with two full-length side rails (rarely an appropriate measure)? Do many of the residents appear lethargic and "zombied out"? Do you see many staff members, especially at meal time? Are the staff members assisting residents (with walking, eating, transferring from place to place)?

Either during or after the tour, seek out and speak to staff members. Approach at least two nurses and three nursing assistants and ask them how they like working at the facility and how long they have been there. Ask how the management treats the staff. Ask how often the facility uses "agency staff" (temporary staffing from outside companies). Extensive use of agency staff may suggest problems with adequate staffing and consistency in staffing. Ask if they feel the facility has enough staff (nurses and nursing assistants). Perhaps, most important of all, ask a nursing assistant (not the admissions person) how many residents she takes care of and on which shift (day, evening, or night—the number will vary depending on the shift). Take notes and compare them later with the suggested staffing ratios discussed below.

If the staff is happy, treated well by the management, and consists of enough personnel to do the job, chances are the care will be good and the residents will be happy and treated well. The opposite is likely to be true if the staff is unhappy, unstable, and insufficient to do the work.

During a visit to the facility, seek out people who are visiting residents. These are usually family members. Most often, they can be found during mealtimes. As stated earlier, *there is no better source of information about a facility than the family of a resident.* Ask how long their loved one or friend has been at the facility. Ask what they think of the place, the staff, and the management. Ask them whom they go to if they have a problem or need, and ask if their problems or needs get addressed. Ask them if they would recommend the facility for your loved one. Remember, no facility or person is perfect and can please everyone. So always ask more than one family or visitor.

NURSING HOME BEST-CARE PRACTICES

There are basic prerequisites that are needed for providing good care and for achieving consistently good ratings on the key quality measures on the Nursing Home Compare website.

First and foremost is leadership. The ownership and management of the facility must be active and involved. This includes the board, the corporate executives, the administrator, and the director of nursing (DON). Quality improvement comes from the top down. Only the leadership can set the goals of an organization, and only the leadership can provide the tools needed to achieve these goals.

Next is adequate staffing with consistent assignment. On the first shift there should be one CNA to no more than eight residents. On the second shift, there should be one CNA to no more than nine residents; and on the third shift, one CNA to no more than sixteen residents.

Consistent assignment is where the same CNA cares for the same residents five out of seven days a week. This is absolutely essential to knowing the resident, to providing person-centered care, and to minimizing behavioral symptoms. A facility that is inadequately staffed and that has a lot of staff turnover is much less likely to have implemented consistent assignment. Next, communication between the family, the staff, the administrator, and the DON is vital, especially whenever there is a change in condition.

A good weight-loss-prevention program starts with assistance with eating. The needs of the dementia patient change over time and are very different depending on the stage of the disease—early, middle, or advanced. There should be three distinct dining programs. The first is for high-functioning residents who eat with minimal assistance. The second is geared toward people in the middle stages of dementia. These residents are able to feed themselves but tend to forget to finish eating, get distracted and wander away, or act in inappropriate ways (playing with food or pushing things off the table). These residents need extensive cueing, step-by-step instruction, directing, and encouragement by staff members, who use a host of assistive techniques. This type of program requires a ratio of one staff member to three residents and lasts for up to ninety minutes or as long as needed. The third program is geared toward people in the late stages of dementia who require extensive to total assistance with eating. This program requires a ratio of approximately one staff member to two or two and a half residents.

Identifying and accommodating the resident's food preferences is critical. A best-practices facility will have a special menu of foods for people with weight loss. Such foods would include gravies, juices, milks, baked goods, hot cereals, mashed potatoes, and other items that are packed with sugar, butter, margarine, cream, half and half, condensed milk, dry milk solids, and so on. High-calorie and high-protein supplements, drinks, milkshakes, puddings, and snacks should be provided throughout the day and night.

The skincare program should be multifaceted. Proper hydration, nutrition, and weight-gain programs, proper vitamin and nutrient intake, good incontinence care, good exercise and range-of-motion programs, regular body repositioning and turning—all of which require adequate staffing—are essential to the avoidance of skin breakdown. Each resident must be assessed on at least a quarterly basis to determine the risk of skin breakdown and to identify necessary preventive measures.

If possible, skin breakdown must be recognized and treated at its earliest stage—an unopened, persistent reddened area. Once a sore is open, a nurse specially trained as a certified continence wound ostomy care nurse (CWOCN) or enterostomal therapist (ET) needs to be involved. The ET and facility nursing staff should be familiar with the different treatments appropriate for treating and healing the various types and stages of wounds. In addition to this level of expertise, a best-practices facility will have a sufficient number of specialized pressure-relieving mattress systems. They range from high-density foam mattresses to motorized low-air-loss mattresses to motorized alternating-air-pressure mattresses. The motorized alternating-air-pressure mattresses are expensive but not prohibitive. They are extremely effective in preventing pressure sores in people at high risk for them and in healing pressure sores that have developed. A facility's arsenal against bedsores will also include a variety of pressure-relieving gel and foam cushions for pressure relief, pads, heel cushions, and other products.

A best-practices facility will have activities and socialization programs that seek to maximize psychosocial functioning by providing enriching, nurturing, and satisfying experiences for residents with dementia. As with dining, the psychosocial needs of people with dementia vary significantly over the course of the illness. A facility should offer three different levels of activity programs, each, at least, twice daily. The first level should be geared to the nondemented residents but should include one activity each day that is open to the entire resident community.

The second level should be geared to those in the early and middle stages of a dementing illness. The aim of this level is to maintain and encourage socialization and interaction with others through a variety of ability-appropriate, meaningful, and enjoyable activities. These should be conducted with smaller groups of people who are still verbal and communicative. A skilled program leader, who goes with the flow of the conversation and provides reassurance and affirmation, can do wonders in restoring self-confidence and preserving the skills needed for communication and social interaction.

The third level of programming is for those in the late stages of dementia who are generally immobile and nonverbal. The focus of this programming is sensory stimulation through a variety of activities including things like music therapy and aromatherapy. Residents with advanced dementia often respond especially well to music. Music therapy, together with various sensory-stimulation activities (including spending time outside in the garden, feeling the warm sun and breeze and smelling the flowers), aim to engage and involve the individual and to promote an individual's awareness of self and the environment.

A critical element is staff training. Training in dementia care should be provided at the time of orientation and thereafter, at least annually. Topics should include: how to communicate with people with dementia, how to determine the needs of a confused or nonverbal resident, how to analyze and respond to changes in mood or behavior, how to respond to extreme behavioral symptoms, and how to provide activities of daily living (ADL) care to a confused or resistive person.

Effective-care-plan meetings are also an important part of nursing home best practices. The care-plan meeting is the periodic meeting where the family or friends of the resident meet with the facility's management team to discuss the condition and care of the resident. It should include the director of nursing, the administrator, a social worker, activities department staff, and the dietary director. One can learn an enormous amount by observing the care-plan meeting. To observe a meeting (as an outside visitor), you would need to get permission from the facility and from the family/responsible party at the meeting. If the facility staff at the meeting demonstrate that they know the resident, her current condition, her preferences as far as activities and meals, and any issues regarding her care and daily living, that is a good indication that person-centered care is being practiced. If the key personnel mentioned above are not even present, or if the staff doesn't seem to know the resident's personal needs, the opposite is probably true.

Finally, it is important to note that at least two thirds to three quarters, and often a higher proportion, of nursing home residents have their care paid for by Medicaid. Adequate Medicaid payment rates are absolutely critical for providing the kind of best practices and programs recommended and described in this chapter. There is no question that recent Medicaid cuts and any future reductions threaten the long-term viability of providing such care.

Conclusion

The caregiver of a person with dementia should use the suggested guidelines to identify whether a condition exists that requires care that cannot reasonably be provided at home. If such a condition exists, the caregiver should follow the suggested investigation process to identify whether a best-practices facility exists nearby and whether admission is possible. The search for a best-practices facility is not necessarily an easy one. Doing the research, seeking referrals, looking for the important signs, and asking the right questions all take time and effort, and there is no guarantee of admission. But while so much of life with a dementia disease is beyond the caregiver's control, the tools outlined above (by highlighting what to look for and what to avoid) can inform and empower the caregiver and put him or her back in control.

THE ASSISTED LIVING OPTION

For people in the early and middle stages of dementia, and their families, an assisted living facility can provide a secure and beneficial environment. A good facility can be a safe haven that can help a person maintain his or her highest practical level of independence, socialization, and well-being. In general, a good facility will provide physical safety and security, socialization and companionship, meaningful activity, and assistance with activities of daily living. There is, however, significant variation in the scope of programming and services provided by assisted living facilities. There have been a number of recent studies and investigative documentaries on inadequate care and staffing at assisted living facilities. The lack of laws, regulation, oversight by inspectors or regulators, and public reporting of facility-specific resident health conditions make it very difficult to find a good assisted living facility.

The hallmark of most new assisted living facilities is their residential, homelike atmosphere and decor. Most people feel more comfortable in a residential, noninstitutional setting. While the decor and atmosphere can be important, far more important is the number and training of staff. The need for assistance with ADLs such as dressing, bathing, eating, and toileting is a major reason for placement in an assisted living facility. It is this critical element of service that varies most widely among assisted living facilities.[14] The marketing information of many facilities promotes the concept of "aging in place." The reality of "aging in place" can be much different than what is presented in a marketing brochure. Many do not provide or even offer the supports, services, and staff members that are needed to care for people as they decline and near death.

Unlike with nursing homes, there is no federal law governing assisted living facilities, and very few states have laws regulating them. Indeed, there is no common agreement about what precisely is meant by *assisted living* and the definition varies tremendously.[15] Most states with laws on assisted living have either very minimal requirements or none at all regarding the minimum of number of staff required to be on duty or for staff training in topics like elder care, dementia care, medication administration, abuse, and so on.

For assisted living consumers, in most states, there are not only inadequate protections as far as meaningful minimum staffing requirements but also the risks associated with medication administration by non-nurse personnel. While there is usually a nurse on staff, most of the care is provided by personal-care attendants who are unlicensed and uncertified. The multitask worker is another hallmark of assisted living care. A personal-care attendant is usually a combination of housekeeper, laundry aide, meal preparer, meal server, activities leader, and medication administrator, *as well as* the provider of ADL care (assistance with dressing, eating, toileting, transferring, etc.). There are a number of drugs that are commonly taken by the elderly that require vigilant monitoring for negative side effects. There are many drugs that require testing immediately before the medication is given (e.g., blood-sugar and blood-pressure levels) or on a periodic (weekly, monthly, quarterly) basis. Close attention must be paid to the results of these tests before administration of the medication. Staff members who are not nurses may not be trained or experienced in this.

Since dementia entails a progressive decline over time in cognitive, self-care, and physical abilities, it is very important to understand the scope of services provided by a particular facility. Once a person reaches a point where he needs extensive or total care by staff for toileting, eating, dressing, and/or transferring, it takes a lot more time to care for that one person. The facility needs to provide this additional staff. Since there are no publicly reported data similar to that for nursing homes, the best source of information about whether an assisted living facility is providing adequate staffing are the people who have or have had loved ones in that facility.

For a person in the early stages of dementia, it is important to maintain physical safety. The home in which he or she lived safely may now present opportunities for injury. Working safely with knives and appliances may be an insurmountable challenge for the formerly expert chef or homemaker. A walk or drive to a nearby store or friend's house may result in an unintended journey far off course.

One of the most important things to look for when considering placement of a person with early-stage FTD, or anyone with dementia who is physically strong and can ambulate easily, is the presence of an effective mechanical system that automatically prevents a resident from leaving the building. A person with FTD may be younger, healthier, and far more mobile than most older people who have dementia. A person with early-stage FTD might have no problem exiting the family home and walking, taking the bus, or driving to another city or destination. There are a number of automatic door-locking and delayed egress systems that are widely used in nursing facilities that work effectively to keep residents with dementia from wandering or exiting from the facility.

A good assisted living facility for people with dementia provides a safe environment that is tailored to the needs and limitations of the residents. A good facility will have:

- a continuous indoor walking or wandering circuit and an enclosed outdoor courtyard or garden

- an automatic door-locking system that prevents unescorted egress
- a special bracelet worn by a resident that will trigger the exit doors to lock, except in case of a fire emergency
- a centrally located residential-style kitchen with all the makings of a home kitchen equipped with special safety features (switches and locks, etc.) that restrict the use of sharp items and cooking appliances so that they can be used only with the supervision of a staff member
- a conveniently located residential-style laundry room similarly equipped with safety features
- a safety-proofed woodworking or craft shop that can be very therapeutic and enjoyable for residents who are accustomed to these activities
- a supportive social atmosphere and a daily routine that is tailored to the needs and abilities of the cognitively impaired
- a daily schedule of activities geared toward the residents' lifetime work and leisure experience and preferences, each modified to accommodate the residents' needs or limitations
- a host of activities that promote group interaction, discussion, and community that helps residents to exercise their social and communication skills

It is absolutely critical for those responsible for placing someone in an assisted living facility to recognize signs of significant decline in functioning and to recognize the need for appropriate interventions. The responsible party must be vigilant in determining whether the assisted living facility resident's needs are being met or whether another care setting is appropriate.

To determine if a person's needs are being adequately met in an assisted living facility, the responsible party should use the same analysis described in the previous section on determining if nursing home placement is appropriate.

Other conditions or treatments that may require a greater level of expertise than might typically be found at an assisted living facility are respiratory/oxygen treatments, wound care, colostomy/ostomy care, injections, catheterization, IV medications, tube feeding, and physical, occupational, or speech therapy. If a special therapeutic diet or special food consistency (e.g., pureed or mechanical soft food, thickened liquids) is necessary, a dietician's input and oversight may be necessary.

It is important to know in advance if the facility charges additional fees if more assistance with ADL care is needed, particularly whether there is an additional charge for incontinence care. The cost for private-duty aides or nursing personnel is borne by the resident and is in addition to the basic monthly fee for the assisted living facility.

Before considering assisted living, it is important to read, watch, and consider the recent studies and investigative documentaries on assisted living. Catherine Hawes, former director of the Program on Aging and Long-Term Care Policy at Texas A&M University, has done extensive research into assisted living. She was part of a series coproduced by the PBS show *Frontline* and the investigative nonprofit ProPublica. The series, titled "Life and Death in Assisted Living," premiered July 30, 2013, and is available for viewing online.[16] It featured four programs exposing shocking and inadequate care at assisted living facilities across the country. Catherine Hawes's work and the "Life and Death in Assisted Living" series today harken back loudly to 1986 when Dr. Hawes was a member of the Institute of Medicine (IOM) panel whose published report exposed the horrible care being suffered by nursing home residents at the time. That IOM study led to the Nursing Home Reform Act of 1987, which brought significant reforms.

An additional excellent resource on assisted living is the report *Best Practices in Assisted Living: Considering Potential Reforms for California* by Eric Carlson and Gwen Orlowski[17] of the National Senior Citizen Law Center.

When looking for a good assisted living facility, some of the resources identified in the previous section on finding a good nursing home apply as well. The local chapter of the Alzheimer's Association, especially participants in the chapter's caregiver support groups, can be very helpful. Also, you can check with the ombudsman in your county's area agency on aging, and the National Consumer Voice for Quality Long Term Care.

The suggestions in the previous section on what to look for and what and whom to ask during a visit to a nursing home should be followed precisely when visiting an assisted living facility, too.

Conclusion

For the most part, assisted living remains an option only for those who can afford it. A facility designed for people with dementia can be an ideal setting, providing a comfortable, noninstitutional environment where activities and routines are tailored to the abilities of the residents. Safety, monitoring, and assistance with medications and most activities of daily living can be provided in a familiar, supportive, residential atmosphere.

Because of the variation in the level of services provided by different assisted living facilities, the responsible party must continually monitor for changes in condition that require additional assistance with care and the implementation of appropriate interventions. The responsible party must also look for specific signs of decline and determine whether the services provided by the facility have been increased to include the interventions needed to ensure the resident's highest level of physical and psychosocial functioning. If the resident's needs have increased but staff support and assistance has not, and/ or avoidable conditions have developed, it is time to consider placement in another setting.

NOTES

1. The ownership information links are also valuable and will help you determine whether the facility is for-profit or not-for-profit, and whether or not it is part of a chain of nursing homes. It may also tell you if it is being managed by a management company that is part of a chain (in large, publicly traded companies, the management company often shares a similar name to the parent entity).

2. Centers for Medicare & Medicaid Services, "Medicare.gov," www.Medicare.gov/nursinghomecompare (accessed December 24, 2013).

3. Ibid.

4. Kim Painter, "Doctors: Anti-Psychotic Meds Overused for Dementia, Kids", *USA Today*, September 23, 2013.

5. American Medical Directors Association (AMDA), "Five Things Physicians & Patients Should Question," http://www.choosingwisely.org/doctor-patient-lists/amda-dedicated-to-long-term-care-medicine (accessed December 24, 2013).

6. May 2011 Report of the Inspector General of the US Department of Health & Human Services.

7. In January 2009, $1.4 billion was paid by Eli Lilly & Co. to resolve claims of improper marketing of Zyprexa (US Department of Justice press release, January 15, 2009, http://www.justice.gov/opa/pr/2009/January/09-civ-038.html); in November 2009, Omnicare reached a settlement with US Department of Justice for $98 million (US Department of Justice press release, November 3, 2009, http://www.justice.gov/opa/pr/2009/November/09-civ-1186.html); in May 2012, Abbott Laboratories agreed to pay federal and state governments $1.6 billion (M. Schmidt and K. Thomas, "Abbott Settles Marketing Lawsuit," *New York Times*, May 8, 2012, p. B1, http://www.nytimes.com/2012/05/08/business/abbott-to-pay-1-6-billion-over-illegal-marketing.html); in July 2012, Glaxo paid $3 billion in a fraud settlement (M. Schmidt and K. Thomas, "Glaxo Agrees to Pay $3 Billion in Fraud Settlement," *New York Times*, July 2, 2012, http://www.nytimes.com/2012/07/03/business/glaxosmithkline-agrees-to-pay-3-billion-in-fraud-settlement.html); in August

2012, Janssen Pharmaceuticals, a division of Johnson & Johnson, settled multistate litigation for $181 million (NY State Attorney General press release, August 30, 2012, http://www.ag.ny.gov/press-release/ag-schneiderman-settles-181-million-deceptive-marketing-case-janssen-pharmaceuticals); and in November 2014, Johnson & Johnson agreed to pay $2.2 billion in fines (US Department of Justice press release November 4, 2014, "Johnson & Johnson to Pay More Than $2.2 Billion to Resolve Criminal and Civil Investigations," http://www.justice.gov/opa/pr/2013/November/13-ag-1170.html).

    8. Gwynedd Square Nursing Center (Lansdale, PA) has consistently had among the lowest rates of antipsychotic use in the United States for over fifteen years. As of the quarter ended December 20, 2013, the national average for use of antipsychotics in long-stay residents was 20.6 percent. For the same period, use of antipsychotics at Gwynedd Square Nursing Center was 8.5 percent. "CASPER Report MDS 3.0 Facility Level Quality Measure Report" for Gwynedd Square Nursing Center, Run Date: January 2, 2014. US Department of Health and Human Services, Centers for Medicare and Medicaid Services website online CASPER Report, www.cms.gov/.

    9. Lucette Lagnado, "Nursing Homes' Drug Use Falls," *Wall Street Journal*, August 26, 2013.

    10. "CASPER Report MDS 3.0 Facility Level Quality Measure Report" for Gwynedd Square Nursing Center, Run Date: January 2, 2014. US Department of Health and Human Services, Centers for Medicare and Medicaid Services website online CASPER Report, www.cms.gov/.

    11. Alzheimer's Association, www.alz.org.

    12. The Association for Frontotemporal Degeneration, www.theaftd.org.

    13. The National Consumer Voice for Quality and Long Term Care, www.theconsumervoice.org, (202) 332-2275.

    14. Catherine Hawes, Miriam Rose, and Charles D. Phillips, *A National Study of Assisted Living for the Frail Elderly—Results of a National Survey of Facilities* (Myers Research Institute, December 1999), pp. 9–11, 17–18, 54–62; . Catherine Hawes and Charles D. Phillips, *High Service or High Privacy Assisted Living Facilities, Their Residents and Staff: Results from a National Survey* (US Department of Health and Human Services, Texas A&M University, Miriam Rose, Myers Research Institute, November 2000), pp. 15–17.

    15. Catherine Hawes, *Frontline*/ProPublica interview, July 29, 2013, http://www.pbs.org/wgbh/pages/frontline/social-issues/life-and-death-in-assisted-living/catherine-hawes-assisted-living-is-a-ticking-time-bomb/.

    16. "Life and Death in Assisted Living, Parts 1–4," by A. C. Thompson, ProPublica, and Jonathan Jones; produced by *Frontline* in association with ProPublica; series aired July 2013.

    17. Eric Carlson and Gwen Orlowski, *Best Practices in Assisted Living: Considering Potential Reforms for California*, special report (National Senior Citizens Law Center, February 2014).

CHAPTER 21

BY THE HANDS OF OTHERS

Creating Helpful Support Networks

Helen-Ann Comstock

Responding to the challenge of caring for someone with frontotemporal degeneration (FTD) is never easy; it is demanding, frustrating, and stressful. Caregivers face the constant task of balancing the needs of the patient with their own needs and often those of other family members as well. It's easy to feel overwhelmed. Caregiving requires a lot of individual effort, but it cannot be handled alone. Other people must be drawn in. By working together and sharing responsibilities, you and they can make life better for the person with frontotemporal degeneration and for you, the caregiver. It is important, even lifesaving, to share the responsibility of caring and to develop your own support network. Having a support network has been shown to have "direct and stress-buffering effects"[1] on well-being. A support network allows you to provide needed assistance to the person with FTD while at the same time keeping a balance in other aspects of your life.

SETTING UP A SUPPORT NETWORK

The key to successfully coping with FTD is planning and establishing a support network. Here are the steps to follow.

1. ***Educate yourself about the disease and its progression***. Knowledge of the disease will help you to understand how the disease affects your family member's behavior. It will help you to know what to expect over the course of the disease. Educating yourself about the disease is absolutely critical. Start by contacting the Association for Frontotem-

351

poral Degeneration (AFTD), a nationwide nonprofit organization specifically devoted to providing information and support to those coping
with FTD. In addition, a resource list for information specific to FTD
is at the end of this chapter and at the end of this book. (See chapters 1
through 9 for more information on understanding FTD.)

2. ***Understand what is happening to your family member. This is the
   key to learning how to cope with the disease.*** Think for a moment
   about the fact that your family member is losing his ability to cope
   with everyday living. He is losing his ability to be in control of his life.
   He still has wants and needs, but he is unable to express these desires
   or fulfill them himself. He is constantly failing to perform in a world
   where he used to be able to do everything. That's very scary! And
   each person is an individual and will react differently to this situation.
   Some become anxious and withdraw. Some express their frustration
   by striking out or running off. Some say impolite or even rude or crude
   things. Some exhibit inappropriate social or sexual behaviors. Family
   life is seriously disrupted by FTD. This is why it is so important to
   learn about the disease and ways to cope with it.

   Caregivers who view a patient's memory and behavioral problems as a direct consequence of the disease generally are less bothered by them than caregivers who continue to view such problems as
   being in the patient's control. It's important to realize that the person
   with dementia is not in control of his behavior. It is the caregiver who
   is in control and who needs to change and adapt, because the person
   with dementia can't. Understanding the disease will aid you in making
   plans for care, and you will become a better caregiver.

3. ***Tell your family and friends about the diagnosis and what it means.***
   Family and friends need to understand what is happening to your loved
   one if you are to have their support and help. Provide them with information about the disease: Give them a brochure or a fact sheet. This
   will help them to see why your loved one's behavior has changed. It
   will help them to realize that there is a neurological reason for the
   changes in behavior. They will learn that the changes are due to the
   disease and that your loved one has no control over the changes that
   are taking place, nor is she able to control her behavior.

   Most people will find that what is happening to your family member
   is painful and frightening. Therefore, do not be hurt or surprised if they

do not jump right in and offer to help. They need time to adjust to the situation. Give them time to learn and understand about the disease and, generally, they will overcome their fears and be supportive. However, be tolerant of those who are not able to overcome their discomfort and who may never be able to visit with your family member or assist with her care. They may offer to help in other ways that are useful to you, the caregiver, and thus become part of your support network.

4. *Ask for help.* It can't be stressed enough how very important it is to draw family members and friends into your support network. Don't be too proud or timid to ask for their help. Caring for someone with frontotemporal degeneration is never easy. You need all the help you can get! Not only will you, the caregiver, benefit from the support of family members and friends, your loved one will also, and so will your family.

In her helpful book, *Dear Aunt S: How to Ask for Help from Family and Friends in Time of Crisis*, Marion Cohen, PhD, writes, "Mostly I had to arrive at the mind-set that it was a crisis we were going through, that it was appropriate to ask for help, and that I had a right to do so—the right to gather a support system."[2] She also points out that asking for help is a commitment toward fulfilling your responsibility toward the ill person, as he has a right to more people helping him.

When you are planning to ask for help, be sure to think about all the people who might be able to provide various kinds of help. Include (1) people with whom you live; (2) family/relatives; (3) friends; (4) people from work or school; (5) people from clubs, organizations, or religious groups; (6) neighbors; and (7) agencies or other formal service providers.[3]

You can go about asking for help in different ways. In my situation, we were living in California when my husband was diagnosed with FTD and all our family members were living on the East Coast, so I needed to depend on friends for help. I had a wine-and-cheese party and invited all our friends. During the party I spoke briefly about my husband's diagnosis and gave out an information sheet. I said that even though my husband was losing his ability to do many things, he still needed companionship and stimulation, and I needed a break from twenty-four-hours-a-day caregiving. I asked them to help on a regular basis (it's important to have a regular commitment) in any way they could, such as taking my husband for walks, playing card games, doing puzzles, and working on reading skills or math problems (he was a math professor). At the end of the evening, twenty-five people (working professionals as well as community volunteers) each committed to spend one hour a week with my husband. One friend even came up with her own idea to help: She saved her errands and took my husband along in her car once a week while she ran her errands. He loved the ride in the car and her company, even though he was unable to converse.

This support network helped us in so many ways. It kept us from the isolation that so many families experience when coping with FTD. It provided my husband with companionship. It gave me some breaks, which allowed me to go to the grocery store, take a walk on my own, visit a friend, and so on. And, since our volunteers mostly were parents of our children's friends, it helped their children to have a better understanding of what was happening to our family. Of course, as the disease progressed and my husband lost his ability to speak and his attention span dropped to less than five minutes, changes needed to be made in the program. By that time, walks, rides in the car, and simple games were the most useful. Daycare became a helpful option. It was a place where my husband could be part of the activities, even though he could not participate in them, and it was a service that gave me some respite.

Now, you may not be comfortable with having a wine-and-cheese party or some other sort of gathering to set up your support network. In her book, Dr. Cohen outlines another way to set up a support network. She suggests the following: Write "asking-for-help" letters. She gives very detailed suggestions about how to do this, as well as how to arrange a family meeting. Writing letters (or e-mails, if you prefer) allows you to tell others about your situation without interruption, and it allows the recipient the time and space to reflect and to get used to the idea. You can offer specific suggestions for how the letter recipient can help: Visit with your family member, drive him to daycare, help with finding resources, invite the caregiver for something fun, include both caregiver and patient in informal gatherings, and so on. Use your creativity; the list of options will vary with each family situation.

In asking for help, try to find a good friend or family member who will take on the asking role for you—someone to act as your advocate. People will be more comfortable talking with a third party. They'll feel greater freedom to ask questions and reveal their fears and discomfort about helping. Your advocate can be invaluable.

5. **Join a support group.** A support group is another important piece of your support network. Joining a support group gives you the opportunity to meet other people who are experiencing the same problems and griefs as you are. Support groups also provide information about FTD and local resources. There is much you can learn from the experiences of other members and their sympathetic understanding of your situation. Support groups specific to FTD are the most helpful, but they are available only in limited areas. Contact the Association for Frontotemporal Degeneration for the location of FTD-specific support groups, or check with your local Alzheimer's Association chapter or local medical center to see if they have an FTD-specific support group.

   If you are unable to locate an FTD-specific support group, try an Alzheimer's support group. You still will learn about local resources and find companionship from group members.

   If you are unable to leave your family member to attend a support-group meeting, or if there is no nearby support group, check with the Association for Frontotemporal Degeneration about AFTD's telephone support group or join an on-line support group. Or, ask if you can be linked up to another caregiver who will become your telephone buddy. I found such an arrangement extremely helpful when I was unable to leave my husband to attend a support-group meeting. Being a telephone buddy is a two-way arrangement. Telephone buddies offer each other support and helpful suggestions during difficult times, but they also share amusing incidents or poignant moments. Having a telephone buddy is the next best thing to having a sympathetic friend stop by for a cup of coffee or a glass of wine.

6. *Make use of respite resources.* Adult daycare provides benefits to the person with FTD and eases the caregiving burden. It allows the caregiver time to return to work or take care of personal needs. It gives the person with FTD an opportunity for socialization and stimulation. In-home or overnight institutional respite gives the caregiver and/or family an opportunity for much-needed relief.

7. *Take care of yourself.* Caregiver members of the FTD support group of the Orange County (CA) chapter of the Alzheimer's Association were asked to answer the question, "What's the most important piece

of advice you would give to someone who has just become a caregiver for a person with FTD?" Overwhelmingly, their response was: *"The first thing to do is take care of yourself."* Here's what they suggest to accomplish this: Keep up spiritual, social, and community activities; exercise; be open to talking with a therapist knowledgeable about FTD; give yourself permission to be "selfish." And learn, learn, learn! Learn to be patient; learn that your relationship with the family member with FTD will change; learn to lower your expectations of what the person with FTD can do (but always keep in mind that she is an adult, not a child), learn about the disease; learn to accept help; learn that it is all right and healthy to laugh. Keep your sense of humor!

To this excellent advice from experienced caregivers, I would add, *learn to remember love.* The person with FTD may not remember much. Eventually she may not seem to know you or respond to anything. She may not show pain or fear or loneliness, but I believe she experiences them. She may not remember your gentle touch, kind words, or hugs, but I believe she feels them. She may no longer be able to do anything. *But I believe she still remembers love and feels your loving care.*

Follow these seven steps to set up a support network for yourself so that you will be able to give that loving care.

RESOURCES

Note that *frontotemporal degeneration* (FTD), which this book uses as the most current term to describe the group of frontotemporal syndromes, may be referred to as *frontotemporal dementia* by resources that have not yet adopted this nomenclature.

Organizations and Medical Centers

The Association for Frontotemporal Degeneration (AFTD), Radnor Station Building 2, Suite 320, 290 King of Prussia Road, Radnor, PA. 267-514-7221. Helpline: 866-507-7222. www.theaftd.org. This is a nationwide nonprofit organization whose mission is to promote and fund research into finding the cause and cure for frontotemporal degeneration; to provide information, education, and support to persons diagnosed with FTD and their families and caregivers; and to educate physicians and allied health professionals about FTD. AFTD provides a toll-free telephone helpline, in-person and telephone support groups, and informational materials, including booklets, books, and DVDs.

Lewy Body Dementia Association, 912 Killian Road, Liburn, GA 30047. 404-935-6444 or 800-LEWYSOS (539-9767). Caregiver link: 800-539-9767. P.O. Box 451429, Atlanta, GA 31145-9429. www.lewybodydementia.org. The Lewy Body Dementia Association was founded to promote research into conquering the disease while assisting those who are affected by it today.

WE MOVE (Worldwide Education and Awareness for Movement Disorders), 204 West 84th Street, New York, NY 10024. 212-875-8312. www. wemove.org. This organization offers information on corticobasal degeneration and other movement disorders.

ALS Association (ALSA), 1275 K Street NW, Suite 250, Washington, DC 20005. 202-407-8580 or 800-782-4747. www.alsa.org. The association's nationwide network of chapters provides comprehensive patient services and support to the ALS community. On the home page, type in "frontotemporal dementia" for information about the overlap between FTD and ALS.

CurePSP, Foundation for PSP, CBD and Related Brain Diseases, 11350 McCormick Road, Suite 906, Hunt Valley, MD 21031. 800-457-4777. www .curepsp.org. An association dedicated to increasing awareness of progressive supranuclear palsy, corticobasal degeneration, and related disorders and providing support, education and hope for persons with PSP, CBD and their families.

Alzheimer's Association (USA), 225 N. Michigan Ave., FL 17, Chicago, IL 60601. National helpline 800-272-3900. www.alz.org. The association publishes a variety of useful brochures (ask for *Related Disorders*, among others). Some Alzheimer's Association chapters maintain FTD support groups, lists of daycare centers, in-home care providers, nursing homes, and information about drugs, clinical trials, research, and care tips. Many association chapters also offer family caregiver training, and this is most valuable as you cope with caring for your family member. I especially urge you to arrange to participate in caregiver training, although it is geared toward Alzheimer's, because much of the information and many of the care tips are helpful for FTD as well.

In addition to the United States Alzheimer's Association and its many chapters, excellent information is available from international Alzheimer's associations or societies.

Alzheimer's Society, United Kingdom, Devon, Gordon House, 58 St. Katharine's Way, London E1W 1LB10 Greencoat Pl., London SW1P 1PH UK. Look for this organization's information Sheet, "What is frontotemporal dementia (including Pick's disease)?" The website has a special section, "Younger People with Dementia," with information designed for younger people with dementia, their families, and their caregivers. The online forum has twenty-four-hour help and support. www.alzheimers.org.uk.

Alzheimer's Australia, 1 Frewin Place, Scullin, ACT 2614 P.O. Box 4019, Hawker ACT 2614, Australia Helpline 1-800-100-500. This organization offers excellent help notes specific to Pick's disease and frontal lobe dementia, plus a reading list. www.fightdementia.org.au.

ADEAR (Alzheimer's Disease Education and Research), National Institute on Aging, P.O. Box 8250, Silver Spring, MD 20907-8250. 800-438-4380. ADEAR's website will help you find current, comprehensive information and resources from the National Institute on Aging (NIA). www.nia.nih.gov/Alzheimers. Under "Publications," click on "Connections." Volume 9, number4, focuses on frontotemporal dementia. Volume 10, numbers 1 and 2, have excellent information on "Driving and Dementia."

NINDS (National Institute of Neurological Disorders and Stroke), National Institutes of Health, 31 Center Dr., Bethesda, MD 20892. www.ninds.nih.gov. Click on "Disorders," then "frontotemporal dementia," and get the "Frontotemporal Dementia Information" page. There also are fact sheets on FTD subtypes and information about related health initiatives. Topics include: Pick's disease, dementia with Lewy bodies, progressive supranuclear palsy, and corticobasal degeneration.

Dementia Research Centre (DRC), Group, United Kingdom, the National Hospital for Neurology and Neurosurgery, Queen Square, London WC1N 3BG, UK. www.dementia.ion.ucl.ac.uk. The Frontotemporal Dementia Support Group (formerly Pick's Disease Support Group) is particularly directed toward caregivers who are coping with behavioral changes in a partner, family member, or friend as a result of frontotemporal degeneration. Click on "CANDID" (Counseling ANd Diagnosis In Dementia) for a wealth of information specific to FTD: Pick's disease support group, fact sheets, articles, books, a newsletter, and so on. Or go directly to CANDID's website, www.pdsg.org.uk.

Family Caregiver Alliance, 785 Market Street, Suite 750, San Francisco, CA 94103. 415-434-3388 or 800 445-8106. www.caregiver.org. Founded in

1977, this was the first community-based nonprofit organization in the United States to address the needs of families and friends providing long-term care at home. It offers fact sheets on various dementias, as well as caregiver issues, statistics, and demographics. On the home page, type in "frontotemporal dementia" for a list of relevant articles.

National Organization for Rare Disorders, Inc. (NORD), 55 Kenosia Avenue, P.O. Box 1968, Danbury, CT 06813-1968. 203-744-0100 or 800-999-6673. www.rarediseases.org. Search the "Rare Diseases Database—Alphabetical Listing," scroll down to "Corticobasal," "Pick's disease," etc., for brief information about the disease and information about organizations offering help. There is a small charge for full-text reports.

Defeat Dementia is an open Facebook group under the auspices of the University of California San Francisco (UCSF) Memory and Aging Center. The group deals with issues related to FTD, Alzheimer's and related dementias.

Website for Caregivers—marymac missions (marymacmissions.com) is a website designed to help caregivers remember to care for themselves as well as their loved one. Mary MacDonald provides tips, breathing exercises, and encouraging words for those feeling the stress and strain of caregiving.

Medical Centers. If you obtained the diagnosis at a university medical center, you will be able to obtain information from the center. Some centers also offer family consultations and maintain support groups.

Other Caregiver Support Options

Lotsa Helping Hands

Lotsa Helping Hands powers free online caring communities that provide tools to organize daily life during times of medical crisis or caregiver exhaustion. There are more than sixty thousand "Private Communities" that are at work supporting caregivers across the United States, and recently an "Open Community" model has been launched to connect caregivers, individuals, and families who need help with those who want to lend a hand. www.lotsahelping hands.com.

The Well Spouse Association (WSA)

This is a nonprofit self-help and volunteer-based organization whose mission is to provide peer emotional support and information to the husbands, wives, and partners of the chronically ill and/or disabled. WSA is the only national organization that focuses exclusively on spousal caregivers. WSA offers local area support groups, mentors, respite weekends, an online forum, and more. 1-800-838-0879. www.wellspouse.org.

Eldercare Locator

The Eldercare Locator is a public service of the US Administration on Aging. It is a nationwide service that connects older Americans and their caregivers with sources of information on senior services. The service links those who need assistance with state and local area agencies on aging and community-based organizations that serve older adults and their caregivers. You may speak to an Eldercare Locator information specialist by calling toll-free at 1-800-677-1116 on weekdays, from 9:00 a.m. to 8:00 p.m. (ET). Spanish-speaking information specialists are on duty. Online chat is available, too. www.eldercare.gov.

Area Agencies on Aging (US)

These agencies provide many helpful long-term-care services to patients and families. You may apply for state and federal financial aid (Medicaid) for home care and nursing home care through your local area agency on aging. Listings for area agencies on aging are located under "Guide to Human Services" in the blue pages of the telephone directory. Website search at www.aoa.gov.

PubMed

PubMed, a service of the National Library of Medicine, National Institutes of Health, provides access to MEDLINE citations and includes links to many sites providing full-text articles and other related resources, at www.ncbi.nlm.nih.gov. Click on "PubMed," then search for Pick's disease, frontotemporal dementia, Lewy body, etc.

Books

In addition to the present book, *What If It's Not Alzheimer's?* 3rd ed., the AFTD website has an extensive list of books, booklets, essay collections and memoirs. www.theaftd.org.

Lipton, Anne, and Cindy D. Marshall, *The Common Sense Guide to Dementia for Clinicians and Caregivers* Written by a neurologist and psychiatrist who have cared for thousands of patients and their families, this guide espouses general principles of dementia care that apply across the stages and spectrum of non-Alzheimer's types of dementia as well as Alzheimer's disease. Publisher: Springer, 2013. Available at: Amazon.com/medicine/neurology/book/978-1-4614-4612-5.

Erb, Clinton A., *Losing Lou-Ann*. An inspiring account of a spouse caring for his wife with Pick's disease. Publisher: Holistic Education, 1996.

Kertesz, Andrew, and David G. Munoz, *Pick's Disease and Pick Complex*. The first book devoted to Pick's disease and its clinical and pathological manifestations. A comprehensive reference that clarifies Pick's diagnosis compared to other forms of dementia. Publisher: Wiley-Liss, 1998.

Kertesz, Andrew, *The Banana Lady and Other Stories of Curious Behavior and Speech*. Nineteen lives are chronicled as told by caregivers, and it is followed by excellent tips for caregivers, a useful glossary of terms, plus FTD references. Publisher: Trafford Publishing, 2006. To order, contact www.trafford.com/06-1883.

Booklets

Three very helpful booklets are available online or may be ordered through the Association for Frontotemporal Degeneration (AFTD). Contact info@theaftd.org.

(1) *A Guide for Managing a New Diagnosis—The Doctor Thinks It's FTD. Now What?* This was developed by AFTD as a publication to help individuals and families take a strategic approach to a diagnosis of FTD and prepare for the changes it brings.

(2) *Understanding the Genetic of FTD: A Guide for Patients and Their Families*. This was created by AFTD in collaboration with the University of Pennsylvania Center for Neurodegenerative Disease Research to provide current and reliable information on the role that genetics play in FTD, the genes that have been associated with hereditary FTD, and genetic testing.

(3) *What about the Kids? Written and Produced by the AFTD Task Force on Families with Children*. This is a sensitive, practical guide for parents to help their children deal with a parent who has FTD.

The Pick's Disease Support Group (PDSG) has published a booklet containing the personal experiences of caregivers coping with a number of conditions. For details on how to order print copies, e-mail info@pdsg.org.uk.

Frontotemporal Disorders: Information for Patients, Families, and Caregivers. This is a consumer-friendly booklet produced by the National Institute on Aging (NIA). The free, thirty-page booklet explains the disorders, causes, symptoms, and management in layman's terms. To order copies, call 1-800-438-4380.

Farmer, Jennifer M., MS, CGC, and Susan L.-J. Dickinson, MS, CGC, *The Genetics of FTD—Should You Worry?* (Association for Frontotemporal Dementias, 2006). This is available to download from the association's website (www.theAFTD.org), or contact the AFTD office for a print copy.

DVDs

It Is What It Is

This is a powerful, eighteen-minute film developed by AFTD to increase understanding. The film chronicles four families as they confront FTD. By telling their stories, these families reflect experiences common to many and become harbingers of hope. The DVD is accompanied by a twelve-page informational booklet (free to download) on frontotemporal degeneration. Produced by the Association for Frontotemporal Degeneration, 2011. Contact www.theaftd.org to order.

Disordered

This three-part documentary on frontotemporal degeneration (FTD) shows how the lives of three patients have changed and how this has affected the people around them. The filmmakers: Klaas Jansma is a psychologist involved in the Dutch National Steering Committee for Young People with Dementia and Pieter Wolswijk is a geriatric psychologist and freelance filmmaker. This documentary is an initiative of the Intercollegiate Group of Geriatric Psychologists in the Arnhelm Region, the Netherlands. To order, contact Klaas Jansma via e-mail at krjansma@hotmail.com.

Planning for Hope—Living with Frontotemporal Disease

This is a moving documentary created by Susan Grant, who is diagnosed with FTD, to bring attention to this terminal disease. Six families share their heart-wrenching stories of perpetual grieving amid financial struggles and caring for their loved ones. Sharing another aspect of hope, professionals explore financial and estate planning for FTD victims and their families. The film provides hope for the future as science is moving at a fast pace. For more information about the film, contact www.theaftd.org.

Publications and Articles

Many excellent publications and articles are in print and can be found online by typing "Pick's disease," "frontotemporal dementia," "frontotemporal degeneration," "FTD," "PPA," or other key words into a search engine. AFTD has archived relevant articles on its website, www.theaftd.org. Search under "News & Events" and" FTD in the News."

NOTES

1. Elizabeth M. Tracy and James K. Whittaker, "The Social Network Map: Assessing Social Support in Clinical Practice, Families in Society," *Journal of Contemporary Human Services* (1990).

2. Marion Cohen, PhD, *Dear Aunt S: How to Ask for Help from Family and Friends in Time of Crisis* (Brooklyn, NY: Center for Thanatology Research, 2003).

3. Tracy and Whittaker, "Social Network Map."

CHAPTER 22

MONEY MATTERS

Securing Financial and Legal Readiness

Paul L. Feldman, Esq.

INTRODUCTION

Planning for the financial and legal consequences of a family member with frontotemporal degeneration (FTD) is a formidable challenge because of the many complex and difficult issues that must be addressed.

The issues range from legal matters when your family member becomes unable to make those types of decisions for himself, to financial considerations over how the cost of care (either at home or in an institutionalized setting) will be met. Financial issues involve strategies for taking full advantage of all insurance- and government-funded programs for the direct cost of care. Also, indirect issues include ways of replacing lost income, maximizing tax deductions, and developing strategies for preserving assets for the future needs of any remaining family members.

Since FTD is a progressive, degenerative disease that leads to gradual loss of decision-making functioning, these issues intensify as the level of functioning of the individual declines. The difficulty of developing a plan can vary tremendously depending on course of the illness and the particular strengths and adaptability of the social and family network the caregiver has to draw upon. Moreover, the steps taken can also be dictated by whether the family member with FTD is married or single, and if the principal caregiver is an adult child or some other relative. Since FTD often strikes at relatively young ages, the financial strategies for meeting the costs of care can also differ depending on whether or not the person (and the spouse, if married) is under the age of sixty-five, or in some instances, under the age of sixty.

This chapter will attempt to lay out the principal legal and financial issues that must be faced in caring for someone with FTD. The goal of this chapter is to provide strategies for seeking out resources to help develop a customized care plan that works for you and your family. It will identify core programs that will be helpful and pinpoint some of the obstacles that you may have to overcome due to the uniqueness of FTD when applying for these programs. A thorough review of this chapter should establish a solid foundation upon which you can draw to seek the individualized advice you will need.

No one person can provide all the information you will need to make these decisions. One reality of our healthcare system is that there is no case manager. Each caregiver must put together what is best for him and his loved one depending on his own needs, and for what he and his loved one may qualify. Caregivers should be aware that estate lawyers and certified financial planners, while competent within their own spheres of expertise, may not be adequately versed in the complexities you are likely to be faced with in this situation. Some of the best professionals available practice in the area now known as elder law. One should be particularly cautious about information picked up from other caregivers or lay people.

While this information can be useful starting points, caregivers and other family members must be careful not to be lulled into believing that the financial information being volunteered is the best or only option. Many individualized factors that are particular to one situation may be inappropriate for your circumstances. Caregivers need to be mindful that these are areas where small differences can dictate large differences in how one plans for these eventualities.

GENERAL RESOURCES

A good first step should be to contact your local chapter of the Association for Frontotemporal Degeneration (AFTD) or Alzheimer's Association. Be aware, however, that there are vast differences in the size and sophistication of local chapters. Many of the programs and legal steps that are needed for FTD are the same as for Alzheimer's, so contacting these organizations can still be an important first step. If your local chapter does not have what you need, don't hesitate to contact a larger chapter in a more urbanized area. Since many programs are state specific, your first priority should be to contact other chapters within your state, then larger chapters in other states. If you don't find what you're looking for through AFTD or the Alzheimer's Association, consider branching out by calling or reviewing the websites of chapters of other neurological degenerative diseases such as Parkinson's disease or multiple sclerosis.

While these diseases may be different, many of the caregiving issues are similar enough to be useful. There are also various caregiver associations such as the Family Caregiver Alliance, the Well Spouse Foundation, or the National Family Caregivers Association.

SURROGATE DECISION MAKING

Unlike other illnesses, all dementias, not just FTD, render the individual incapable of handling her own affairs. These may be financial or legal in nature and can range from something as simple as endorsing a check to something as serious as end-of-life issues. There are a number of legal instruments designed to cover these contingencies, the most common of which is a durable power of attorney, but healthcare directives and a living will can also be employed. These instruments transfer to someone else the legal authority for acting in the best interest of the person while she is still alive but incapacitated. A will and a trust are legal instruments for passing property to others after the person dies, though trusts can sometimes be used to provide for the person financially while she is still alive. All of these legal instruments are largely governed by state law and should be executed in the state in which you reside. It is strongly suggested that you seek an attorney licensed in your state who regularly practices in elder law. If any of these documents are already in place, an attorney in the state in which you are now residing should review them. The attorney should ensure that the documents are compatible with current state laws and applicable to your current situation. Because of the degenerative nature of FTD, it is important that these legal documents get put into place as soon as possible. Some families, as the disease progresses, may move from one state to another (for instance, to be near other family members). It is important that these legal instruments be reviewed by an appropriate attorney in the new state in which the family now resides.

VOLUNTARY ARRANGEMENTS

Durable Power of Attorney

The most common voluntary arrangement that an individual with FTD establishes is one controlled by a durable power of attorney (POA), either for financial purposes and/or for medical purposes (including end-of-life-care decision making). The document designates someone else (or several individuals) to be the agent to make decisions in the specific areas authorized by the document. A properly drawn document that designates only one agent should have a successor designated if the primary individual cannot provide the appropriate assistance.

The document should list certain authority for the agent to make decisions. The authority given would be for such things as selling or transferring real estate, making banking decisions, entering a safe deposit box, filing tax returns, and having the ability to handle pension and Social Security, as well as any other area for which the individual can no longer make decisions. Especially important is the ability to undertake financial planning to deal with the issues involved with government entitlements, principally Medical Assistance (known in many states as Medicaid).

It is helpful to have several (at least four) original copies of this document executed since someone being asked to rely on this document (such as a title company involved in a real-estate transaction) will often wish to retain an original. It is also helpful when executing a general POA that you obtain forms from the bank at which your family member's primary checking account is located. Once the forms from the financial institution are obtained and executed, it is sometimes easier to exercise one's authority under a POA already registered.

There is a difference between being listed on a bank account as a power of attorney, which means that you have the ability to access the account, and being listed as a joint owner. A joint owner also has the ability to access the account, but at the death of one of the joint owners, the account is owned by the surviving joint owner and is not controlled by the will of the deceased individual with FTD.

In some states, there is a tax benefit to having it owned jointly if your family member with FTD predeceases you. In the unlikely event that you predecease your family member and the account was jointly owned, your family member might be taxed on his own money. In the case of a spouse, most joint accounts, except for the one into which the pension or Social Security checks of your family member with FTD is directly deposited, should be changed to the name of the well spouse alone, or the well spouse with another family member such as an adult child.

Handling of a Social Security check can be done without a power of attorney by utilizing the procedure established by the Social Security Administration to become the representative payee. This is exclusively a federal program administered under extensive federal regulations. An individual can authorize someone to be the representative payee to receive that individual's check to be deposited into an account in the name of the representative payee and administered for the benefit of the recipient. The regulations also provide that if the individual cannot voluntarily authorize someone to be the representative payee, after a physician certifies that the recipient is unable to handle his own check, Social Security can designate an individual to serve in such position from a prioritized list of those who are eligible. This can be done by direct deposit (checks can even be directly deposited to a nursing home).

A general POA can provide your agent the authority to make medical-care decisions or withhold authorizing certain medical-care decisions (or withdrawing consent after having previously authorized a medical decision). You can separate the authority to make medical-care decisions from the authority to make financial decisions, similar to separating the guardianship of a person from the guardianship of an estate.

Living Will

If you have a medical POA, it can also provide for end-of-life-care decisions in the nature of a "living will" (legally known as an advance directive). One can have a living will and a medical power of attorney (with different decision makers). The most important aspect is making sure that the healthcare provider knows of the existence of this document. This document will express the intentions of your family member at a time when he or she cannot express them him- or herself.

As the health of a family member declines, these documents should be conveniently located so they can be retrieved on short notice. Caregivers need to be aware that ambulance crews in most states, as paraprofessionals, cannot legally follow healthcare directives because they are not under the direct supervision of a physician until they reach the hospital. Even emergency rooms may be reluctant to follow the directives. Caregivers need to assert themselves if faced with this situation by presenting a copy of the directives and insisting the instructions be followed.

Trusts

Another voluntary arrangement to handle just the financial affairs of an individual with FTD is the establishment of a trust. A trust is a legal arrangement between several individuals. The first, the one who sets it up (usually done by the impaired individual or a family member under a POA), is known as the settlor or grantor. The person managing the fund is known as the trustee, and the person who benefits from the trust is known as the lifetime beneficiary. Upon the death of the lifetime beneficiary, the trust acts as a will and passes whatever assets remain in the trust to the designated remainder beneficiaries. A trust is generally used only when there are significant assets or special circumstances, such as the financial support of more than one person, which would justify the expense incurred in administering a trust, including the bookkeeping and/or the extra tax returns that would have to be prepared.

In the case of a spouse, a preexisting will needs to be updated so that, in the unlikely event the well spouse dies, the estate will not transfer to the impaired spouse with FTD. (Even with an updated will, it is prudent to remove the name of the impaired spouse from joint ownership of a home and financial accounts to cover this possibility.) In such a circumstance, setting up an unfunded trust is ideal. In an unfunded living trust, no assets need be transferred. Only upon death (or disability, if so specified in the trust document) would assets be transferred. The trust can be drawn up to specify how the assets would be used to care for the impaired spouse with FTD.

In rare instances, when the individual suffering from FTD either refuses to plan or has reached a point where she is unable to plan, the family or caregiver may be left with no alternative but to go to court to declare the person to be incapacitated. The process by which to do so is covered in the next section.

INVOLUNTARY ARRANGEMENTS

One of the major challenges of FTD is that a person can be very high functioning in some areas while experiencing severe deficits in others. This often occurs in the early stages of the disease. Such a person may be able to function but without appropriate judgment.

In this case, the caregiver may establish a guardianship or conservatorship in a court proceeding. A guardianship is established by going to a lawyer to prepare a petition or a complaint to be filed in the trial division of your state court system (sometimes known as the orphans' court or surrogate court, depending on the state) requesting a hearing in front of a judge. Medical testimony is presented and, depending on the specific jurisdiction, the alleged incapacitated person may or may not be required to attend the hearing. Also depending on the jurisdiction, an attorney for the alleged incapacitated person sometimes must be appointed to represent the interests of the person. This attorney is different from the attorney representing the individual who is petitioning the court as the interests of the petitioning individual sometimes differ.

If the judge decides that the individual is unable to receive and evaluate information effectively and make appropriate decisions based on that information, that judge may appoint either a limited or a plenary guardian to be responsible for financial and/or personal decisions. If, for example, you were to file to appoint a guardian to handle only the finances at a time when your family member can still make medical decisions, you might be required to file again later to have a guardian appointed for making medical decisions when the disease progresses further. Even if the individual is relatively high functioning and able to express his opposition to being defined as incapacitated, the judge can find that the individual's executive functioning (i.e., decision making) is impaired to such an extent that a guardian is still warranted. The court will then have supervision over the financial decisions that must be made. All of the voluntary or involuntary arrangements established to address this issue each have advantages and disadvantages. If pursuing a guardianship becomes necessary, one should have a clear understanding of the restrictions and procedures before proceeding to establish one.

The guardianship provisions are usually separate and distinct from regulations when a commitment, either involuntary or voluntary, is needed under a state's Mental Health Act. If an individual is so impaired and his actions are so likely to pose an immediate risk of harm, either to himself or to others, a person could be temporarily admitted to a psychiatric-care facility to prevent harm. Since this can be an immediate detainment by the local health department, an individual must be given a hearing within a very short time after the commitment (usually three to five days). These involuntary commitments under the Mental Health Act can be extended for short periods of time and also converted to a voluntary commitment, should the individual understand the immediate need for care. A commitment under the Mental Health Act is not an alternative to proceeding under the guardianship provisions of state law, since the goal of the former is treatment and the goal of the latter is decision making. It should be noted that these steps are rarely undertaken. By the time commitment becomes necessary, the person generally is so impaired that these issues become moot.

ISSUES AFFECTING INCOME

Income-Related Sources

An individual with FTD eventually will become incapacitated and unable to work. If the individual has already retired, he may be receiving "old age retirement benefits" under the Social Security Act, which would not be effected by his incapacity. However, one must be of a certain age (currently it's being raised from sixty-five to sixty-seven) to receive normal benefits ("normal retirement age"). One can retire sooner, as early as sixty-two, but at reduced benefits. If one is over normal retirement age and receiving Social Security, she is already eligible for Medicare.

If a person is younger than normal retirement age and has generally worked twenty quarters (five years) in the past ten years prior to the onset of the disability, the individual will be eligible for Social Security Disability. Two years after qualifying for Social Security Disability, an individual is entitled to Medicare. Federal law governs all these programs. Social Security Disability and old age retirement benefits are not dependent on one's other resources (such as the well spouse's income or pension). The amount received depends solely on the amount earned in previous years and the presence of any dependent children under the age of sixteen. The extra allocation for dependent children generally stops as each child turns sixteen. To qualify, you must provide documentation of the diagnosis that the person is ill and not mentally capable of applying for him- or herself. Your loved one need not be present when you apply, but you do have to go in person to a local Social Security office. Social Security intake workers will help you. They will go back retroactively to when the disease first affected your loved one's employment status (which shortens the twenty-four-month wait for when the person becomes eligible for Medicare). Sometimes examinations by one of Social Security's own designated physicians is required, but this is usually waived in the case of Alzheimer's and FTD. Since FTD disorders are so rare, it is a good idea to include a letter from your loved one's physician describing the disorder and emphasizing the degenerative nature of the illness. To find out more, contact your local Social Security office or check online at www.ssa.gov.

If an individual must leave work because of his incapacity, he is likely to be eligible for any disability coverage his employer may have. (Sometimes individuals may have left work—or even been fired—long before a diagnosis is made. Legally, it may be possible to go back and try to claim the disability benefit, though this could be difficult to do.) This coverage sometimes contains a Social Security offset clause limiting the total combined benefits from the employer's coverage and Social Security to no more than 70 percent of the employee's former income. Your family member may own an individual disability-income policy of his own. This is most often the case for certain professionals and self-employed individuals. Contact the agent representing the insurer to see about filing a claim. Some disability-income policies are written in such a way that they cover you if you cannot perform the duties of your "own occupation."

Others are more restrictive and only provide coverage if you cannot work at all. Obviously, which type it is can affect how soon your loved one will be declared eligible.

If an individual is unable to work and is disabled but does not have a sufficient work record to qualify for Social Security Disability, then that person can qualify for Supplemental Security Income (SSI), which provides income up to minimum poverty levels, which is slightly in excess of $710 a month as of 2013 (and is raised every year). If that is the case, an individual will also qualify for Medicaid, which is a federal program administered by individual states. One source that may be able to be tapped for income is an individual retirement account (IRA). The normal penalty imposed for early withdrawals on those under the age of fifty-nine and one-half is waived if the person is disabled.

Expense-Related Considerations—Deductibility

There are some income-tax consequences about which an individual should be aware. It is likely that one will incur expenses for nursing home care, personal care in a facility, or companion care at home (depending on the level of functioning that the individual with FTD is able to achieve). These are considered to be medical expenses, which are deductible for income-tax purposes to the extent that they exceed 7.5 percent of your adjusted gross income. Having a good accountant to do this end-of-the-year planning (prior to the end of the year) will pay for itself.

Expense-Related Considerations—Dependent Care Allowance

This program is most often used as a tax credit for parents with children in some type of childcare arrangement, but it can also be used by any wage earner caring for a disabled family member. Under the provisions of the dependent-care allowance, you are allowed to set aside up to $5,000 if married, or $2,500 if single, of earned income to pay for the costs in caring for a disabled dependent living in your home. The money set aside is not subject to federal income tax and possibly state income tax, depending on the state in which you reside. (Note that the money spent on care from the amount set aside can still go toward satisfying the 7.5 percent medical-expense deductible.) Check with your employer to see if this benefit is offered.

COVERING THE COST OF MEDICAL CARE

It is difficult to provide a blanket description of how the expenses of caring for your loved one at home will be covered. So much depends on the particular type of expenditure, the provisions of your health plan, and unfortunately, all too often, technicalities. The problem is that the type of treatment most often called for to care for someone with dementia does not fit the traditional "medical model" for which these plans were designed. The fact that it is FTD often only compounds the problem further. For most people, it is a question of what will be covered and how well. The two main coverage sources for those under sixty-five are private health insurance (primarily through an employer) and eventually Medicare (once the twenty-four-month waiting period after qualifying for Social Security Disability ends). For those already sixty-five or over, it most likely will be Medicare and a standard Medigap policy. Someone without enough prior work experience to qualify for the minimum Social Security Disability may also qualify for Supplemental Security Disability Income (SSDI), depending on asset and income limitations. If one qualifies for SSDI, then she will also qualify for Medicaid, a comprehensive healthcare program for those with low income.

For Those under Normal Retirement Age

The main coverage will be group health insurance, either through the employer of the individual with FTD or the spouse's employer. If it is the former, coverage may continue if the individual qualifies for disability income through that employer. If not, coverage will generally continue for up to twenty-four months under COBRA after the person leaves employment. However, while COBRA ensures that coverage continues, the family must pay the full premium (i.e., the employer's share as well as the employee's). This can be a substantial amount (these premiums can, however, be counted as a deductible medical expense as discussed earlier). When COBRA coverage ceases after twenty-four months, the person (and any children under the age of sixteen) will be covered under Medicare if he qualified for Social Security Disability twenty-four months earlier.

Unless the spouse has coverage through his own place of employment, the well spouse may be left without coverage. There are no good solutions to this. A spouse in this situation should check into the professional associations she belongs to or could join. If either person is fifty or over, they can join AARP and obtain coverage through one of these organizations.

In terms of the types of expenses, doctor's visits, lab tests, and prescriptions are usually covered under private health insurance. A professional therapist for the person with FTD is probably covered (a psychiatrist is likely to be called upon to prescribe medications that will help control the behaviors associated with a person with a dementia). Hospitalization is likely to be covered. However, the type of hospitalization a person with FTD is most likely to need will be in an inpatient psychiatric facility, and that may or may not be covered. If it is covered, there are stricter limitations than for a regular hospitalization. What is not likely to be covered is the use of an adult daycare facility and a home health aide. Medicare only covers a home health aide if skilled care or physical, occupational, or speech therapy is also required. Skilled care means a nurse needs to perform medical procedures like dress a wound or change a catheter.

In January 2006, legislation was passed that helps to offset the costs of a Medicare recipient, who is not covered by another credible drug plan, with basic and catastrophic prescription drug costs, once enrolled under a Part D plan. Currently, standard coverage usually provides for an up-front deductible ($325) and then the Medicare recipient pays 25 percent and Part D pays 75 percent of the next $2,970 of costs incurred. After $2,970 of drug costs, there is a gap in coverage, generally referred to as the "donut hole." During this payment stage, the recipient receives a discount on brand-name drugs and pays a percentage of the costs of generic drugs.

After there has been $4,750 of out-of-pocket, uncovered prescription costs, the catastrophic coverage kicks in, and the Medicare recipient pays either $2.00 for generic drugs and $5.00 for brand-name drugs or 5 percent of the cost of the prescription, whichever is greater.

There are many different Medicare Part D–approved insurers that provide greater coverage and thorough research should be undertaken before enrolling. One must evaluate the drugs you are taking against the covered list of formularies of the plan and other features, such as the monthly premium, whether the annual deductible is waived, or if there are any caps on any particular drug. You are required to enroll when you first become eligible, or you are assessed a 1 percent per month premium penalty. Additional information and advice as to all of the many different aspects of Part D may be obtained online at www. medicare.gov or by calling 1-800-Medicare.

For Those at Normal Retirement Age

The principal sources of coverage are likely to be Medicare and Medigap. Again, doctor's visits, lab work, and hospitalization (with restrictions on psychiatric admissions) will be covered. Home health care and adult care typically will not (unless as noted above for skilled care or physical, occupational, or speech therapy). Important exceptions to this are waiver programs and the Medicare Life Care Program.

Exceptions under Medicare That Provide Broader Coverage

Under its Life Care Program, Medicare will underwrite the cost of adult daycare programs, if there is a skilled component. Such programs have a very large component of skilled care, such as counseling and other therapy, which is provided for individuals with FTD and enables them to remain at home longer. This program recognizes that keeping an individual healthy and at home is often not only less expensive but often a better option than placing her somewhere without the benefit of appropriate care suited to her dementia program. Also, some states have what is known as a waiver program to permit Medicaid to underwrite the cost of care at home, provided the other criteria necessary to establish eligibility have been met. Although this program does not provide twenty-four-hour care, it can provide up to approximately eight hours of care. Combining that with an adult daycare program might allow the impaired individual to be managed at home longer. However, there are waiting lists of individuals who wish to enroll for this program, and one should plan to apply for the waiver program at least six months to one year ahead of the time that you anticipate you will need it.

Other Sources of Coverage

There are at least two other possible sources of coverage beyond private health insurance, Medicare, and Medicaid. One is long-term-care policies. These policies for long-term care have begun to be more widely sold in the past few years. Many of these policies expressly include coverage for a person with cognitive deficits. If the family member with FTD is fortunate enough to be covered under such a policy, it can also provide coverage for home health care, for example, adult daycare and a home health aide (without needing skilled care). There may also be some limited state-funded programs. Your local Alzheimer's chapter may be your best source for finding out about these state-specific programs.

CAREGIVER-RELATED ISSUES

Caring for a person with FTD can be very taxing and time-consuming. Some caregivers try to hold down a job and take care of their loved one at the same time. There are two options caregivers can turn to for some relief.

Family Care Leave

Family members who are working for public agencies or private-sector employers with fifty or more employees are eligible for leave under the Family Medical Leave Act (FMLA). To be eligible you must have worked for your employer for at least twelve months and have worked one thousand hours in the previous six months. You must be related to the family member with FTD but cannot be an "in-law." You do not have to be living with the FTD sufferer. You are allowed up to twelve weeks off work without pay. You are guaranteed your job or one equivalent when you return. You keep your benefits, but for employer-provided health insurance you must continue to pay the employee share. You do not have to take all twelve weeks at once. You must work this out with your employer. Employers require thirty days' notice. Some states have their own family-care leave programs that may be more generous than the federal program.

Respite Care

Sometimes caregivers need a break. Either they are exhausted or they have needs of their own that must be met. To deal with this difficult circumstance, they can turn to respite care. Respite care is placing the patient with FTD in a nursing home or similar overnight-supervised setting for a limited period, typically a few days or a week or two. Normally, this is not covered by any insurance because it is not medically necessary. However, some long-term-care policies do provide for this and a few states have state-funded programs to help defray the costs. Your local Alzheimer's Association chapter can tell you whether there are any such programs in your state.

Genetic Testing

The vast majority of frontotemporal dementia cases are nonfamilial, meaning that the condition is not inherited. In those cases that do involve a genetic component, however, family members of FTD patients are confronted with the daunting prospect of genetic testing.

The issue of genetic testing is best contemplated in consultation with a professional genetics counselor. (See chapter 3.) Besides involving very personal issues, the question of genetic testing raises legal issues as well.

All impacted family members need to be aware that the results of their genetic tests may become a permanent part of their medical records and could later affect their insurability for health, life, disability, and long-term-care policies. Employability may even be impacted. All told, how this information is used—if at all—varies by state, by type of insurance, and by insurer (not just for FTD but for other genetically identifiable diseases as well).

As is to be expected, state and federal laws are evolving as genetic testing for all sorts of disorders becomes more widespread. For now, families need to be mindful of the personal and financial risks inherent in choosing to be tested.

COVERING THE COST OF INSTITUTIONAL CARE

Medicare does not cover nursing home care except under limited circumstances, nor do most private health-insurance plans. If the family has purchased a separate long-term-care policy before the onset of the illness, some coverage will be possible. Even then, unless the most generous options were selected, the policy may not be enough to cover an extended long-term stay. What do families do? The answer is that the government steps in through Medicaid. Medicaid is a federal- and state-funded program that covers nursing-home costs for those without the means to pay.

When Medicare Does Pay

Two conditions must be met before Medicare will pay for nursing home care. First, the level of care required must be skilled nursing care, or physical or speech therapy. Second, the family member must have been hospitalized for at least three days prior to being discharged to a nursing home. Even under these limited circumstances, Medicare (along with most Medigap policies) will still only pay for up to one hundred days of care. In other words, Medicare is set up to facilitate recovery following a hospitalization and not for the kind of long-term institutionalization someone with dementia typically requires. Please note that this program will only pay for care in a certified facility.

Medicaid Eligibility

There are at least four levels of progressively intensive types of institutionalized care: minor supervised assisted living, custodial care, intermediate care, and skilled care. As previously stated, Medicare will only pay for skilled nursing home care and then only under certain circumstances. Medicaid does not require prior hospitalization and also covers intermediate in addition to skilled care. The regulations governing the financial requirements for eligibility for Medicaid are very strict. While this is a federal program (with matching funds from the state), many of the limits governing eligibility are set by each state. Therefore, it is important to work with an elder-care attorney or some other expert who is knowledgeable about the limits in your state. It is also important that this be done as far in advance as possible to maximize the funds the family has available and to provide the kind of detailed documentation of the family's finances the application process will later require.

To qualify for Medicaid, the program looks at the person's income and assets. If the person's income is less than the cost of the nursing home and the person has insufficient "available" assets to cover the cost of care, then Medicaid will pay. Some states have income restrictions over which a person does not qualify. How the program looks at those assets and income depends on whether or not the person is married.

A single institutionalized individual is entitled to keep a minimum of assets for his or her spending needs, which is approximately $2,000 or $8,000 (the amount can vary between or even within a state depending on technicalities, plus the levels themselves can vary between states). Individuals with more than the allowed assets will have to "spend down" their funds to reach this level before Medicaid will begin paying. In addition, any income they have, such as Social Security or a pension, will go toward offsetting the amount Medicaid must pay—less than $35 per month (or $45, again depending on the state), which is set aside for personal, nonmedical expenses such as a haircut or clothes.

There are some key assets that are exempt and not counted as part of the minimum assets to be retained for the individual. Medicaid allows the family member to set aside up to approximately $12,500 in prepaid funeral expenses (again, these levels can be set differently in different states). You can establish "an irrevocable burial reserve" by going to a funeral director directly and prepaying for the arrangements, or you can establish a restricted account at your local bank. Although you would not be able to access this money, neither would you be required to spend these monies on your family member's medical care.

If the family member is married, a different set of rules govern assets and income. These rules are intended to leave the "community spouse" with enough money to meet his or her expenses. The community spouse is entitled to keep as much income as he or she earns. Also, the community spouse is entitled to an additional amount of the institutionalized spouse's income, if the community spouse's income is below a specified minimum amount (approximately $1,938.75 per month plus the shelter costs of the spouse living in the community in excess of $568 per month). Whatever income the community spouse cannot retain will all go to the nursing home except for $35 (or $45) a month.

The community spouse is also entitled to keep assets up to $115,920 (not counting the house, a car, and certain other exempt assets explained later). If the combined assets of both spouses (regardless of whose name these assets are in) exceed $115,920 (the amount is adjusted each year for inflation), they must "spend down" to the $115,920 level before Medicaid will begin paying nursing home charges.

If the couple's combined assets exceed $115,920, there are several alternatives to spending the excess that will help preserve the family's assets. It is legitimate to spend excess assets on (1) paying down the mortgage since the house is excluded, (2) a home improvement because the house is excluded, or (3) a car. Under the Deficit Reduction Act of 2006 (the DRA), there is a penalty if money is transferred to someone else (e.g., another family member). What Medicaid does under the DRA is to delay the date it will begin paying nursing-home costs measured by the amount transferred (the disqualified period) and, most important, this period does not begin until the person becomes "otherwise eligible," which means not until you have spent down. The change in the law under the DRA effectively precludes any gifting if it is not done at least five years prior to applying for Medicaid. Whatever steps are taken will have to be documented when the time comes to apply, so careful record keeping of any such transactions is required. As part of the application process, family records will be scrutinized for up to sixty months before the date of application. It is important that family members begin to keep detailed records of all expenditures in anticipation of this review. A rough guideline would be documentation for any expenditure over $500, but this is only a rule of thumb. Medicaid reserves the right to scrutinize an expense of any amount.

Some transfers are exempt for Medicaid purposes. If a child has been living at home for two years or more with the principal goal of taking care of the FTD parent so that he or she can remain within the community, that gift of a principal residence to that child would not have any effect on the Medicaid-eligibility process. However, one must have a POA that authorizes such transactions when parents cannot take this action themselves.

Excluded Assets

Some assets are exempt and some assets can be declared "unavailable"—which is essentially the same, since those assets are not counted. Rules don't exist for each and every asset that exists. The way something gets counted can be open to interpretation. States may count assets in different ways. There can even be variations within a state depending on how one Medicaid office interprets the rules versus another. In some states, an individual retirement account (IRA) (or any other type of qualified retirement plan, such as a 401k) owned by the community spouse is exempt. Unless the assets are minimal and simple, an elder-care lawyer should be retained. Such attorneys can develop a plan for addressing these highly complex issues based on the assets and the requirements of the particular state.

The primary asset that is excluded in all states is the residence in which the community spouse resides. If the family member being institutionalized is single and the family wishes to retain his residence for his possible return, they can. However, because of a change in the Medicaid laws, which now provides for an estate recovery program, the state would place a lien on the property. Therefore, if your family member lives alone and he cannot remain at home, the house should be sold.

If the house is not sold, the Medicaid estate-recovery lien is calculated based on the amount of money that Medicaid has paid under the program. However, this amount is only assessed against the probate estate in some states, and against any asset (including nonprobate assets, such as a jointly owned residence) in other states. This lien is then considered along with your family member's other creditors and satisfied from those remaining assets. Again, this applies only if the family member is single. If he is married, the residence of the community spouse is untouched as long as the title to the house is in the name of the surviving spouse only. If jointly owned (with right of survivorship or tenants in the entirety) and the community spouse survives the institutionalized spouse, it is also not touched.

OTHER OPTIONS

Sometimes families are committed to keeping their loved one at home. This is not always possible for everyone, since the costs can be staggering. There are a couple of options for freeing up assets to help cover the costs. These options deplete the assets of the family and should only be pursued as a last resort. If the homeowner is sixty-five or over, it is possible to get a reverse mortgage. This frees up the equity in the home while allowing the person to continue to live there. Some mortgage holders limit the amount of equity available to be drawn upon. When the person (and her spouse, if married) dies (or, if not married, transfers to a nursing home), ownership of the house goes to the bank holding the reverse mortgage. Any equity that is left goes to the beneficiaries. If the equity gets used up, the person (and spouse) can still remain in the home for as long as he or she lives.

Another option is to draw on any life insurance the person may have. Some policies sold in the last ten years have what is called an "accelerated death benefit." Under this provision, the insurance company will advance a portion of death proceeds (usually around 70 percent) for use by the insured. The remainder is then payable to the beneficiary upon death. Generally this cannot be exercised until the person has only six or twelve months to live. The time allowed varies between insurance companies. If the policy does not have this provision, there are independent companies that will "buy" the policy and name themselves as the beneficiary and advance a portion of the death benefit. The purchasing company then assumes responsibility for all future premiums. Generally, these companies don't have limits on how long the person is expected to live before they will do this. In return for taking the risk that the individual will live a long time, the company keeps the remainder. Sometimes this can be as much as 50 percent or more of the death benefit. This device is called a "viatical settlement." See your insurance agent as well as an elder-care lawyer for advice before entering into any such controversial agreement.

CONCLUSION

The legal and financial issues for a family dealing with FTD are formidable. There are no easy answers. What there is, is a complex maze of programs and legalities to be faced. Unfortunately, our healthcare system is based on a medical model, not one suited to dementia, let alone a form of dementia most health-care providers have not dealt with before. It is like fitting a square peg into a round hole. Family members are strongly encouraged to seek help from legal and financial professionals familiar with the issues described in this chapter.

Many of the issues are filled with technicalities. One misstep can cause delays, angst, and sometimes thousands of dollars. For instance, failure to spend down to below $115,920 by even one dollar can mean a delay before qualifying for Medicaid. This can mean additional nursing home costs that must be paid by the family. Many of these issues are governed at the state level (and sometimes can even vary within a state from county to county, district to district). This presents a compelling reason to engage a knowledgeable professional familiar with your area. Finally, some things like a living will and record keeping in anticipation of filing for Medicaid need to be undertaken as soon as possible.

Hopefully this chapter has provided the necessary signposts for caregivers to make their way through the maze.

RESOURCES

To locate an elder-care lawyer near you, contact:

- the Local Bar Association: check your local telephone directory or conduct an Internet search for this information
- the National Academy of Elder Care Lawyers: 520-881-4005, www .naela.com
- the National Association of Medicaid Directors: www.medicaiddirectors .org, click on "state directors tabs" and "map links" to find names and state Medicaid websites

PART 4

CARING FOR YOURSELF

CHAPTER 23

A DAILY BREAK

Respite and Personal Care for the Caregiver

Vivian E. Greenberg, ACSW, LCSW

UNDERSTANDING CAREGIVING

Caregiving and *caregiver* are just about household terms today. There are books and conferences for caregivers. There are support groups for caregivers. And there are organizations like the National Family Caregiver's Association that advocate and lobby for them. Because people are living longer, with more chronic and disabling illness, all this public awareness is a good thing. Unless caregivers take care of themselves, paying attention to their own needs for emotional and physical well-being, they will, to quote Boen Hallum of the Central Ohio Parkinson Society, "become an extinct species."[1] And then, who will be left to take care of the increasing numbers of elderly and disabled individuals?

While the words *caregiver* and *caregiving* basically describe what the job is all about, they do not do justice to the range of emotions that flood the caregiver. Almost academic in tone, these words seems to convey the message that giving care is some kind of cerebral exercise. Just know what to do, and the caregiver will be okay. Not so!

Caregiving is a complex process. It is a mixture of dark and light emotions that are normal. The guilt, shame, anger, sadness, confusion, and powerlessness that surface at one time or another come with the territory. Caregivers need to know this crucial fact. They need to know, as well, that in no way does harboring these feelings indicate that they are bad people or poor caregivers.

What these darker emotions accomplish, however, is to create stress and to obscure the lighter emotions that caregiving does hold. The joy of making a difference in someone's life, the competence of being able to do things you thought you could never do, and the empowerment of learning the healthcare system lose their value in the wake of darker emotions.

Caregivers, eager to provide the best care possible to the person they love, all too frequently forget that they too have a life that must be lived and interests and dreams that should be pursued. It is not unusual that in their zeal to be the best and do it all, they lose their own personal identity, not only becoming an extension of the person they care for but also becoming ill themselves. The line they tread between self and other is a fine and slippery one.

What caregivers—and all of us—should be taught in our moral and religious lessons is that self-love is considerably different from selfishness or self-centeredness. Or as Shakespeare so eloquently put it in his drama *Henry V*, "Self-love is not so vile a sin as self-neglect."[2]

All caregiving is hard and stressful. In caring for someone with frontotemporal degeneration (FTD), the challenges are different and perhaps even more exasperating. The three crucial elements that make caregiving the trial it is are (1) the unpredictability of the patient's behavior, in that the caregiver has no idea what will trigger it; (2) the bizarre nature of the behavior itself—lack of inhibition, compulsivity, aggression, or impulsiveness; and (3) the lack of empathy and emotion in the patient, which on a daily basis can leave the caregiver feeling demoralized, unappreciated, and irrelevant.

Given the presence of these factors, caregivers of FTD patients are at high risk for depression, moodiness, sleeplessness, and chronic anxiety, plus physical ailments like high blood pressure, gastrointestinal problems, back ache, and chronic pain. The energy involved both in being on constant alert for the triggers of inappropriate behaviors and in managing them once they happen is enough to wipe out ten caregivers, let alone one. How, for example, does one deal with someone who is compelled to wash his hands or brush his teeth every hour? Or someone who is compelled to walk around in circles? What must it be like for the caregiver who must constantly walk on eggshells because she is never quite sure when she will be embarrassed by some inappropriate action or word?

And, as if all of the above were not enough to burn out the most capable caregiver, consider how painful it is to care for someone whose emotional range is a flat line. How does one relate to a person on a daily basis who cannot register a smile, a laugh, or a tad of excitement? How does one relate to someone whose mood cannot be figured out because his facial expression is always the same?

Add to this cauldron of stress the fact that the person who is being cared for is not the person he once was. Behaviors, attitudes, affect, and values are opposite of what they were. It is as if the person you once lived with and had a relationship with is now a stranger. It is as if that earlier person is dead. You may find yourself crying a lot, either in anger or in grief.

The fact is that you are mourning, grieving for the loss of the person you once knew. The anger and grief are normal. They must have an outlet for expression, or else they will weigh you down in bitterness and remorse. Friends help, but grief counseling is better. The point is, you must get support! Remember too that it is okay to punch pillows, cry, and talk to others, as much as you need to. To deny the grief or to push away the feelings by being perpetually busy will not take you through the process to the other side, where you can feel release and acceptance.

WHAT IS RESPITE?

All caregivers must get respite. Defined literally, *respite* means a short interval of rest or relief. Since each of us is different in habits, tastes, and interests, what is respite for one may not be respite for the other. Consequently, sources of respite are varied. Some of the more common are:

- taking a walk
- visiting friends
- sitting at a café with a newspaper and coffee
- working out at a gym
- playing cards or games like bridge or checkers
- sports, like tennis, bowling, shooting baskets, and golfing
- meditation
- dancing
- lunching with friends
- movies with friends

Other caregivers report that respite for them is watching the sunset or the leaves fall, being with grandchildren, going to the library, or shopping. Whatever relaxes or brings peace of mind or physical or mental enjoyment to the caregiver is respite.

Of note, as well, is that your area agency on aging has funds for caregiver respite. Each county has different eligibility requirements, so call to find out what they are. In addition, two other resources are the Caregiver Action Network (formerly the National Family Caregivers Association) www.caregiveraction.org/ and Arch National Respite Network www.archrespite.org, offering information and referral services for respite services nationwide. The Association for Frontotemporal Degeneration (AFTD) offers grants for caregivers. You can also check with your local Alzheimer's Association to see if they have funding available. While the costs of home care are frequently high, you must remember that those who come to help out serve two people—not just the patient but the caregiver, too.

Caregivers must escape from the confinement and isolation of providing care. For caregivers of FTD patients, however, being with others is a number one imperative. A chat room on the computer may be helpful, but it is not enough. Caregivers must get out and be with people they can see, touch, talk to, and hear. Human connection is what will make them feel they have a life and identity outside of the world of caregiving. Human connection will give their lives meaning and purpose.

It is not surprising that results of studies on caregivers of FTD patients suggest that when caregivers pay attention to their needs for social support and respite early on, not only is their quality of life enhanced but so is that of the patient. Indeed, institutionalization may even be delayed.

What it all comes down to, again to quote Boen Hallum, is that "what is good for the caregiver will be ultimately good for the patient."[3] If the caregiver is replenished, he will have more within him to give. He will return to his caregiving duties a more patient and more empathic caregiver.

Edward M. Hallowell, MD, author of *Connection* and professor of psychiatry at Harvard Medical School, tells us that connection is the single most important factor in having a satisfying life. The unique and healing comforts of connection cannot be found anywhere else. He goes on to state that social isolation is a higher predictor of death than the commonly accepted dangers of cigarettes, obesity, and high cholesterol. That frequency of visits with friends and number of meetings attended (social, religious, political) are what create contentment and meaning in life. That human connection, being with others, has the magical property to make us feel better.

KNOWING WHEN YOU NEED RESPITE

The big question remaining is, how do you know when you need respite? Ideally, of course, respite should be thought about and put into place before a crisis happens. Home health aides, neighbors, friends, and daycare programs should all be known about and put into use. A network of support services should be at your fingertips: names and numbers all posted on the refrigerator. This, however, is rarely the case.

The signs of stress are not bashful about making themselves known, but caregivers often deny or ignore their persistent messages. One caregiver said that she thought she was managing just fine, until her dentist told her she was grinding down her teeth in her sleep. Another thought he needed no help whatsoever until he started falling asleep in his car on the way home from work. Yet another, who was referred for counseling by her dermatologist, suffered from a stress-related eczema characterized by itching, redness, and inflammation.

Other stress-related disorders are: headaches, back aches, stomach problems, and high blood pressure. Depression and anxiety run rampant among those giving care to loved ones. Inability to sleep, poor appetite, and loss of energy are symptoms of depression. Inability to concentrate and panic attacks, characterized by rapid heartbeat and fast breathing, are some of the signs of anxiety.

Although caregivers may not know when they are edging into the terrain of burnout, the persons they are caring for will. Irritability, impatience, resentment, shortness of temper, the feeling that "I'd rather be anyplace but here," all will affect the caregiving relationship. When care is not being given with a full heart, the patient knows that something is not right. The patient knows the caregiver isn't emotionally there. And it is that "quality," in contrast to "quantity," of care that matters most.

Remember, the effectiveness of your caregiving is in direct proportion to its quality. The underpinning of quality care cannot be anger, guilt, or resentment.

Caregivers, you must take care of yourselves! Eat well, get enough sleep, and push yourself to exercise. A fifteen-minute walk every day can make an enormous difference in your mood and attitude. Rent a movie that will make you laugh and laugh, and laugh some more. Norman Cousins, in his uplifting book, *Anatomy of an Illness*, has proven to us that laughter is the magic potion to heal ailing minds and bodies.

So, FTD caregivers, get out there! You are valuable people, first to yourselves, then to your patient. Don't forget who you are. You will lose control over your lives and become resentful caregivers. So visit friends, play cards, go to meetings and luncheons. Gather "warm fuzzies" wherever you can. You, more than anyone, know about the cruel tricks life can play. There's not a minute to lose!

NOTES

1. Boen Hallum, *Parkinson's Disease: A Caregiver's Observation* (Columbus: Central Ohio Parkinson Society, 1998).
2. Shakespeare, *Henry V*, act 2, scene 4.
3. Hallum, *Parkinson's Disease*.

CHAPTER 24

FROM LOSS TO LIFE

Managing Emotions and Grief

Rev. David Cotton

"I just can't stand to see him suffer like that!" How many times have we heard someone utter those words about a loved one? They seem so common that we don't really even stop to consider what is really being said. "I can't stand to see her suffer like that." The pain of illness is plural pain. The ripple effect of illness reaches out from patient to spouse to children to family to friends to colleagues, and on and on in ever-widening circles. Family and friends experience pain just like the patient, sometimes even more. As chaplain in an acute-care hospital, I often hear family members exclaim that they can't bear to see their loved one suffer. When the patient is either sedated or comatose, the only real suffering is on the part of those who are caregivers.

When the illness is frontotemporal degeneration (FTD), the stakes are even higher than with other physical ailments because the situation is more complicated. The pain experienced by family and friends of the patient is the pain of grief. We must be willing to let go of the notion that grieving means that a person has died. Grieving results from loss, and yes, from the little deaths that loss introduces into our lives.

LOSS ALONG THE WAY

Caregivers of those with FTD are faced with a devastating array of losses with which they must learn to cope if they are to survive the onslaught of this progressive, incurable disease. Their loved one is still there, still a part of life in the relationship and the family, but he is not the same. The dramatic changes in personality have the effect of making the patient a different person, sometimes gradually, sometimes rapidly, before the very eyes of those closest. The first significant loss that must be grieved, then, is the loss of self—the loss of the person who used to be there before the condition took that self away and created a new personality and a new person inside the same body.

From witty and communicative to nonverbal, from socially adept to totally uninhibited, from intelligent and productive to irrational and disinterested, from caring and compassionate to angry and self-centered, frontotemporal dementia is the insidious destruction of a person and the unwelcome appearance of a new one. Having a different person in the same body, in the same relationship, can be very confusing and disorienting to the caregiver. This is especially true when the disease comes on so slowly and subtly that it is difficult to tell whether the change is due to emotional and psychological changes instead of physical deterioration of the brain. Often, irritation and resentment can build in response to personality changes. These feelings can sometimes germinate long before the caregiver's awareness and understanding that his or her loved one's changes are due to FTD. These changes are not the product of negative attitudes or emotions and not the fault of the FTD sufferer. The result may be a sense of guilt over the expression of anger or frustration when it is realized that the cause was physical and not emotional. This guilt often mixes with the inevitable sadness at losing someone while she is still physically present.

The caregiver, having lost the person who used to be there, in turn grieves the second loss—the loss of the relationship that used to exist. The conversation that used to be so meaningful is no longer possible. The emotional support of a trusted spouse is gone. Physical intimacy, once so important, is no longer present. The social life as a couple is over for good. The spouse as caregiver has lost not only a person but also a partner.

This loss, though, is not limited to the marriage relationship. Parents see the order of the world turned upside down when they must bid good-bye to the child they know and love while that child is still alive! Siblings lose a part of their lives, someone who "was always supposed to be there," and siblings are forced to face their own mortality and vulnerability as they wonder, "Am I next?" Friends and coworkers, too, face the reality of loss as they see the familiar and the comfortable slip away, only to be replaced by confusion and awkwardness. All relationships are impacted by the losses caused by frontotemporal dementia.

Grieving the loss of the relationship carries with it strong feelings of loneliness and isolation. The first person you greet in the morning, the one you seek out for advice and approval, the one with whom you share everything, the person with whom you fell in love is gone, and no one else feels it like you do. The sense of isolation becomes even deeper when the caregiver realizes that so few people understand even the basics of FTD. This lack of understanding often results in faulty comparisons with and improper identification of fronto-temporal dementia as Alzheimer's disease, leading to further frustration and isolation.

Perhaps an equally difficult third loss is the loss of personal freedom for caregivers. They may need to quit their jobs in order to adequately care for their loved one. Time away from home is limited by the constant demands of caregiving. Networks of friends and acquaintances break down as the caregiver is swallowed up more and more by increasing responsibilities. This loss of personal freedom can lead to feelings of anger as the question "Why me?" inevitably arises. And then the guilt usually is not far behind as images of selfishness descend upon the psyche of the caregiver.

Economic considerations engender a fourth experience of loss as well. The earning power of the person with FTD is lost; at the same time, the financial demands for professional assistance are on the rise. The loss of the status quo is a present reality, and the loss of the future that had been planned and dreamed of sends the ripples of loss far into the course of time.

OWNING YOUR GRIEF

So how do caregivers cope with this nightmarish collection of losses? How can they deal with the grief that washes over them and threatens to sweep them away? First, caregivers must "own their grief" and accept it as an integral part of the experience they are facing. Owning our grief means allowing ourselves to feel sad, to feel discouraged, and yes, even to feel sorry for ourselves. Owning our grief means that we are willing to accept that each person's grieving has elements of similarity, but that each person's grief is unique, to time, personality, circumstances, and so many other factors that make feelings so difficult to quantify and put into a formula.

Owning our grief means that we learn not to feel guilty about grieving and that we understand grieving not as right or wrong, proper or improper. Grief is just an uninvited yet omnipresent companion with caregivers on the journey of caring for one who suffers from FTD. And owning our grief means that we do not allow anyone else to make us feel guilty, intentionally or unintentionally. No one understands, no one can understand, the pain of dealing with this disease. You can describe your nightmare to someone else, but no one is capable of experiencing the emotions that are yours and yours alone. This is especially true for a nightmare from which you never wake up.

This journey of care and grief does not flow on a steady or predictable curve. There are no reliable stages through which we must move. As caregivers, it is crucial that we not place arbitrary timetables and limits on our feelings of grief over the losses we have sustained. "It's been three months, six months, or six years; the number doesn't matter! I or you should be done with the crying and grieving by now and moving on with life." We all hear messages like this, both from ourselves and from those around us.

Owning our grief means affirming our own individual timetable, which, as mentioned above, is not a steady curve. Grief is much more like a roller-coaster ride than a climb up an inclined plane. FTD caregivers are especially aware of this. They are facing the reality of adjusting to the their loved one's changed behaviors and lost abilities, only to wake up and find that those behaviors and abilities have changed again, necessitating a new set of coping strategies and skills. Each loss brings with it the companion of grief. The only way to survive that grief is to own it and face it and hold on for whatever lies around the next curve.

Owning our grief reaches past ourselves and enters the lives of those around us, recognizing that they too are grieving. Children, brothers and sisters, parents, friends and colleagues; all feel the loss of the person they knew. As a practitioner, experience has confirmed that often the most difficult aspect for grieving families is the capacity to allow others to grieve in their own distinct way. Unfortunately, the first impulse is to judge that others are not grieving appropriately if their expression and experience do not match our own. As we learned that grief is unique to us, so we must allow each person affected by the loss to grieve in his individual way. We can own our grief by allowing others the right to own theirs.

A Child's Grief

Children certainly face some aspects of grieving that are particular to their situation. One important issue is the role reversal between parent and child.

As the patient's abilities for self-care decline, the children find themselves more and more in the role of parent for one who should be caring for them. The resulting confusion and perhaps anger may produce feelings of guilt and resentment. It is important to be sensitive to their needs during this time and to give them permission to own their feelings.

As the disease progresses and inhibitions fall away, bizarre behavior may result in embarrassment for younger children of an FTD sufferer. Children may withdraw or vent their anger and frustration at the primary caregiver. This is a time to call in outside resources to assist in dealing with the panoply of emotions that accompany having a parent with FTD. If children are in school, be sure to notify administration, teachers, and counselors so they are aware of the situation at home and can be sensitive to changes in affect or behavior. In addition, a counselor from outside the family can be extremely helpful because the children will have the freedom to express frustrations that they may not share with a close family member who is also grieving.

There may be problems at school due to a number of reasons. Children experiencing such basic, life-changing upheavals at home may question the priority and importance adults put on grades, homework, and school atten-dance, no matter whether they are in elementary school or graduate school. Children's sense of priorities may be drastically affected by the loss of the parent they once knew and depended on. Readjustment will require patient listening and measured reactions that stress the importance of maintaining a life separate from the reality of the disease.

One source of difficulty with children is the question of how much infor-mation to share. Do they need to know everything? Will they just be weighed down even more by the burden of dealing with the details? Each situation is different and varies with family dynamics, ages of the children, personalities, and so on, but in general it is best to share the truth as much as possible.

Often, when the truth is shared, the response from the children is either silence or far less than had been anticipated. What's the answer? Listen, listen, and listen some more. Give them time to collect their thoughts. Give them permission to be mixed up and reaffirm that you want to hear what they are thinking and feeling even if they don't understand it themselves. Don't assume you know what they are thinking and feeling. Open yourself up and share your feelings with them. It's the best way to make them feel comfortable that they can trust you with their feelings.

The loss and reaction to it are different but just as devastating for older children. In their late teens and twenties, the establishment of an adult relationship with their parents is a major accomplishment. Yet for those who have a parent suffering from FTD, the entire process is short-circuited. Older children may have a distorted impression of their responsibilities in the face of serious illness and may feel the need to "fix" the situation.

At this age level, plans are put on hold and lives are interrupted at just the time when they were supposed to blossom in independence and self-sufficiency. Their wings are put away for later, their role becomes caregiver (for both parents), the resentment inevitably surfaces, and the resulting guilt can be devastating and debilitating. Older children still need their parents, and their reaction to loss must not be underestimated.

A Parent's Grief

For the parents of an FTD sufferer, the world has been turned upside down. A child with neurodegenerative illness—this is not the way things are supposed to work! Anger and fear collide as thoughts and feelings tumble around inside. Parents and other family members may stay away in order to hide feelings they are ashamed to admit are present. Visits may be short, and conversation may revolve around meaningless topics unrelated to the situation. However frustrating this behavior may be, patience and tolerance are the order of the day. Confrontations will only result in driving family members farther away. Honest sharing of one's own struggles and conflicting emotions may be the best prescription for opening up parents and other family members to face their feelings and own their grief.

Declaring War and Calling in the Reserves

Finally, owning our grief means admitting that we need help and seeking that help wherever it can be found. Recently in the intensive-care unit here at the hospital, I was with a family when the doctor came to talk with them about the sudden onset of a life-threatening condition. "We are now at war!" the physician exclaimed to the family, assuring them that all resources at our disposal would be thrown into the battle when and if needed.

As a primary caregiver for someone with FTD, it's time to declare war and call out the reserves. When people offer to assist in a particular way, let them! Have a list of helpful jobs from which they can choose when people say,

"If there's something I can do . . ." It's normal to want to do everything your-self, but why should you? Your family and friends love you and care about you, and they want to be a part of this area of your life. They want to reach out to help the patient and help you. The battle is huge and the stakes are high. This is the time to muster all the forces you can to give you some time to sleep, some time to get out of the house, some time to care for yourself. (For more information see chapter 20.)

FOUR STEPS TO EMOTIONAL HEALTH

How does one move through the rough, rocky, uneven terrain of grief and along toward emotional health? Consider this four-step model, a process that will not only enable caregivers to survive the experience of facing FTD but also empower them to grow stronger and more confident. The four steps to emotional health are reimage, refocus, remember, and refresh.

1. Reimage

This requires the caregiver to move from what used to be to what is, from what should be to what can be. There is a powerful urge to avoid the reality of the new situation and to expend a great deal of time and energy trying to maintain the illusion that things can still be the way they used to be. To reimage is to let go of the desire to live in the past and to face the present with open eyes and an open mind, accepting the truth. You are loving someone, living with someone, looking at someone who has become somebody else. This requires a tremendous supply of courage to keep going forward.

No, it's not fair that FTD has invaded your loved one, your family, your life. Life should be different, but life is not about "should." Life just is. Rei-maging calls us to live in the now. It is difficult to put away the dreams of what should be, but living in the present is liberating and freeing. Reimaging allows us to appreciate the beauty of today. It calls us to see the good, to find the humor, to appreciate the blessing of a phone call from a friend, the gift of a radiant sunset, the delicacy of a rose, the brightness of a smile. Reimaging is the foundation for future growth that each of the next three steps can build upon.

2. Refocus

Caring for a loved one with FTD can become such an overwhelming job that one's entire life is swallowed up, and the disease becomes the only thing in sight. Refocusing calls upon the caregiver to see past the disease. First, it is important to remember that the disease and the person are different and distinct. We must learn to focus on the person, seeing so much more than the disease.

In the same way, caregivers are called to look past the disease and see themselves apart from its ravages. Caregivers, too, run the risk of defining their own lives by the disease, allowing it to shape and fashion them as it has the victim. The caregiver, then, becomes a secondary victim. Refocusing beckons us to see our lives and to see ourselves as so much bigger than any disease. Of course, FTD is a segment of our life, and its impact is profound. But emotional health comes when we refocus and see the big picture of life where there is health as well as disease, courage as well as fear, stability as well as unpredictability, laughter as well as tears, faith as well as doubt. It's what we choose to focus on that creates the picture of our life. Refocusing means realizing that there is a choice and that only we can make it. To refocus is to choose the positive, the good, and the healthy as our focal points and to train our eyes and our hearts to see the good amid the bad.

3. Remember

Even though it may seem that FTD has stolen a person away from you, there is so much that the disease cannot touch, so much it cannot take from you, unless you let it! FTD cannot take away the past, the precious memories of time you once shared. It cannot take away the love you experience, the love that will last a lifetime. This ugly disease cannot take away your faith, in God and in yourself, faith that there is a power so much greater than this or any disease, faith that you can not only survive, but overcome. Give yourself permission to remember the good times you shared: how you met, important life transitions, times of laughter and lightness. Remember what brought you to where you are now, and savor the precious memories.

4. Refresh

The essence of refreshing is taking care of yourself. It's so easy to become consumed with caregiving for another that caregiving for yourself gets neglected or left behind altogether. Refresh calls us to create an oasis of health in the midst of the desert of disease.

How do we create an oasis? First, we need to get help. The FTD caregiver needs professional, physical, emotional, and spiritual assistance to make the soul a place that blossoms and grows. Sometimes the obstacles to obtaining professional help may seem overwhelming. Insurance is reluctant to pay for help in the home and notoriously unwilling to pay for professional counseling for the caregiver. But don't be discouraged! Home nursing, home health aides to assist with personal care, social workers, and so on, may not be offered, but they often are available to those willing to negotiate the tortuous route of paperwork and red tape. Therapy for the caregiver is not at the top of most insurance companies' list of necessary provisions, but for the determined, persistence often can bring the payoff of a specific number of paid sessions with a professional counselor or therapist. Ask a friend to help with the insurance forms and phone calls instead of feeling you have to do it all yourself.

If at the end of the process you find you cannot procure the services of professionals, don't give up. Refreshment can be found in other places as well. Be creative. Check with your local congregation to see if it sponsors volunteers who might come to your home to help with care or to give you some time away from the demands of caregiving. Consult with a local dementia organization or support-group chapter to obtain information on assistance available in your area. If you can't afford professional therapy, check to see if there is a group of other caregivers with whom you can meet and share your experiences while learning from the journeys of others. Sometimes it's comforting to know that others are facing the same trials and troubles that you are, even if they don't have all the answers. (For more information on support networks, see chapter 20.)

In addition, refresh means that you are willing to acknowledge that you need practical, physical help. This is the time to call on extended family, friends, neighbors, congregants—whoever can give you a helping hand. Raking the leaves, cleaning the gutters, mowing the lawn, shoveling the walk, fixing a lamp, and the like, these are the chores that detract from your quality of life when caregiving prevents you from getting around to them. Others may not be comfortable with providing direct patient care, and you may not be comfortable with that either. But there are many people in your circle of family and friends who would be willing to assist you with a specific job, either as a one-time help or on a regular basis. They win, you win, and your loved one wins. Others ease their frustration and feelings of helplessness by pitching in. You are able to find time for yourself to relax and to refresh your body, mind, and soul. Your loved one has the benefit of your being able to spend more concentrated "together time" instead of being pulled away by so many distractions. Let go, and let others help!

A seminary professor of mine once said, "Life is what you do with fifteen minutes." This statement has had a profound effect on my life, as I have realized and have helped others to realize that refresh doesn't have to mean a vacation to the tropics or even a day at the spa. Refresh can and does mean grabbing a few moments of peace and tranquility when you can. It means intentionally making time for emotional rest and relaxation, building these times into the day where and when you can.

As a caregiver for someone with FTD, of course the opportunities for a vacation in the traditional sense of the word are few and far between, if not impossible. To refresh, however, is to believe in and to practice the art of the possible. A cup of tea in the sunshine, a daily devotional reading, writing a journal entry, praying or meditating in a designated spot, walking in the yard or the garden, calling a friend for support. These are opportunities to refresh yourself. Taking time for yourself is not selfish. On the contrary, times of refreshment will make you a better caregiver because you will be more patient and more able to handle the next crisis, which will inevitably arise. Take fifteen minutes for yourself . . . and refresh!

In addition to body and mind, refresh applies to the spirit, to the soul. It's so tempting to look at this time of caregiving as merely a time of destruction: of a person, of a relationship, of a dream. But this time can also be a period of creation, a time of development for your soul and your relationship to God. The Judeo-Christian tradition recognizes the concept of *shalom*, a word that is normally translated as "peace" but that signifies so much more. The truer, deeper meaning involves health and, perhaps even more fully, may be described as wholeness.

Wholeness, completeness, how can this be possible when you are losing someone? To answer this question, we must step outside ourselves and turn for answers to something greater than ourselves, something greater than the problem, greater than the disease. If you are religious, the structures are already in place. Consult your clergy and make him or her a part of the solution. Seek out spiritual resources in books, tapes, even on television. Find out if your local congregation sponsors prayer groups, support groups, study groups, and the like, that will get you in touch with others who share your faith and who can share your journey with you and pray for you.

Feelings of anger or disappointment with God are natural at a time such as this. I tell people with whom I work that it's okay to have those feelings, for a time. "It's an okay place to visit, but you don't want to live there," is my phrase. If you are religious, if you have been religious, don't try to fight this battle without the strength and courage and power and peace that only your faith and your God can provide. The prophet Isaiah talks of God's redeeming acts as bringing "times of refreshing," and these times can be yours, too. Just reach out.

All persons are not religious, but all are spiritual. If you fall into this category, don't neglect the spirituality that can bring wholeness and health. Don't be afraid to take time to look inside, to go deep into your secret, spiritual places to find the meaning that this life event holds for you. Merely operating on a surface level will never get you to the places where your spirit can bring you peace and tranquility. Just as it is important to go inside, it is equally critical to go outside yourself. Look beyond yourself to a higher power in order to gain perspective, which we cannot have from our point of view in the midst of the problem. Allow your spirit to probe deeply inside and to soar unfettered outside, and you will find where you need to go the next time you need to refresh.

SEEING THE WHOLE

Perhaps you may be wondering whether you will ever get over the trauma of caring for and ultimately losing someone who is a victim of FTD. In many years of counseling with hundreds of families facing grief and loss, I can assure you that you need not worry about "getting over it." That isn't the task you must complete. Instead of getting over it, which seems impossible because it is, those who are experiencing a great loss need to "get on with it."

"Getting on with it" simply means getting on with life: as it is, each minute, each hour, each day. Getting on with life involves "owning your grief" as you learn that loss is a component of your life and the lives of those close to you and to your loved one.

A friend completing her master's degree in art from New York University used a unique perspective for her final show. Every work of art she produced, from canvases to plaster figures to metal sculptures, had a hole in it. But instead of being just an empty space, the hole was incorporated into each work of art so that the hole was part of the whole. And the whole was still beautiful!

Living with grief and loss is a daily exercise in living life with a hole in it. Through "owning our grief" and through seeking emotional, physical, and spiritual health in the fourfold plan of reimage, refocus, remember, and refresh, we can see life as bigger than the hole left by frontotemporal dementia. We can learn to see the beauty of life again, the beauty of the whole.

CONTRIBUTORS

PREFACE

Susan L.-J. Dickinson, MS, CGC
Executive Director
The Association for Frontotemporal Degeneration
Radnor, Pennsylvania

CHAPTER 1

Martin Rossor, MD, FRCP, FMedSci
Professor of Clinical Neurology
UCL Institute of Neurology
Director, NIHR Dementias and Neurodegenerative Diseases Clinical Research
  Network
Director, NIHR Queen Square Dementia Biomedical Research Unit
Queen Square, London, United Kingdom

CHAPTER 2

Murray Grossman, MD, EdD
Associate Professor of Neurology and Psychiatry
Department of Neurology
Director, Penn Frontotemporal Degeneration Center
University of Pennsylvania Perelman School of Medicine
Philadelphia, Pennsylvania

CHAPTER 3

Elisabeth McCarty Wood, MS
Certified Genetic Counselor
Center for Neurodegenerative Disease Research
University of Pennsylvania Perelman School of Medicine
Philadelphia, Pennsylvania

CHAPTER 4

Carol F. Lippa, MD
Professor and Interim Chair
Department of Neurology
Director, Memory Disorders Program
Drexel University College of Medicine
Philadelphia, Pennsylvania

Kate J. Bowen
Research Coordinator
Department of Neurology
Drexel University College of Medicine
Philadelphia, Pennsylvania

CHAPTER 5

Richard J. Caselli, MD
Professor of Neurology
Department of Neurology
Mayo Clinic
Scottsdale, Arizona

Roy Yaari, MD, MAS
Neurologist, Dementia Specialist
Banner Alzheimer's Institute

Investigator, Arizona Alzheimer's Disease Consortium
Phoenix, Arizona

CHAPTER 6

Keith M. Robinson, MD
Chief of Rehabilitation
Philadelphia Veterans Affairs Medical Center
Associate Professor of Physical Medicine and Rehabilitation
University of Pennsylvania Perelman School of Medicine
Philadelphia, Pennsylvania

Amy P. Lustig, PhD, MPH, CCC-SLP
Speech-Language Pathologist
Philadelphia Veterans Affairs Medical Center
Philadelphia, Pennsylvania

CHAPTER 7

Carol F. Lippa, MD
Professor and Interim Chair
Department of Neurology
Director, Memory Disorders Program
Drexel University College of Medicine
Philadelphia, Pennsylvania

Kate J. Bowen
Research Coordinator
Department of Neurology
Drexel University College of Medicine
Philadelphia, Pennsylvania

CHAPTER 8

David J. Irwin, MD
Instructor of Neurology
Department of Neurology, Frontotemporal Degeneration Center
Center for Neurodegenerative Disease Research
University of Pennsylvania Perelman School of Medicine
Philadelphia, Pennsylvania

Elisabeth McCarty Wood, MS
Certified Genetic Counselor
Center for Neurodegenerative Disease Research
University of Pennsylvania Perelman School of Medicine
Philadelphia, Pennsylvania

Virginia M.-Y. Lee, PhD
Professor, Department of Pathology and Laboratory Medicine
Director, Center for Neurodegenerative Disease Research
University of Pennsylvania Perelman School of Medicine
Philadelphia, Pennsylvania

John Q. Trojanowski, MD, PhD
William Maul Measey-Truman G. Schnabel Jr., MD, Professor of Geriatric
    Medicine and Gerontology
Director, Institute on Aging
Director, Alzheimer's Disease Core Center
Director, Udall Parkinson's Research Center
Codirector, Center for Neurodegenerative Disease Research and Marian S.
    Ware Alzheimer Drug Discovery Program
Professor, Department of Pathology and Laboratory Medicine
University of Pennsylvania Perelman School of Medicine
Philadelphia, Pennsylvania

CHAPTER 9

David S. Knopman, MD
Professor of Neurology
Mayo Clinic
Rochester, Minnesota

PART 2 INTRODUCTION

Sharon S. Denny, MA
Program Director
The Association for Frontotemporal Degeneration
Radnor, Pennsylvania

CHAPTER 10

Amy P. Lustig, PhD, MPH, CCC-SLP
Speech-Language Pathologist
Philadelphia Veterans Affairs Medical Center
Philadelphia, Pennsylvania

CHAPTER 11

Heather Cianci, PT, MS, GCS
The Dan Aaron Parkinson's Rehabilitation Center at Pennsylvania Hospital
Good Shepherd Penn Partners
Philadelphia, Pennsylvania

CHAPTER 12

Lisa Ann Fagan, MS, OTR/L
Rehabilitation Consultant

Philadelphia, Pennsylvania
Visiting Instructor, Department of Occupational Therapy & Occupational
    Science
Towson University
Towson, Maryland

CHAPTER 13

Lisa Ann Fagan, MS, OTR/L
Rehabilitation Consultant
Philadelphia, Pennsylvania
Visiting Instructor, Department of Occupational Therapy & Occupational
    Science
Towson University
Towson, Maryland

CHAPTER 14

Lisa Ann Fagan, MS, OTR/L
Rehabilitation Consultant
Philadelphia, Pennsylvania
Visiting Instructor, Department of Occupational Therapy & Occupational
    Science
Towson University
Towson, Maryland

CHAPTER 15

Katherine P. Rankin, PhD
Associate Professor of Neuropsychology
The Memory and Aging Center
Department of Neurology
University of California–San Francisco
San Francisco, California

CHAPTER 16

Lauren M. Massimo, PhD, AGNP-BC
Nurse Practitioner
Penn Frontotemporal Degeneration Center
University of Pennsylvania Perelman School of Medicine
Philadelphia, Pennsylvania

Geri R. Hall, PhD, ARNP, GCNS-BC, FAAN
Advanced Practice Nurse
Banner Alzheimer's Institute
Phoenix, Arizona

CHAPTER 17

Bruce L. Miller, MD
A. W. and Mary Clausen Distinguished Professor of Neurology
Director, Memory and Aging Center
Adjunct Professor in Psychiatry
Department of Neurology
University of California San Francisco
San Francisco, California
Medical Director, John Douglas French Foundation for Alzheimer's Disease
Los Angeles, CA

Rosalie Gearhart, RN, MS, CS
Administrative Nurse and Clinical Nurse Specialist
Associate Clinical Professor
Memory and Aging Center
Department of Neurology
University of California San Francisco
San Francisco, California

CHAPTER 18

Maribeth Gallagher, DNP, PMHNP-BC, FAAN
Dementia Program Director
Hospice of the Valley
Scottsdale, Arizona

Jeannette Castellane
BA Psychology
Gerontology Certification
Allentown, Pennsylvania

CHAPTER 19

Darby Morhardt, PhD, LCSW
Associate Professor and Director, Education
Cognitive Neurology and Alzheimer's Disease Center
Northwestern University Feinberg School of Medicine
Chicago, Illinois

Mary O'Hara, AM, LCSW
Social Worker
Assistant Director of Education
Cognitive Neurology and Alzheimer's Disease Center
Northwestern University Feinberg School of Medicine
Chicago, Illinois

CHAPTER 20

Morris J. Kaplan, Esq., NHA
Chief Executive Officer
Gwynedd Square Nursing Center
Lansdale, Pennsylvania

CHAPTER 21

Helen-Ann Comstock
Founder, The Association for Frontotemporal Degeneration
Former Pick's disease caregiver, 1978–1984
Executive Director, Alzheimer's Association Southeastern Pennsylvania Chapter, 1985–2000
Perkasie, Pennsylvania

CHAPTER 22

Paul L. Feldman, Esq.
Feldman & Feldman Attorneys at Law
Philadelphia, Pennsylvania
Specializing in Elder Law

CHAPTER 23

Vivian E. Greenberg, ACSW, LCSW
Author, lecturer, consultant, freelance writer, and columnist
Private Practice
Pennington, New Jersey

CHAPTER 24

Rev. David Cotton
Coordinator of Pastoral Care
Jersey Shore Medical Center
Neptune, New Jersey

ABOUT THE EDITORS

Lisa Radin and her son, Gary Radin, provided complete care for their husband and father Neil Radin over a four-year period after he was diagnosed with frontotemporal degeneration (FTD). Based on this firsthand experience with a devastating and terminal illness, they compiled this collection of expert articles on FTD and dementia. In 1998, following Neil's death, they founded the Neil L. Radin Caregivers Relief Foundation based in New Jersey, and in 1999 were involved in planning the first Multidisciplinary Conference on Pick's Disease and Frontotemporal Dementia in Philadelphia. In 2000, Lisa also helped organize the Frontotemporal Dementia and Pick's Disease Criteria Conference at the National Institutes of Health in Bethesda, Maryland. In 2003, she became a founding member of the Association for Frontotemporal Degeneration and is currently a special-events consultant for the Alzheimer's Association Delaware Valley chapter. Gary and Lisa continue to support fundraising efforts for these organizations, speak about their experience as caregiver's and are both facilitators for support groups serving those in need.

RESOURCES

ADAPTING THE HOME ENVIRONMENT

Ageless Design, 916-412-9390, www.agelessdesigns.net. Information on dementia-specific home modifications.

American Association for Retired Persons (AARP), 888-687-2277. www.aarp.org. Under "search," type in "home modifications."

American Occupational Therapy Association, Inc., 301-652- 6611; 800-377-8555 (TDD). www.aota.org. Information on home modification and how to contact an occupational therapist.

Institute for Human Centered Design (IHCD) (Formally Adaptive Environments Center,. 617-695-1225 (V/TTY). www.humancentereddesign.org. Home-modification resources.

LifeEase, 800-966-5119 (within USA) or 603-938-5116 (outside of USA). www.lifease.com. Home-evaluation information.

National Resource Center on Supportive Housing and Home Modifications, University of Southern California, Andrus Gerontology Center, (213) 740-1364. http:/gero.usc.edu/nrcshhm. Home modification information.

The Alzheimer's Store™, 800-752-3238. www.alzstore.com. Products designed for people with dementia and their caregivers.

AREA AGENCIES ON AGING (US)

These agencies provide many helpful long-term-care services to patients and families. You may apply for state and federal financial aid (Medicaid) for home care and nursing home care through your local area agency on aging. Listings for area agencies on aging are located under "Guide to Human Services" in the blue pages of the telephone directory. www.n4a.org. Go to the "About" menu and to "AAA's/Title VI."

CAREGIVER'S ORGANIZATIONS

Caregiver Action Network (Formally National Family Caregivers Association), 2000 M St. NW, Suite 400 Washington, DC, 20036. 202-772-5050. www.caregiveraction.org. A nonprofit organization providing education, peer support, and resources to family caregivers across the country free of charge.

Family Caregiver Alliance, 785 Market St., Ste. 750, San Francisco, CA, 94103. 415-434-3388 or 800-445-8106. www.caregiver.org. Fact sheets on various dementias, as well as caregiver issues, statistics and demographics.

Well Spouse Foundation, 63 W. Main St., Ste. H, Freehold, NJ, 07728. 800-838-0879. www.wellspouse.org. Gives support to wives, husbands, and partners of the chronically ill and/or disabled.

EATING UTENSILS AND THICKENERS

AliMed Inc., 800-225-2610. www.alimed.com. Makes pureed food and has feeding equipment.

Bruce Medical Supplies, 800-225-8446. www.brucemedical.com. Has eating and drinking utensils.

SimplyThick, LLC, 800-205-7115. www.simplythick.com. Gel used for thickening foods and drinks.

Thick-It®: Kent Precision Foods, Inc., 800-442-5242. www.precision-foods.com. Dry powder used for thickening foods and drinks. Gives link to regional sales representatives and available locations.

ELDER-CARE LAWYERS

The Eldercare Locator is a public service of the US Administration on Aging. It is a nationwide service that connects older Americans and their caregivers with sources of information on senior services. The service links those who need assistance with state and local area agencies on aging and community-based organizations that serve older adults and their caregivers.

You may speak to an Eldercare Locator information specialist by calling toll-free 800-677-1116 on weekdays, from 9:00 a.m. to 8:00 p.m. (ET). Spanish-speaking information specialists are on duty. www.eldercare.gov.

EXERCISE EQUIPMENT

TheraBand™, The Hygenic Corporation, 800-321-213. www.thera-band.com.
Over the Door Pulleys, PrePak Products, Inc., 800-544-7527. www
.prepakproducts.com.

GENETICS

Genetic Alliance, Inc.: 4301 Connecticut Ave. NW, Suite 404, Wash-
ington, DC, 20008-2369. 202-966-5557. www.geneticalliance.org.
The alliance supports individuals with genetic conditions and their fami-
lies, educates the public, and advocates for consumer-informed public policies.
The Genetics of FTD: Should You Worry? A brochure written by Susan
Dickinson and Jennifer Farmer. Available through the Association for Frontotemporal Dementias: 609-970-9157 or 866-507-7222. www.theaftd.org.
National Human Genome Research Institute: www.genome.gov. The
National Human Genome Research Institute leads the Human Genome Project
for the National Institutes of Health, conducts cutting-edge research in its laboratories, and supports genomic science worldwide. This website contains a
lot of useful information for the layperson about the Human Genome Project,
genetic research, and genetic conditions and testing.
National Society of Genetic Counselors, Inc., 312-321-6834. www.nsgc
.org.
The NSGC is the national professional organization for genetic counselors. Use the "Find a Counselor" link to find a genetic counselor by either
geographic location or field of specialty. This website also has a "Family
History Tool" to help individuals and families collect and store their family-
history information.
US Surgeon General's Family History Initiative: www.hhs.gov.
Familyhistory or www.familyhistory.hhs.gov/fhh-web/home.action. An online
program titled "My Family Health Portrait" is available as a free download
through the Family History Initiative. This website also contains resources
and frequently asked questions pertaining to family-history risks for many
different health conditions.

MEDICAID

www.medicaid.org.

MEDICAL CENTERS AND ORGANIZATIONS

If you obtained the diagnosis at a university medical center, you should be able to obtain information from the center. Some centers also offer family consultations and maintain support groups.

The Association for Frontotemporal Dementias (AFTD), Radnor Station Building 2, Suite 320, 290 King of Prussia Road, Radnor, PA. 267-514-7221 or 866-507-7222. ww.theaftd.org. The nationwide nonprofit organization whose mission is to promote and fund research into finding the cause and cure for frontotemporal degeneration; to provide information, education, and support to persons diagnosed with FTD and their families and caregivers; and to educate physicians and allied health professionals about FTD. Toll-free telephone helpline, informational materials, telephone support groups.

Lewy Body Dementia Association, 912 Killian Rd, Liburn, GA, 30047. 404-935-6444 (national office). Caregiver Link: 800-LEWYSOS (539-9767). P.O. Box 451429, Atlanta, GA, 31145-9429. www.lewybodydementia.org. The Lewy Body Dementia Association was founded to promote research into conquering the disease while assisting those who are affected by it today.

WE MOVE (Worldwide Education and Awareness for Movement Disorders), 204 West 84th Street, New York, NY, 10024. 212-875-8312. www.wemove.org. Information on corticobasal degeneration and other movement disorders.

ALS Association (ALSA), 1275 K Street NW, Suite 250, Washington, DC, 20005. 202-407-8580 or 800-782-4747. www.alsa.org. The association's nationwide network of chapters provides comprehensive patient services and support to the ALS community. On the home page, type in "frontotemporal dementia" for information about the overlap between FTD and ALS.

CurePSP, Foundation for PSP, CBD and Related Brain Diseases, 11350 McCormick Road, Suite 906, Hunt Valley, MD, 21031, 800-457-4777. www.curepsp.org. An association dedicated to increasing awareness of progressive supranuclear palsy, corticobasal degeneration, and related disorders and providing support, education and hope for persons with PSP, CBD and their families.

Alzheimer's Association (USA), 225 N. Michigan Ave., Fl. 17, Chicago, IL, 60601. National helpline: 800-272-3900. www.alz.org. The association publishes a variety of useful brochures (ask for *Related Disorders*, among others). Some Alzheimer's Association chapters maintain FTD support groups, lists of daycare centers, in-home care providers, nursing homes, and information about drugs, clinical trials, research, and care tips. Many association chapters also offer family caregiver training, and this is most valuable as you cope with caring for your family member. Although caregiver training is geared toward Alzheimer's, much of the information and many of the care tips are helpful for FTD as well.

In addition to the United States Alzheimer's Association and its many chapters, excellent information is available from international Alzheimer's associations or societies.

Alzheimer's Society, United Kingdom, Gordon House, 10 Greencoat Pl., London SW1P 1PH UK. Information Sheet, "What Is Frontotemporal Dementia (Including Pick's Disease)?" The website has a special section, "Younger People with Dementia," with information designed for younger people with dementia, their families, and their caregivers. www.alzheimers. org.uk.

Alzheimer's Australia, 1 Frewin Place, Scullin, ACT 2614 P.O. Box 4019, Hawker ACT 2614, Australia helpline: 800-100-500.

Excellent help notes specific to Pick's disease and frontal lobe dementia, plus a reading list. www.fightdementia.org.au.

ADEAR (Alzheimer's Disease Education and Research), National Institute on Aging, P.O. Box 8250, Silver Spring, MD, 20907-8250. 800-438-4380. ADEAR's website will help you find current, comprehensive information and resources from the National Institute on Aging (NIA). www.nia.nih. gov/Alzheimers. Under "Publications" click on "Connections." Vol. 9, no. 4, focuses on frontotemporal dementia. Vol. 10, nos. 1–2 have excellent information on "Driving and Dementia."

NINDS (National Institute of Neurological Disorders and Stroke), National Institutes of Health, 31 Center Dr., Bethesda, MD, 20892. www. ninds.nih.gov. Click on "Disorders," then "frontotemporal dementia," and get the "Frontotemporal Dementia Information" page. There also are fact sheets on Pick's disease, dementia with Lewy bodies, progressive supranuclear palsy, and corticobasal degeneration.

Dementia Research Center, United Kingdom, the National Hospital for Neurology and Neurosurgery, Queen Square, London WC1N 3BG, UK. www. dementia.ion.ucl.ac.uk. Click on "CANDID (Counseling ANd Diagnosis In Dementia)" for a wealth of information specific to FTD: Pick's disease support group, fact sheets, articles, books, newsletter. Or go directly to CANDID's website, www.pdsg.org.uk.

Family Caregiver Alliance, 785 Market Street, Suite 750, San Francisco, CA, 94103. 415-434-3388 or 800 445-8106. www.caregiver.org. Founded in 1977, the first community-based nonprofit organization in the United States to address the needs of families and friends providing long-term care at home. Fact sheets on various dementias, as well as caregiver issues, statistics, and demographics. On the home page, type in "frontotemporal dementia" for a list of relevant articles.

Lotsa Helping Hands, www.lotsahelpinghands.com. This organization powers free online caring communities that provide tools to organize daily life during times of medical crisis or caregiver exhaustion. There are more than sixty thousand "Private Communities" that are at work supporting caregivers across the United States, and recently an "Open Community" model has been launched to connect caregivers, individuals, and families who need help with those who want to lend a hand.

National Aphasia Association, 350 Seventh Avenue, Suite 902 New York, NY, 10001. 212-267-2814 or 800-922-4622. www.aphasia.org. It is a nonprofit organization that promotes public education, research, rehabilitation, and support services to assist people with aphasia and their families.

National Organization for Rare Disorders, Inc. (NORD), 55 Kenosia Avenue, P.O. Box 1968, Danbury, CT, 06813-1968. 203-744-0100 or 800-999-6673. www.rarediseases.org. Search "Rare Diseases Database—Alphabetical Listing," scroll down to "Corticobasal," "Pick's disease," etc., for brief information about the disease and information about organizations offering help. There is a small charge for full-text reports.

NURSING HOME AND ASSISTED LIVING

CMS, formerly the Health Care Financing Administration/HCFA, is the federal agency that oversees all nursing home care and Medicare and Medicaid funding. Centers for Medicare and Medicaid Services, 7500 Security Blvd., Baltimore, MD, 21244-1850. 877-267-2323. www.cms.hhs.gov.

Consumer Consortium on Assisted Living, 2342 Oak St., Falls Church, VA, 22046. 703-533-8121. www.ccal.org.

The National Consumer Voice (Formally National Citizens Coalition for Nursing Home Reform). 1001 Connecticut Avenue, NW, Suite 42, Washington, DC, 20036. 202-332-2275; TTY 301-296-5650. www.theconsumer-voice.org.

SPEECH AND HEARING

ASHA: American Speech and Hearing Association, 2200 Research Boulevard, Rockville, MD, 20850-3289. 800-638-8255. www.asha.org.

WEBSITES

Alzheimer's Research Forum, www.alzforum.org. Founded in 1996 to create an online scientific community dedicated to developing treatments and preventions for Alzheimer's disease.

PubMed, a service of the National Library of Medicine, National Institutes of Health, provides access to MEDLINE citations and includes links to many sites providing full-text articles and other related resources, www.ncbi.nlm.nih.gov. Click on "PubMed"; search on PubMed for Pick's disease, frontotemporal dementia, Lewy body, etc.

SUGGESTED READING
AND DVDs

GENERAL INFORMATION

Books

Doernberg, M. *Stolen Mind: The Slow Disappearance of Ray Doernberg*. Chapel Hill, NC: Algonquin Books, 1989. A personal story.

Erb, C. A. Losing Lou-Ann. Brandon, VT: Holistic Education, 1996. A personal story.

Kertesz, Andrew, *The Banana Lady and Other Stories of Curious Behavior and Speech*. Victoria, BC, Canada: Trafford Publishing, 2006. To order, contact www.trafford.com/06-1883.

Mace, N., and P. Rabins. *The 36-Hour Day*. Rev. ed. Baltimore, MD: Johns Hopkins University Press, 1991.

DVDs

It Is What It Is—A powerful, eighteen-minute film by AFTD to increase understanding. It chronicles four families as they confront FTD. By telling their stories, these families reflect experiences common to many and become a harbinger of hope. The DVD is accompanied by a twelve-page informational booklet on FTD. Produced by the Association for Frontotemporal Degeneration, 2011. Order online: www.theaftd.org or call 866-507-7222.

Planning for Hope–Living with Frontotemporal Disease is a moving documentary created by Susan Grant, who is diagnosed with FTD, to bring attention to this terminal disease. Six families share their heart-wrenching stories of perpetual grieving, amidst financial struggles and caring for their loved ones. Sharing another aspect of hope, professionals explore financial and estate planning for FTD victims and their families. Today, there is no single known cause, treatment, or cure for FTD. However, the film provides hope for the future as science is moving at a fast pace. Order online: www. FTDPlanningForHope.com.

Disordered by Klaas Jansma and Pieter Wolswijk—This three-part documentary on frontotemporal degeneration (FTD) shows how the lives of three patients have changed and how this has affected the people around them. Klaas Jansma is a psychologist involved in the Dutch National Steering Committee for Young People with Dementia. Pieter Wolswijk is a geriatric psychologist and freelance filmmaker. This documentary is an initiative of the Intercollegiate Group of Geriatric Psychologists in the Arnhem Region, the Netherlands. Order online: contact Klaas Jansma via e-mail at krjansma@ hotmail.com.

Websites

The Association for Frontotemporal Degeneration (AFTD)
    Main website: www.theaftd.org.
    AFTD Kids and Teens: www.aftdkidsandteens.org.
Alzheimer's Association: www.alz.org.

Many of the Alzheimer's Disease Research Centers throughout the United States have a website with FTD modules rich in information including:

Northwestern University: www.brain.northwestern.edu/dementia.
University of Pennsylvania: www.ftd.med.upenn.edu/our-center.
Mayo Clinic: www.mayoclinic.org/frontotemporal-dementia.
University of California, San Francisco: www.memory.ucsf.edu/ftd.

MEDICAL FOCUS

Articles

(The following articles were written for the medical community)

Boxer A. L., M. Gold, E. Huey, et al. "The Advantages of Frontotemporal Degeneration Drug Development (Part 2 of Frontotemporal Degeneration: The Next Therapeutic Frontier)." *Alzheimer's & Dementia* 9, no. 2

(March 2013): 189–98. doi: 10.1016/j.jalz.2012.03.003. Epub available October 10, 2012. Review. PubMed PMID: 23062850; PubMed Central PMCID: PMC3562382.

Boxer A. L., M. Gold, E. Huey, et al. "Frontotemporal Degeneration, the Next Therapeutic Frontier: Molecules and Animal Models for Frontotemporal Degeneration Drug Development." *Alzheimer's & Dementia* 9, no. 2 (March 2013): 176–88. doi: 10.1016/j.jalz.2012.03.002. Epub available October 5, 2012. Review. PubMed PMID: 23043900; PubMed Central PMCID: PMC3542408.

Grossman, M., "Primary Progressive Aphasia: Clinical-Pathological Correlations." *Nature Reviews Neurology* 6 (2010): 88–97.

Rabinovici G. D., B. L. Miller. "Frontotemporal Lobar Degeneration: Epidemiology, Pathophysiology, Diagnosis and Management." *CNS Drugs* 24, no. 5 (May 2010): 375–98. doi: 10.2165/11533100-000000000-00000. Review. PubMed PMID: 20369906; PubMed Central PMCID: PMC2916644.

Rascovsky K., M. Grossman. "Clinical Diagnostic Criteria and Classification Controversies in Frontotemporal Lobar Degeneration." *International Review of Psychiatry* 25, no. 2 (April 2013): 145–58. doi: 0.3109/09540261.2013.763341. Review. PubMed PMID: 23611345; PubMed Central PMCID: PMC3906583.

Whitwell J. L., K. A. Joseph. "Recent Advances in the Imaging of Frontotemporal Dementia." *Current Neurology and Neuroscience Reports* 12, no. 6 (December 2012): 715–23. doi: 10.1007/s11910-012-0317-0. Review. PubMed PMID: 23015371; PubMed Central PMCID:PMC3492940.

Books

Beinfield, H., and E. Korngold. *Between Heaven and Earth: A Guide to Chinese Medicine.* New York: Ballantine, 1992.

Byock, Ira. *The Best Care Possible: A Physician's Quest to Transform Care through the End of Life.* New York: Avery/Penguin, 2012.

Kaptchuk, T. *The Web That Has No Weaver: Understanding Chinese Medicine.* 2d ed. Lincolnwood, IL: Contemporary Books, 2000.

Kertesz, A., and D. G. Munoz, eds. *Pick's Disease and Pick Complex.* Chichester, UK: Wiley-Liss, 1998.

Lipton, A., and C. Marshall. *The Common Sense Guide to Dementia for Clinicians and Caregivers.* New York: Springer, 2013.

Booklets

A Guide for Managing a New Diagnosis—The Doctor Thinks It's FTD. Now What? is a publication from AFTD that helps individuals and families take a strategic approach to a diagnosis of FTD and prepare for the changes it brings. Contact info@theaftd.org to request the printed booklet.

Understanding the Genetics of FTD: A Guide for Patients and Their Families. In collaboration with AFTD, the University of Pennsylvania Center for Neurodegenerative Disease Research has created a booklet of current and reliable information on the role that genetics plays in FTD, the genes that have been associated with hereditary FTD, and genetic testing. Contact info@theaftd.org to request the printed booklet.

Frontotemporal Disorders: Information for Patients, Families, and Caregivers is a consumer-friendly booklet published by National Institute on Aging. The free, thirty-page booklet, which includes contributions from AFTD, explains the disorders, causes, symptoms, and management in layman's terms. To order copies, call: 800-438-4380.

Publications

Alzheimer's Care Quarterly, July/September 2005 issue on "Atypical Dementias." Published by Lippincott Wilkins Williams, Carol Bowlby Sifton, ed. This issue focuses on frontotemporal dementia, with a variety of articles about FTD written for the lay public, including one by an FTD patient. www.ovid.com.

Alzheimer Disease and Associated Disorders 19, suppl. 1, October/December 2005, Murray Grossman, ed. Contains articles from the July 2004 FTD Symposia. www.alzheimer journal.com. Click on "Archive" and scroll to the supplement.

The Pick's Disease Support Group (PDSG) has published a booklet containing the personal experiences of caregivers coping with a number of conditions. For details on how to order print copies, e-mail info@pdsg.org.uk.

Website

Comart, J., and A. Mahler. "How to Talk to Families about Advanced Dementia: A Guide for Health Care Professionals." Hebrew Senior Life. 2013.

Retrieved from http://www.hebrewseniorlife.org/workfiles/IFAR/DementiaGuide
ForProfs.pdf.

MANAGING DAILY CARE

Books

Achilles, E. *Dysphagia Cookbook.* Nashville, TN: Cumberland House, 2004.

Alzheimer's Association. *Activity Programming for Persons with Dementia: A Sourcebook.* Chicago: Alzheimer's Association, 1995.

Dunn, H. *Hard Choices for Loving People: CPR, Artificial Feeding, Comfort Measures Only, and the Elderly Patient.* 5th ed. Landsdowne, VA: A and A Publishers, 2009. To order, visit www. hankdunn.com or call 1-855-232-4265.

Perrin, T., and H. May. *Well-Being in Dementia: An Occupational Approach for Therapists and Careers.* Edinburgh, UK: Churchill Livingstone, 2000.

Zgola, J. M. *Doing Things: A Guide to Programming Activities for Persons with Alzheimer's Disease and Related Disorders.* Baltimore, MD: Johns Hopkins University Press, 1987.

Booklet

Palliative care dementia booklet from Institute for Aging Research.

Mitchell, S., A. Catic, J. L. Givens J. Knopp, J. Moran. *Advanced Dementia: A Guide for Families.* 2011. Institute for Aging Research. Available to download online at www.hebrewseniorlife.org/workfiles/IFAR/Palliative _Care_Dementia_Booklet.pdf.

CAREGIVER RESOURCES

Books

Cohen, Marion. *Dear Aunt S: How to Ask for Help from Family and Friends in Time of Crisis.* Brooklyn, NY: Center for Thanatology Research, 2003.

Richards, Marty. *Caresharing.* Woodstock, VT: SkyLight Paths, 2008.

Booklet

What about the Kids? The AFTD Task Force on Families with Children has written and produced a new tool for parents with young children and teens. *What about the Kids?* is a sensitive, practical guide for parents to help their children deal with a parent who has FTD. Contact info@theaftd.org to request the printed booklet.

CARING FOR YOURSELF

Books

Kushner, H. S. *When Bad Things Happen to Good People.* New York: Schocken, 1981.
Lewis, C. S. *A Grief Observed.* New York: HarperOne, 2001.

INDEX